Pharmacology and Pharmacokinetics

Fogarty International Center Proceedings No. 20

Pharmacology and Pharmacokinetics

Edited by
Torsten Teorell
Institute of Physiology and Medical Biophysics
University of Uppsala
Uppsala, Sweden
and
Fogarty International Center
National Institutes of Health
Bethesda, Maryland

Robert L. Dedrick
Biomedical Engineering and Instrumentation Branch
Division of Research Services
National Institutes of Health
Bethesda, Maryland

and

Peter G. Condliffe
Laboratory of Nutrition and Endocrinology
National Institute of Arthritis, Metabolism, and Digestive Diseases
National Institutes of Health
Bethesda, Maryland

PLENUM PRESS · NEW YORK—LONDON

Library of Congress Cataloging in Publication Data

Main entry under title:

Pharmacology and pharmacokinetics.

"Proceedings of an international conference sponsored by the John E. Fogarty International Center for Advanced Study in the Health Sciences, National Institutes of Health, Bethesda, Maryland, October 30–November 1, 1972."

Includes bibliographical references.

1. Pharmacology—Congresses. I. Teorell, Torsten, ed. II. Dedrick, Robert L., ed. III. Condliffe, Peter G., 1922- ed. IV. John E. Fogarty International Center for Advanced Study in the Health Sciences. [DNLM: 1. Kinetics—Congresses. 2. Pharmacology—Congresses. QV4 P5362 1972]

RM21.P48   615'.7   73-81090
ISBN 0-306-30744-8

Proceedings of an international conference held at the John E. Fogarty International Center for Advanced Study in the Health Sciences, National Institutes of Health, Bethesda, Maryland, October 30–November 1, 1972

Published in 1974 by Plenum Press, New York
A Division of Plenum Publishing Corporation
227 West 17th Street, New York, N. Y. 10011

United Kingdom edition published by Plenum Press, London
A Division of Plenum Publishing Company, Ltd.
4a Lower John Street, London W1R 3PD, England

All rights reserved

Printed in the United States of America

Preface

This collection of papers by leading pharmacokineticists and pharmacologists is the proceedings of a conference held at the John E. Fogarty International Center for Advanced Study in the Health Sciences, National Institutes of Health, October 30 to November 1, 1972. As part of its advanced study program, the Center conducts workshops, seminars, and conferences on topics related to the biomedical interests of the Scholars-in-Residence.

Professor Torsten Teorell came to the Center in 1970 as one of the first Scholars. In 1971 and 1972, he spent several months at the Center devoting his attention to contemporary problems in the application of pharmacokinetics to experimental and clinical pharmacology. As one of the founders of pharmacokinetics, Professor Teorell has made many contributions to the field since he first presented a formal multicompartment model for the analysis of drug action and drug metabolism in 1937 (Teorell, 1937). Since the appearance of his original paper, pharmacodynamics, or pharmacokinetics, has become increasingly important as a tool for the study of drug action in patients. The translation of experimental pharmacological findings into therapeutic regimens is today increasingly dependent on adequate models of drug action. The purpose of the conference, of which this book is the proceedings, was to discuss contemporary findings in this important biomedical research field.

The conference program was designed by Professor Teorell with the help of a small committee which included Drs. Edward R. Garrett, Sidney Riegelman, Julius Axelrod, Mones Berman, and the late Daniel H. Efron. Professor Teorell also consulted other scientists including Dr. John A. Wagner concerning the program. We are indebted to these people for their assistance in arranging the program.

Professor Teorell held the Chair of Physiology at Uppsala University from 1940 until his retirement in 1972. During this period his laboratory became well known as a center for research on membrane permeability and for the quantitative study of the transport of materials across membranes in biological systems.

In the year of his retirement from the administration of a productive research department but not from scientific research, it is with great pleasure that I pay tribute to this distinguished scientist in behalf of the conference participants and the staff of the Fogarty International Center.

Peter G. Condliffe, Ph.D.
Fogarty International Center

Participants*

Prof. E. J. Ariëns
Pharmacological Institute
University of Nijmegen
Nijmegen, The Netherlands

Dr. K. Frank Austen
Robert B. Brigham Hospital
Parker Hill Avenue
Boston, Massachusetts 02120

Dr. Julius Axelrod
Laboratory of Clinical Sciences
National Institute of Mental Health
Health Services and Mental Health
Administration
Bethesda, Maryland

Dr. Daniel Azarnoff
University of Kansas Medical Center
Rainbow Blvd, at 39th St.
Kansas City, Kansas 66103

Dr. Leslie Z. Benet
University of California
School of Pharmacy
San Francisco Medical Center
San Francisco, California 94122

Dr. Mones Berman
Laboratory of Theoretical Biology
National Cancer Institute
National Institutes of Health
Bethesda, Maryland 20014

Dr. Kenneth B. Bischoff
Director
School of Chemical Engineering
Cornell University
Ithaca, New York 14850

Dr. E. Ann Brown
National Heart and Lung Institute
National Institutes of Health
Bethesda, Maryland 20014

Dr. William E. Bunney
Laboratory of Clinical Science
National Institute of Mental Health
Health Services and Mental Health
Administration
Bethesda, Maryland 20014

Dr. John J. Burns
Vice President for Research
Hoffmann-La Roche, Inc.
Nutley, New Jersey 07110

Dr. Byron Clark
Director, Pharmacology and Toxicology
Programs
National Institute of General Medical
Sciences
National Institutes of Health
Bethesda, Maryland 20014

Dr. Peter G. Condliffe
Laboratory of Nutrition & Endocrinology
National Institute of Arthritis, Metabolism, and
Digestive Diseases
National Institutes of Health
Bethesda, Maryland 20014

Dr. Allan H. Conney
Department of Biochemistry and Drug
Metalbolism
Hoffman-La Roche, Rt. 3 Bldg 86
Nutley, New Jersey 07110

* Affiliations as of the time of the conference

Dr. Richard Crout
Acting Director
Office of Scientific Evaluation
Bureau of Drugs
Food and Drug Administration
Rockville, Maryland 20852

Dr. Robert L. Dedrick
Chief, Chemical Engineering and
 Instrumentation
Division of Research Services
National Institutes of Health
Bethesda, Maryland 20014

Prof. L. Dettli
Medizinische Universitatsklinik
Medical Clinic 2
Burgerspital
Ch 4000 Basel, Switzerland

Dr. Robert L. Dixon
Chief
Pathologic and Physiology Branch
National Institute of Enviromental Health
 Sciences
National Institutes of Health
Research Triangle Park, North Carolina 27709

Dr. Joseph E. Fenstermacher
Laboratory of Chemical Pharmacology
National Cancer Institute
National Institutes of Health
Bethesda, Maryland 20014

Prof. Silvio Garratini
Director
Instituto di Richerche Farmacologiche "Mario
 Negri"
Via Etritrea, 62
20157 Milan, Italy

Dr. Edward R. Garrett
J. Hillis Miller Health Center
University of Florida
College of Pharmacy
Gainesville, Florida 32601

Dr. Edward J. Goetzl
Robert B. Brigham Hospital
125 Parker Hill Avenue
Boston, Massachusetts 02120

Dr. Milo Gibaldi
Department of Pharmaceutics
State University of New York at Buffalo
Buffalo, New York 14214

Dr. James R. Gillette
Laboratory of Chemical Pharmacology
National Heart and Lung Institute
National Institutes of Health
Bethesda, Maryland 20014

Prof. Lars-M. Gunne
Psychiatric Research Center
Ulleraker Hospital
S-750 17 Uppsala, Sweden

Dr. Thomas A. Haley
National Center for Toxicological Research
Food and Drug Administration
Jefferson, Arkansas 72079

Dr. Maureen Harris
Health Scientist Administrator
Fogarty International Center
National Institutes of Health
Bethesda, Maryland 20014

Dr. Peter Hinderling
J. Hillis Miller Health Center
University of Florida
College of Pharmacy
Gainesville, Florida 32601

Dr. William J. Jusko
Asst. Professor of Pharmaceutics
State University of New York at Buffalo
Millard Fillmore Hospital
Buffalo, New York 14209

Dr. Seymour Kety
Department of Psychiatry
Massachusetts General Hospital
Boston, Massachusetts 02114

Dr. Bert N. La Du
New York University Medical Center
Medical Science Building - Room 419
550 First Avenue
New York, New York 10016

Dr. Louis Lemberger
Lilly Laboratory for Clinical Research
Marion County General Hospital
Indianapolis, Indiana 46202

Dr. Gerhard Levy
Department of Pharmaceutics
State University of New York at Buffalo
School of Pharmacy
Buffalo, New York 14214

Participants

Dr. Kenneth Melmon
Department of Clinical Pharmacology
University of California
San Francisco, California 94122

Dr. John H. Nodine
Hahnemann Medical College
Philadelphia, Pennsylvania 19102

Dr. Gabriel L. Plaa
Professor and Chairman
Department of Pharmacology
University of Montreal
Faculty of Medicine
Montreal 101, Canada

Dr. Judith Rapoport
Department of Pediatrics
Georgetown University Medical School
Washington, D. C. 20005

Dr. Stanley I. Rapoport
Laboratory of Neurophysiology
National Institute of Mental Health
Health Services and Mental Health Administration
Bethesda, Maryland 20014

Dr. Sidney Riegelman
Prof. of Pharmacy and Pharmaceutical Chemistry
Chairman, Department of Pharmacy
University of California
San Francisco, California 94122

Mr. Robert Ronfeld
Department of Pharmacy
University of California
School of Pharmacy
San Francisco, California 94122

Dr. Malcolm Rowland
Department of Pharmacy
University of California
San Francisco, California 94122

Dr. Shaun Ruddy
Robert B. Brigham Hospital
125 Parker Hill Avenue
Boston, Massachusetts 02120

Prof. G. Segre, *Conference Chairman*
Department of Pharmacology
University of Siena
Siena, Italy

Dr. Folke Sjöqvist
Professor of Clinical Pharmacology
Karolinska Institute Stockholm
Huddinge University Hospital
S 14186 Huddinge, Sweden

Dr. Louis Sokoloff
Chief, Laboratory of Cerebral Metabolism
National Institute of Mental Health
Health Services and Mental Health Administration
Bethesda, Maryland 20014

Dr. Mathilde Solowey
Special Assistant for Program Development to the Director of BCRC
Division of Cancer Treatment
National Cancer Institute
National Institutes of Health
Bethesda, Maryland 20014

Prof. Torsten Teorell
Institute of Physiology and Medical Biophysics
University of Uppsala
S 75105 Uppsala 1, Sweden

Prof. John R. Vane
Department of Pharmacology
Institute of Basic Medical Sciences
Royal College of Surgeons of England
London, WC2A 3PN, England

Dr. Elliot S. Vesell
Department of Pharmacology
Milton S. Hershey Medical Center
Pennsylvania State University
Hershey, Pennsylvania 17033

Dr. John G. Wagner
Professor of Pharmacy
The University of Michigan
University Hospital
Ann Arbor, Michigan 48104

Dr. R. T. Williams
Professor of Biochemistry
St. Mary's Hospital Medical School
Norfolk Place - Paddington
London, W.2, England

Dr. Per Wistrand
University of Uppsala
Medicinska Fakultet
Box 456
S 75105 Uppsala 1, Sweden

Dr. Daniel S. Zaharko
Laboratory of Chemical Pharmacology
National Cancer Institute
National Institutes of Health
Bethesda, Maryland 20014

Contents

Introduction
         G. Segre 1

Classical Pharmacokinetics to the Frontier
         Edward R. Garrett 3

A Modern View of Pharmacokinetics
         John G. Wagner 27

Translation of Pharmacokinetics to Clinical Medicine
         L. Dettli 69

Effect of Route of Adminstration on Drug Disposition
         S. Riegelman and M. Rowland 87

Interspecies Scaling
         R. T. Williams 105

Animal Scale-Up
         Robert L. Dedrick 117

Drug Metabolism in Normal and Disease States
         A. H. Conney, R. Kuntzman, B. Carver, and E. Pantuck 147

Drug Action: Target Tissue, Dose–Response Relationships, and Receptors
         E. J. Ariëns and A. M. Simonis 163

Pharmacokinetics and Pharmacodynamics of Acetazolamide in Relation to Its Use in the Treatment of Glaucoma
         Per J. Wistrand 191

The Role of the Lungs in the Metabolism of Vasoactive Substances
         John R. Vane 195

The Importance of Tissue Distribution in Pharmacokinetics
         James R. Gillette 209

Physiological and Physical Factors Governing the Initial Stages of
Drug Distribution
Seymour S. Kety 233

Target Organ Modification in Pharmacology: Reversible Osmotic
Opening of the Blood–Brain Barrier by Opening of Tight
Junctions
Stanley I. Rapoport 241

Pharmacogenetics–Single Gene Effects
Bert N. La Du 253

Application of Pharmacokinetic Principles to the Elucidation of
Polygenically Controlled Differences in Drug Response
Elliot S. Vesell 261

Immediate Immunologic Reactions: Noncytolytic Mediator Release
and Cytolytic Cell Destruction
*Edward J. Goetzl, Shaun Ruddy, Daniel J. Stechschulte,
and K. Frank Austen* 281

Pharmacokinetic Studies with Amphetamines: Relationship to
Neuropsychiatric Disorders
Lars-M. Gunne and Erik Änggård 297

A Pharmacokinetic Approach to the Treatment of Depression
Folke Sjöqvist 315

Kinetics of Drug–Drug Interactions
Malcolm Rowland 321

Comparative Pharmacokinetics of the Anticoagulant Effect of
Coumarin Drugs in Man and Rat
Gerhard Levy 339

Pharmacokinetics and Cancer Chemotherapy
Kenneth B. Bischoff 351

Concluding Remarks
Torsten Teorell 369

Index 373

Introduction

These sessions are full of interesting topics related to the development and present status of pharmacokinetics. This conference will deal with the problems and perspectives in the joint field of pharmacology and pharmacokinetics. We are grateful to the Fogarty International Center for organizing this conference and for having invited such distinguished scientists to review the subject and to take part in the discussion. Since its first appearance as a "Grenzgebiet" in Professor Thorell's well-known paper, pharmacokinetics has developed in its theoretical aspects as well as in its practical applications. Its impact in the practical field can be judged by the fact that the European Economic Community requires a careful pharmacokinetic study for every drug put on the market, in particular for antibiotics, chemotherapeutic agents, and contrast media. Even with this interest of the drug companies, one aspect of pharmacokinetics, namely its application to dosage regimen, has not yet been explored as it deserves.

A new discipline is emerging, called Biopharmaceutics, to which a new journal is devoted. And a new field of interest is appearing with the study of the kinetics of the pharmacological effects, on which a recent review appeared in the *Annual Reviews of Pharmacology*, after the review of Pharmacokinetics which appeared in 1968.

Pharmacokinetics has also made an important contribution to the development of new disciplines, such as pharmacogenetics, which derives its first approach from drug kinetics; the study of drug interaction, which is in vogue today, is, in most cases, based on drug kinetics.

Important theoretical developments have occurred even in the short period since the Schering Workshop on Pharmacokinetics held in Berlin in 1969; computer programs, in particular the SAAM of Berman and his group, have steadily improved.

We can rightly say that in this field theory and practice go hand in hand, as the session that now begins will show.

G. Segre

Classical Pharmacokinetics to the Frontier

Edward R. Garrett

The Beehive, College of Pharmacy
J. Hillis Miller Health Center
University of Florida, Gainesville, Florida

The obvious has become apparent within the last decade. It is not only the efficacy of a drug at a site of action that determines the intensity and duration of its pharmacological or chemotherapeutic effect, but the amount of drug that gets there and stays. The net effect of the drug on the body results not only from its action on the receptor site in the biophase but from the action of the body on the drug.

The necessary vital processes of the body delay the transport of drug molecules across membranes, dilute them into various compartments of distribution, transform them into metabolites, and excrete them. The necessary formulation processes of drug manufacture modify the release and availability of the drug molecules to the body's absorption sites, the first steps in their long traverse to the receptor sites of drug action.

Pharmacokinetics is the study of the time courses of absorption distribution, metabolism, and excretion of drug in the intact total organism. The amounts of drug and metabolites in the available compartments in the body such as blood, tissues, and excreta are measured as functions of time and dosage. Kinetic models are established to quantify and predict these dynamic processes for appropriate dosage regimens. The derived constants, and quantifiable concepts, such as apparent volumes of distribution, are related to physiological and clinical reality. These parameters become the focus of attention, abstractions one level above the observed data.

Biopharmaceutics is the design of dosage forms for optimum therapeutic regimens based on the application of pharmacokinetic principles to determine the amounts of drug absorbed, the rates of absorption, and the rates of release from the pharmaceutical formulation in the intact biological system and permit estimates of the "bioavailability" of the drug from the dosage forms. The time course of drug concentrations in the body is compared with the formulations of the drug that have the highest biological availability. These are, if possible, intravenously and orally administered solutions. Comparisons of the bioavailability of the drug from various dosage forms can be made on the basis of the relative amounts of drug and metabolites in the different body compartments as a function of time.

THE MODELS OF PHARMACOKINETICS

The mathematical expressions of pharmacokinetics are based on models that conceive the body as a multicompartmental organism. It is presumed that the drug and/or its metabolites are equitably dispersed in one or several tissues of the body. Any conglomerate which acts as if it is kinetically homogeneous is termed a "compartment." Such a compartment acts as an isotropic fluid in which the molecules of drug that enter are homogeneously dispersed and where the kinetic dependencies of pharmacokinetic processes can be formulated as functions of the amounts or concentrations of drug and metabolites therein.

These compartments are separated by barriers that inhibit the free diffusion of drug among them. The barriers are kinetically definable in that the rate of transport of drug or metabolite across this membrane barrier between compartments is a function of the amounts or concentrations in these compartments.

The simplest postulate is that the rates of transport in either direction are proportional to the amounts or concentrations in the separated hypothetical compartments. If experimental studies as functions of increased dosage indicate that this simple postulate is not entirely valid, then saturable transport or metabolic processes, rate-limited by the capacity of the membrane-barrier or enzyme may be postulated and operationally defined by quantitative mathematical equations which describe the transport as functions of levels of drug in these compartments.

The general operating rule in such pharmacokinetic analysis is to postulate the minimum number of compartments consistent with physiological reality. No absolute claim can be made that more compartments than those chosen are not more valid reflections of the true biological processes. An approach such as this should be parsimonious in its postulates unless experimental evidence dictates that parsimony leads to the denial of reality (Garrett et al., 1960).

BASIC CONCEPTS (Garrett, 1971)

The one-compartment body model considers that the drug amount, F, is homogeneously and rapidly distributed in the total equilibrated volumes of distribution, V_F, and that the sum of its rates, R, of removal is proportional to the concentration, f, in those fluids:

$$R = k_e F = k_e V_f f \tag{1}$$

This model can be represented by

$$F \xrightarrow{k_e} U \tag{2}$$

where F_0 is the initial amount of drug in the body compartment and U_∞ is the total amount that would be excreted at infinite time. The amount F at any time would be the product of the concentration, f, at any time and the apparent volume of distribution, V_F, for the drug in the rapidly equilibrated fluids of distribution. This model requires intravenous administration and extremely rapid equilibration. The apparent elimination rate constant, k_e, can be determined from the slope of semilogarithmic plots of the blood concentration, f, against time, or of the amount of drug not yet excreted, $U_\infty - U$, against time. The apparent volume of distribution of the equilibrated fluids, V_F, is obtainable from the quotient of the dose, F_0, and the concentration, f_0, in the blood extrapolated to zero time. Alternatively, plots of the instantaneous rates of urine excretion, R_U, of unchanged drug against the blood concentration, Eq. (1), permit estimates of renal clearance from the slope, $k_e V_f$. The slopes of semilogarithmic plots of the renal excretion rate against time also permit estimates of the elimination rate constants.

The concept of a biological or metabolic half-life is only valid on the premise of postulated pseudo-steady-state conditions, the relatively instantaneous equilibration of a drug among the tissues and blood of the body where the drug distributions among compartments maintain the same ratios throughout the time courses of metabolism and elimination. In practice this is a type of relative equilibrium, wherein the time course shows a constancy in the ratios of concentrations in the several compartments. The half-life concept, i.e., that the time, $t_{\frac{1}{2}}$, is a constant and independent of the blood concentration when the concentration of the drug in the blood is halved, is also only valid when the rate of drug elimination is directly proportional to the amount in the body and

$$t_{\frac{1}{2}} = -\ln 0.5 / k_e \tag{3}$$

When the drug, F, is eliminated by parallel first-order routes of metabolism to M, biliary excretion to E, urinary excretion to U as

$$F \begin{array}{c} \xrightarrow{k_{F,U}} U \\ \xrightarrow{k_{F,M}} M \\ \xrightarrow{k_{F,E}} E \end{array} \qquad (4)$$

the overall elimination rate constant, k_e, is the sum of the separate rate constants for renal excretion, $k_{F,U}$; for metabolism, $k_{F,M}$; and for biliary excretion, $k_{F,E}$:

$$k_e = k_{F,U} + k_{F,M} + k_{F,E} \qquad (5)$$

The ratios of the amounts formed as metabolites, M, to the amounts renally excreted, U, at any time are in the ratio of the individual rate constants,

$$k_{F,M}/k_{F,U} = M/U = M_\infty/U_\infty \qquad (6)$$

and also

$$k_{F,E}/k_{F,U} = E/U = E_\infty/U_\infty \qquad (7)$$

Under usual conditions, when the rate of distribution in the equilibrated body fluids is fast, relative to the elimination rates, the two-compartment body model which can be visualized with reference to the hydraulic analogy of Fig. 1

$$\text{Tissue } (T) \underset{k_{B,T}}{\overset{k_{T,B}}{\rightleftarrows}} \text{Blood } (B) \xrightarrow{k_{B,U}} \text{Urine } (U) \qquad (8)$$

quickly reduces to the one-compartment body model of Eq. (2), i.e.,

$$\text{Fluids } (F) = \text{Blood } (B) + \text{Tissue } (T) \xrightarrow{k_e} \text{Urine } (U) \qquad (9)$$

and the observed elimination rate constant, k_e, is a function of the intrinsic rate constants (Garrett, 1964, 1969, 1971; Garrett *et al.*, 1960; Garrett and Alway, 1963; Garrett and Gravenstein, 1967):

$$k_e = \frac{k_{B,U}}{1 + k_{B,T}/k_{T,B}} = k_{B,U} \frac{V_B}{V_F} \qquad (10)$$

where V_B/V_F is the fraction of the volumes of distribution that is blood. V_B may be obtained from the extrapolated zero time value, b_0, of the blood concentration vs. time plot before distribution of the intravenously administered dose, D_0.

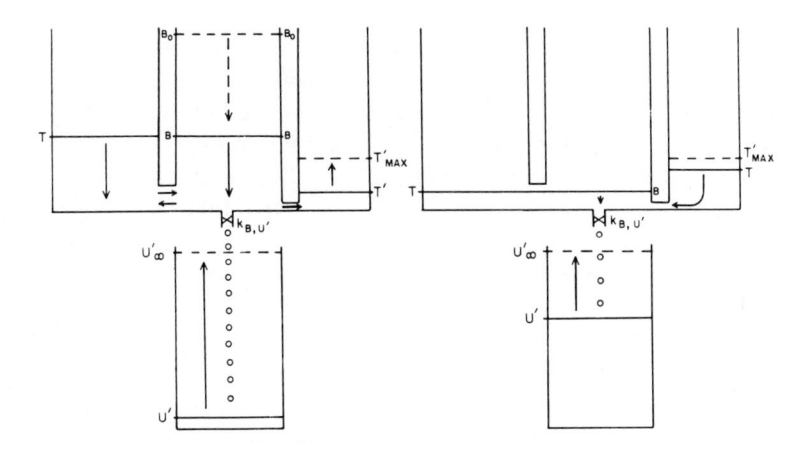

Fig. 1. Hydraulic analogy of the three-compartment body model. B_0 is the level for the amount corresponding to the original dosage in the blood compartment before any equilibration or loss. B is the level for the amount of drug at any time and is drawn in both figures for the conditions when B has equilibrated with the shallow or rapidly equilibrating compartment, T. T' represents the levels of drug in the deep or less rapidly equilibrating tissue compartment and T'_{max} is the maximum value achieved in this compartment for such a dosage, B_0. The sizes of the channels between the blood, B, and tissue compartments, T and T', represent the magnitudes of the transfer rates and the ratio of the widths of the compartments, T/B and T'/B, represent the ratio of the volumes of distributions of the tissue compartments with respect to the blood compartment. The level U' represents the drug eliminated and metabolized, $U' = B_0 - (B + T + T')$ and U'_∞ is the level which would correspond to the amount of drug eliminated or metabolized at infinite time. The left figure represents the time after equilibration of the blood and rapidly equilibrating tissues, T, while the slowly equilibrating compartment tends to increase in amount. It will be noted that in the right figure the subsequent slow release of drug from the slowly equilibrating compartment, T', to the blood compartment, B, will modify and prolong the overall release rate of drug into U'.

The analogy to the two-compartment body model is when the T' compartment does not exist or has insignificant capacity. In the pre-equilibrated state, the level of the shallow T compartment rises rapidly as the level of the central compartment, B, falls. The relatively large size of the channel between these two compartments relative to that for excretion into the U compartment permits the pseudo-steady-state equilibration to be effected between B and T as represented by the ultimate equality of levels in the two compartments. (Figure 11 of Garrett, 1971.)

The only way to estimate the distributive constants, $k_{B,T}$ and $k_{T,B}$, is by acute dosing (i.e., intravenous administration). The only way to be assured that the k_e values obtained from the slopes of semilogarithmic plots of blood concentration against time for oral or depot administration are valid estimates is to confirm that the distributive processes are fast on intravenous dosing.

For many drugs that are not excessively protein bound, V_B is greater than the true blood volume and includes those fluids or tissues from which drug access from the blood is virtually instantaneous.

The apparent volumes of distribution referenced to unbound drug in the plasma have the greatest physiological significance since it is this concentration that provides the gradient for diffusion into other compartments and for metabolic changes. Studies on protein binding and partition into red blood cells should be conducted so that only free and unbound drug in the plasma water should be used in calculating these apparent volumes of distribution. The multicompartmental body model includes "deep" compartments that never equilibrate with the drug in the blood throughout the elimination processes. Such compartments may be bone, fat,

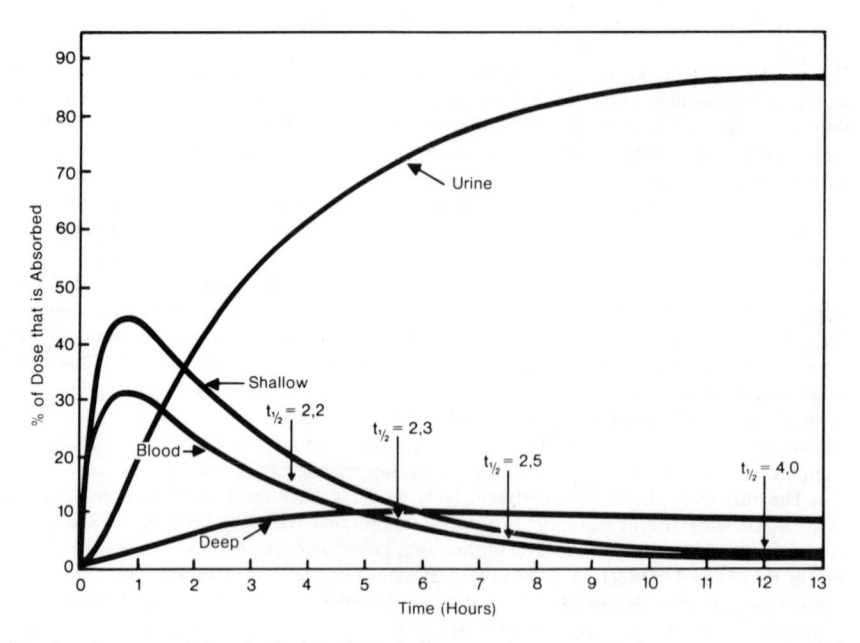

Fig. 2. Amounts of drug in the blood, B, shallow compartment, SC, deep compartment, DC, after first-order absorption from the gastrointestinal tract, GI, as generated by the analog computer for the model

$$\begin{array}{c} SC \\ \Updownarrow \\ GI \rightarrow B \rightarrow U \\ \Updownarrow \\ DC \end{array}$$

with first-order transferences among compartments. SC is a rapidly equilibrating tissue whereas DC is a slowly equilibrating tissue. (Figure 20 of Garrett, 1971.)

eosinophiles, embryos, etc. Their existence allows the body to retain drug for longer periods than the arbitrary half-life estimates made on the basis of a major depletion of drug content in the body would permit.

In practice, the greatest number of compartments that are mathematically obtainable from the analyses of the plasma level–time curves on intravenous dosing is three: the central or instantaneously equilibrated tissues (B), the readily permeable tissue (T), and the slowly permeable tissues (T') or "deep" compartment that never truly equilibrates with the other two (Figs. 1 and 2)

$$T' \rightleftarrows B \rightleftarrows T$$
$$\text{urine} \quad \text{bile} \quad \text{metabolites} \tag{11}$$

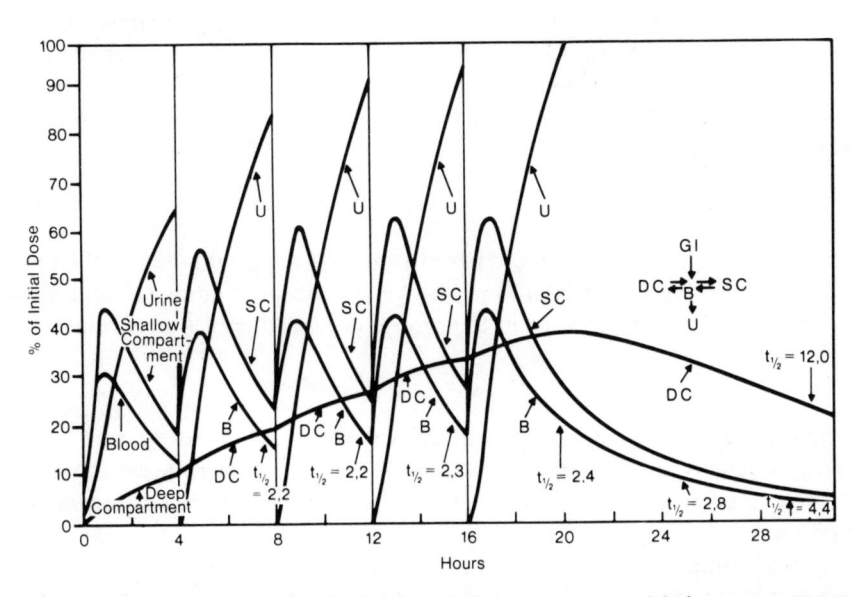

Fig. 3. Curves of amounts of drug in blood, B, shallow compartment, SC, deep compartment, DC, and urine, U, after first-order absorption of drug from the gastrointestinal tract, GI, as generated by the analog computer on repetitive dosing. The model is

$$\begin{array}{c} SC \\ \updownarrow \\ GI \rightarrow B \rightarrow U \\ \updownarrow \\ DC \end{array}$$

The data for the urine, U, are corrected to the zero amount line at each dosing interval for convenience of representation. (Figure 21 of Garrett, 1971.)

Confirmation of the presence of this deep compartment may be obtained from slowed and almost constant terminal rates of elimination or metabolism of drug as monitored by the rate of drug and metabolite appearance in the urine or excreta. A consequence of the presence of a deep compartment of sufficient capacity is that on chronic dosing, the body will accumulate large amounts of such drug. The elimination of significant amounts of such drug, even after termination of its chronic administration will be prolonged and slow (Fig. 3).

OUTLINE OF METHODS OF PHARMACOKINETIC ANALYSES

The first estimates of pharmacokinetic parameters can be obtained by the plotting of the logarithmic values of the concentrations of drug in the blood (b), plasma (p), or free drug in plasma unbound (p_u), against time. A terminal linear slope in a two-compartment body model is indicative of a relatively fast equilibration among tissues with the central compartment and permits the estimation of an overall disposition constant k_e from the slopes in accordance with

$$\ln p_u = -k_e t + \ln p_u' \tag{12}$$

where the extrapolated intercept permits the first approximation of the total apparent volumes of distribution V_D of the equilibrated fluids referenced to the measured concentrations in the central compartment. For example,

$$V_D = V_{p_u} + V_T = D_0/p_u' \tag{13}$$

where D_0 is the dose administered intravenously and where V_{p_u} and V_T are the apparent volumes of distribution of the central and peripheral compartments, respectively, referenced to the unbound drug concentration in the plasma.

An estimate of the apparent volume of distribution of the central compartment may be obtained from the extrapolated intercept of the unbound level of drug in the plasma, $(p_u)_0$, at zero time:

$$V_{p_u} = D_0/(p_u)_0 \tag{14}$$

If the drug is eliminated by urinary excretion in whole or part, if all removal routes are first order, and there is no hold up in the kidney, the terminal straight line of a semilogarithmic plot of drug amount not yet excreted in the urine against time will give a slope of the same k_e value:

$$\ln(U_\infty - U) = -k_e t + \ln U_\infty \tag{15}$$

where U_∞ is the total amount of drug excreted in the urine and U is the cumulative amount excreted at any time, t. The ratio

$$\frac{U_\infty}{D_0 - U_\infty} = \frac{(k_e)_r}{k_e - (k_e)_r} \qquad (16)$$

permits the estimation of the first-order rate constant $(k_e)_r$, for the renal elimination of the intact drug and the sum of the constants, $k_e - (k_e)_r$, for the other routes of drug removal. If the total amounts of metabolites formed are known, the individual rate constant for metabolism can be estimated [see Eqs. (4)–(6)].

The complete semilogarithmic plot of plasma level against time can be analyzed by feathering, i.e., the logarithm of the difference of the antilogarithm of values from the extrapolated terminal semilogarithmic line of slope k_e or β and the actual early values of the plasma level when plotted against time will give a new straight line of slope α, so that the entire blood level curve can be constructed as

$$p_u = Ae^{-\alpha t} + Be^{-\beta t} \qquad (17)$$

and from the A, B, α, and β values the microscopic rate constants for the two-compartment body model [see Eq. (8)] can be calculated from equations given in the literature (Riegelman *et al.*, 1968).

If single feathering does not result in a straight line that accounts for all of the initial time data, the process can be repeated and a three-compartment model should be postulated. Similarly, if the semilogarithmic plot against time of the plasma concentration and the amount of drug unexcreted in the urine does not show a terminal linear slope, a "deep" compartment should be postulated.

An alternative method of estimating k_e from urinary excretion data is from the slope of the plot of the logarithm of the urinary excretion rate (amount excreted in a constant time interval) against time. This method has the advantage that not all of the urine has to be collected.

The renal clearance plot of rate of urinary excretion of drug against the plasma level has a slope representative of the product of the rate constant k_e and the apparent volume of distribution of the equilibrated fluids, provided that the drug is only renally excreted. In the general case where there are other first-order routes of elimination or metabolism, the renal clearance determined from such plots would be multiplied by the fraction of the total drug renally excreted (Garrett, 1970).

If the renal clearance plot is nonlinear, it is indicative of blood-level-dependent pharmacokinetics. This can be attributed to enzyme or blood protein saturation or blood-concentration-dependent renal excretion.

These mathematical and graphical procedures can serve as preliminary estimates of the parameters necessary to describe the dynamic model for the distribution, metabolism, and excretion of the drug and metabolite, and to correlate with pharmacological activity.

Analog computation (Garrett, 1964; Garrett and Alway, 1964; Röpke and Riemann, 1969) is a powerful tool in this process since the techniques of classical mathematics are inadequate when the numbers of compartments considered exceed two or three. Programs now exist for fitting such models by digital computation (Berman *et al.*, 1962) and obtaining statistical estimates of error in the quantitative values of these parameters. However, prior to using the digital computer, it is vital to instruct the program as to the model to be fitted and the anticipated range of values of these parameters. If this is not done, the reiterative procedures of digital computation do not permit solutions for the parameters of the pharmacokinetic model with economic use of computer time. Thus, the prior use of mathematical approximations and analog computer techniques are necessary.

The reliability of a first-order multicompartmental model for the distribution, metabolism, and excretion of a drug can only be tested by varying intravenous dosage within the clinical dose range and determining whether the derived intrinsic rate constants and apparent volumes of distribution are invariant with dose. The apparent elimination or metabolic rate constant will vary with dose when the blood protein (Krüger-Thiemer, 1967), tissues, and enzymic processes are saturable; or when the drug has the property of changing the diffusivity, permeability, or size of distributive compartments as a function of dose.

Protein binding and red-blood cell partition effects can be analyzed *in vitro* (Meyer and Guttman, 1968). The possible time dependence of these processes can be checked. Ultracentrifugal filtration of the blood and plasma aliquots sampled with time can give information as to the time dependence of these processes *in vivo*.

Enzymic saturation can be checked with microsomal preparations *in vitro* or with competitive inhibitors *in vivo*. Metabolite administration concomitant with drug should permit a decision as to whether the enzymic system is product-inhibited. Biliary excretion rates may be monitored as functions of doses. Independent checks of cardiac volume and renal clearance are helpful to assign the dependence of pharmacokinetic parameters on dose.

Concomitant pH monitoring of blood and urine would give evidence of ambient or pH effects that may modify the tubular reabsorption or tissue distribution of the drug and its metabolites. The pH can be controlled by induced alkalinosis or acidosis. Applicable methods are the administration of ammonium chloride or by the control of respiratory rate.

Occasionally, the rate of metabolite appearance does not mirror the loss of drug and may be assigned to storage of metabolite or precursor in an intermediate compartment such as the liver.

The rate of appearance of a compound in the urine may not be consistent with its rate of loss in the body and may imply storage or binding or saturable processes in the kidney.

The phenomenon of enterohepatic circulation may be clarified by monitoring biliary excretion and fecal content simultaneously; or by pharmacokinetic studies with oral administration of the metabolite. The pharmacokinetics of metabolites should be monitored and it must be realized that their volumes of distribution are not those of their drug precursor.

The possibilities of enzymic induction in the intact animal should not be ignored. It can be readily checked by determining blood levels and urinary excretion rates at selected times after repetitive daily administration of the drug at intervals that do not implicate cumulative effects.

BIOAVAILABILITY OF DRUGS FROM DOSAGE FORMS

Pharmacokinetics can be used to determine the biological availability of drug from the dosage form. Although the primary proof of pharmacological or chemotherapeutic availability of a drug at its site of action from its vehicle or formulation is the magnitude and duration of the biological responses, these are difficult to quantify. Assuredly, the next preferred proof of availability is the appearance of the active species in the biophase. Unfortunately, the exact position of this biophase is infrequently known and if known, it is too difficult or small to sample and assay as a function of time.

A secondary proof of availability is the appearance of the drug and its metabolites in the blood, tissues, and excreta of the organism. This is based on the reasonable assumptions that the drug will exercise its action in the body when it does appear and that the biological activity is related to the amounts that do appear.

This is frequently accomplished by comparing the time course of drug concentrations in the body with the most readily available formulations of the drug which are, if possible, intravenously and orally administered solutions. Comparisons of the biological availability of the drug from various dosage forms can be made on the basis of the relative amounts in the different biological compartments as a function of time.

The simplest way to determine the amount of a drug biologically available from a formulation is to measure the amount of drug or its metabolites that are excreted from the body by routes other than those that are simple consequences of the route of administration.

The use of amount excreted as a criterion of relative biological availability depends on the acceptance of the assumption that the amounts of drug and its metabolites that are excreted in the urine are directly proportional to the amount absorbed. The use of the amount of only one metabolite excreted as a criterion of efficacy of absorption, even on the assumption that the percent metabolized by a particular route is constant and independent of dose, is invalid if the drug is metabolized or transformed before absorption. Since fractions of the dose metabolized may differ among individuals, it is always best to use an individual as his own control when comparing total drug or metabolite excreted for estimation of relative biological availabilities of several formulations administered by the same route.

An alternative method of determining the amount of drug absorbed from the formulation is by the application of the Dost principle of corresponding areas (Dost, 1968). If a drug is eliminated from, or metabolized in the body by a first-order process, the area under the plot of the concentration of the drug in the blood against time, A, is directly proportional to the absorbed fraction, γ, of the dose, D_0, and inversely proportional to the overall apparent first-order elimination constant, k_e, the sum of the first-order rate constants of the separate eliminations and metabolisms, and to the apparent equilibrated volume of distribution, V_f of the body:

$$A = \gamma D_0 / V_f k_e \qquad (18)$$

This equation is valid to compare availability of a drug by any route of administration and any order of absorption unless the drug is highly metabolized so that oral absorption would differ from administration by most other routes in that an extremely high concentration of drug would hit the liver on the first pass prior to its dilution with the blood and equilibrating tissues.

Thus, it is best to compare the relative biological availability of drug in various formulations administered by the same route and in the same individual on the presumption that V_f and k_e are invariant.

The application of Eq. (18) to the Dost method of corresponding areas (Dost, 1968) is also limited in that all eliminations and metabolisms must be first order and the pertinent rate constants must be independent of dose (Garrett, 1971).

The *amount* of drug available from a formulation is not the only important factor in determining the bioavailability of the drug from the dosage form.

More important criteria for a dosage regimen in many instances are the *rates* of the drug being made available in the body. It may be desirable to maintain a body level of drug for a desired length of time *below* the maximum level which yields toxicity and *above* the minimum level which exercises no effect against a disease.

The rate of appearance, concentration, and duration of the requisite concentration of the drug in the biophase of drug action must be related to the rate of appearance of the drug in the blood and its rapidly equilibrated tissues. Thus, the parameters that can characterize the latter can be related to the appearance of the drug in the biophase and the desired pharmacological action.

The simplest model to establish for the appearance of a drug in the body from a formulation is the one-compartment body model with first-order release of the amount F in the formulation, first-order absorption of the amount D, and overall first-order transformation of the amount B in the body of apparent volume of distribution V_f into the urine U and metabolites M:

$$F \xrightarrow{k_f} D \xrightarrow{k_a} B \xrightarrow{k_e} U + M \tag{19}$$

where the respective apparent first-order rate constants are k_f, k_a, k_e. In the specific instance when a solution of the drug is administered, k_f is infinite. If, as is generally, but not always, true (penicillin is a classical example of the exception), the drug is absorbed more readily than it is excreted, a plot of the logarithm of the concentration of drug in the blood against time would permit estimation (Dost, 1968) of the overall elimination rate constant, k_e, from the terminal slope (Fig. 4) of such a plot. Successive "feathering" can yield estimates of the first-order rate constants k_a and k_f.

It is surprising how often such a first-order process serves to characterize the absorption process in practice.

The determination of the rate constants, k_a and k_e, by the above specified methods permits the estimation of the blood curve at any time from the expression

$$b = \frac{B}{V_f} = \frac{D_0}{V_f} \frac{k_a}{(k_e - k_a)} (e^{-k_a t} - e^{-k_e t}) \tag{20}$$

when the time duration of a blood level b above a certain desired minimum b_{min} from the administration of a solution of drug, D_0, can be calculated. If the rate of release of the drug from the formulation is the rate-determining

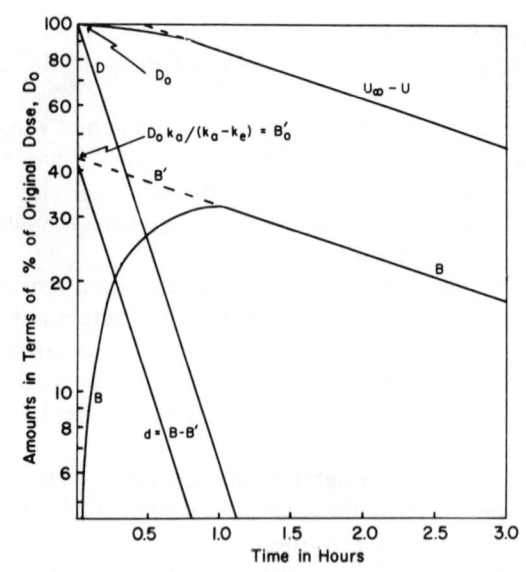

Fig. 4. Semilogarithmic plots of amounts of drug in the blood, $B = bV_f$ and not-yet-excreted into the urine, $U_\infty - U$, in accordance with the model $D \xrightarrow{k_a} B \xrightarrow{k_e} U$. The total dose, D_0, is considered to be absorbed in this example, i.e., $\gamma_a = 1$. The terminal slopes of these plots of $\ln B$ and $\ln(U_\infty - U)$ against time are $-k_e$. "Feathering" gives the difference between the linearly extrapolated values of the terminal data and the real data, i.e., $d = B' - B$ which when plotted semilogarithmically, i.e., as $\ln d$ vs. t produces the straight line with the slope $-k_a$. This would be the same slope that would have been obtained if the drug, D, released by a first-order rate from the absorption site had been plotted as $\ln D$ vs. t. (Figure 16 of Garrett, 1971.)

factor in the absorption then this calculated interval of a blood level above a b_{min} value can serve in the estimation of biological availability of a drug dosage D_0 from various formulations.

Other criteria of biological availability which would fully characterize drug–time appearance curves in the blood on the basis of a sequential first-order model are the maximum blood level, b_{max}, achieved and the time, t_{max}, at which this maximum is reached.

If both the rate of absorption and the rate of release from the dosage form are characterized by first-order rate constants, i.e., k_e and k_f in Eq. (19), respectively, then a further "feathering" of the blood level–time curves permits estimates of the apparent first-order rate constant, k_f, for the *in vitro* release of the drug from the formulation when $k_a \gg k_f$. In practice, practically all formulation release rates [except perhaps from a mass of coated pellets of different thickness of coating (Garrett and Lambert, 1966)] follow apparent first order.

If only data on drug (or metabolite derived from drug) excreted in the urine are available, the ability to fit models is severely limited. The only reasonable model to assume is that given by Eq. (19) with its previously stated underlying assumptions. Nelson (1959, 1960, 1961) derived an expression based on this model.

The absorption rate was expressed as

$$dA/dt = -d(F + D)/dt = d^2 U/dt^2/k_e f + (dU/dt)/f \qquad (21)$$

Thus, if k_e can be obtained from the slope of the linear plot of the terminal data of $\ln(U_\infty - U)$ against time, i.e., after absorption is completed, and if f, the total fraction of absorbed drug that is renally excreted unchanged, is known, all that is necessary to obtain the instantaneous rate of absorption in Eq. (21) is the instantaneous first and second derivatives of the urinary excretion rates of the unchanged drug. The first derivative, dU/dt, is obtainable at any given time from (a) the instantaneous slopes or tangents to the curve of total accumulated drug excreted in the urine against time, or (b) from the amount of drug excreted in a given interval of time. The second derivative, $d^2 U/dt^2$, can be obtained from the tangents to the plot of the instantaneous rates of urinary excretion against time. This method has many limitations. The major one is the difficulty of obtaining accurate urinary excretion data and sufficient numbers of urinary analyses during the drug absorption phase. The taking of second derivatives by such a process is also a risky business.

Equation (21) can be integrated (Wagner and Nelson, 1963 and 1964) so that the amount, A_t, of drug absorbed up to time t can be expressed as

$$A_t = [(dU/dt)/k_e + U]/f \qquad (22)$$

Thus, from the knowledge of the excretion rate, dU/dt, at any time, i.e., the amount excreted per unit time, and the total cumulative amount of drug, U, excreted into the urine up to that time, the amount of drug, A_t, absorbed at any given time can be calculated. This Eq. (22) needs no assumption of order of absorption or of drug release since it determines the overall transfer of F and D to the body B [Eq. (19)] by any process whatsoever, at any time t.

If the same individual is used to compare two different formulations so that the fraction, f, of drug excreted unchanged can be assumed to be constant, fA_t values can be calculated from Eq. (22) without explicit knowledge of f. Thus, the ratios of these values give the relative amounts absorbed, $(A_t)_1/(A_t)_2$, from formulations 1 and 2 at any given time.

Wagner and Nelson (1963, 1964) have also shown that the amount absorbed, A_t, at any time t may be expressed by

$$A_t = V_f\left(b + k_e \int_0^t b\, dt\right) \qquad (23)$$

Thus, the area under the drug concentration in the blood–time curve to a time t, i.e., $\int_0^t b\, dt$, and knowledge of the blood level b at that time permit the estimation of the amount absorbed up to that time. This equation needs no assumption of order of absorption or drug release since it determines the overall transfer of F and D to the body B [Eq. (19)] by any process whatsoever at time t.

If the same individual is used to compare two different formulations so that V_f can be assumed to be constant, A_t/V_f values can be calculated from Eq. (23) without explicit knowledge of V_f. Thus, the ratios of these values give the relative amounts absorbed, $(A_t)_1/(A_t)_2$, from formulations 1 and 2 at any given time.

Similar expressions have been derived for the two-compartment body model by Loo and Riegelman (1968).

These several methods are limited in that they presume first-order removal of drug from the body into the excreta and metabolites; that apparent first-order rate constants of equilibration, elimination, and metabolism are independent of blood level and dose; that there is no storage in an intermediate compartment or lag between the loss from the blood and the appearance in the monitored excreta.

The use of computers can eliminate the restrictions of one- and two-compartment body models and the assumption of first-order eliminations. The exact pharmacokinetic models can be established on the basis of intravenous and oral dosing in solution and the time functions of release from the dosage form that further perturb the monitored drug and metabolite levels in blood, tissue, and excreta can be determined.

PHARMACOKINETICS AND SITES OF DRUG ACTION

The natures of the time courses of biological response and blood level of drug as functions of varying dose permit the characterization of a receptor site occupancy model to describe the availability of the biophase in the complex organism. We may postulate that the biological response is proportional to the occupancy of receptor sites and that it is possible to obtain quantitative estimates of biological responses as a function of time concomitant with blood levels of drug (Fig. 5). Comparisons of the resulting

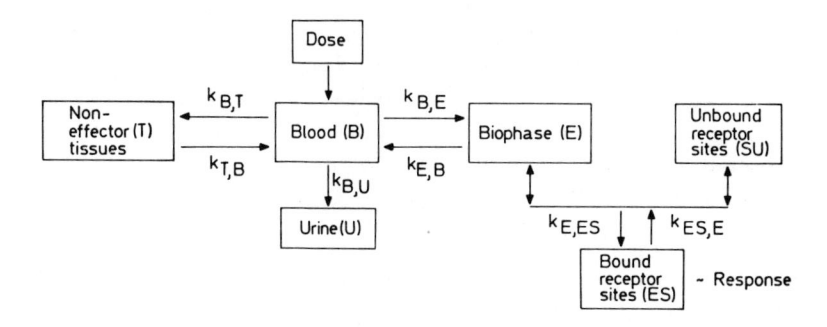

Fig. 5. A model for the effect of drug distribution on pharmacodynamic response.

curves should give insight into the properties of the biophase (deep or shallow) and the effect of blood–tissue equilibration on the time course of drug action as estimated from an apparent half-life in the decay of biological response (Garrett et al., 1967). The biophase is that body compartment in which the receptor sites reside.

If the maximum value of the biological response is not proportional to dosage or is relatively invariant with dose, it may be concluded that affinity of the drug for receptor sites is high, and the receptor sites are relatively saturated for a large range of drug concentrations in the biophase. Increasing dosages would maintain the constant maximum response for increased time intervals. If the onset of the maximum response is time invariant, rapid equilibration of drug with receptor sites may be concluded. If the magnitude of the biological response is proportional to the dose then the affinity of the drug for the receptor sites is low and there are excess numbers of such receptors.

If the decay of the biological response parallels the rapid decay of the blood level of the drug, the biophase is related to the blood level. If the rise and decay of the biological response parallels the content of the equilibrated tissues, the biophase is related to, or equivalent in properties to the rapidly equilibrating tissues.

Observation of a long delay in the maximum biological response manifests the biophase as a deep compartment. The appearance of the maximum response after the blood level of drug has decreased to low amounts of its tissue-equilibrated value is also characteristic. Sustained and time-invariant biological responses are indicative.

If the distribution of drug into a deep compartment can be monitored (pharmacokinetically feasible when the deep compartment has reasonable capacity) and the time course of biological response is similar, then a possible identity of this deep compartment and the biophase may be assumed. The implication is that the rates of equilibration with the receptor sites are fast and no lag period will be observed. If dosage variation shows a linear relation of maximum biological response with dose, low affinities and nonsaturation of receptor sites are indicated. Invariant maximum biological response with increasing doses are indicative of high affinities and saturation of receptor sites.

PHARMACOKINETICS AND CLINICAL METABOLIC PROFILES

The perturbations of magnitudes of pharmacokinetic parameters among individuals challenged with a drug can be used as a diagnostic tool in evaluating the state of dynamic processes, the presence of metabolic diseases and genetic abnormalities, and the failure of physiological functions.

Human beings vary in their rates of absorption, distribution, and metabolism of drugs and even vary in the type and magnitude of the biological response resulting from drug administration. The basic pharmacokinetic pattern for a given drug might be expected to be the same for all humans but the *magnitudes* of the rate constants for absorption, distribution in body compartments, metabolism, and excretion will vary among individuals. Variations in the pharmacokinetic pattern of a drug may be used to indicate the possibility of a deviation in normal biological response to a given drug, the so-called "adverse drug reaction."

A quantitative knowledge of the distributive, metabolic, and excretory patterns of a drug could serve to define the clinical state of the individual, to assess the efficiency of his enzymic processes, to detect abnormalities in metabolism, and to provide an estimate of the operational lean–fat ratio. Pharmacokinetic profiles for appropriate drugs may also allow one to obtain an estimate of the renal, hepatic, and biliary efficiency for the elimination of drugs, membrane transfers or tissue binding of drugs, and the availability of the drug from the dosage form in relation to the gastrointestinal absorption capabilities of the individual. The profile of uptake, distribution, metabolism, and excretion of standard drugs could serve as *in situ* measures of liver, kidney, and hemodynamic function in the individual patient. Optimum magnitudes of dose and regimen optimized for a particular individual can then be readily given by the computer. The patient may be classified on the basis of generalized pharmacokinetic parameters so that the practicing physician can give an individualized therapy on the basis of this classification.

PHARMACOKINETICS AND PREDICTION OF CHRONIC DOSING REGIMENS

Pharmacokinetics can predict an optimum dosage regimen to maintain a blood level of drug between certain maximum and minimum values. The former may be chosen on the basis that higher levels would induce toxicities and the latter on the basis that lower values would be insufficient to maintain desired chemotherapeutic or pharmacological effects. On the assumption of the sequential first-order model of absorption and elimination with rapid equilibration among all bodily compartments, Dost (1968) has derived a series of equations which permit the calculation of concentrations of drug in the blood at any time after doses were administered at uniform intervals. Krüger-Thiemer (1964, 1966) has programed these equations and modifications of them on the digital computer. Dettli (1971) has demonstrated the clinical applications of these individualized dosage regimens.

The rate constants for absorption, distribution, and elimination and the apparent volumes of distribution of these several compartments can be determined from acute dosings as described previously. Curves representative of amounts and concentrations in the various compartments can be generated by the analog computer to predict effects from repetitive dosing at separated intervals. Typical curves are predicted for repetitive dosing at four-hour intervals in Fig. 3 from the parameters derived from the analysis of the acute dosing of Fig. 2 in accordance with the model of Eq. (11) where the drug is absorbed into the blood compartment by a first-order process.

It should be observed that when all tissues are quickly equilibrated with the blood, the apparent half-life, $t_{\frac{1}{2}}$, after the drug is absorbed is constant and independent of the subsequent time.

When a deep compartment is present as in the model of Eq. (11), and the drug is absorbed by a first-order process, the apparent half-life, $t_{\frac{1}{2}}$, after the drug is completely absorbed increases with time (Figs. 2 and 3). When the dose responsible for the curves of Fig. 2 is administered repetitively at four-hour intervals, the possibility of accumulation of large amounts of drug in a slowly equilibrating deep compartment, DC, is graphically shown in the analog computer-generated curves of Fig. 3. The slow release of drug from this compartment manifests itself in an increased apparent half-life of the drug in the body.

If it is postulated that the longer a drug remains in the body, the greater the opportunity for the demonstration of toxicity, comparison of the curves of Figs. 2 and 3 demonstrate that repetitive or sustained dosing may lead to toxic effects that would not be manifested by separated acute dosages.

THE FRONTIERS

This summary of the present status of pharmacokinetics is necessarily superficial. However, it does serve as a basis for considering the frontiers that border on the future.

The clinical applications are apparent. The concomitant determination of pharmacokinetic parameters and correlation with quantified pharmacodynamic effects will permit the prediction of proper dosage regimens for the treatment of disease and minimization of toxicities. This demands the development and use of methods to monitor quantifiable pharmacodynamic parameters as functions of time.

Future pharmacokinetic studies must challenge subjects with various dose levels by various routes of administration so that realistic nonlinear models can be deduced to account for dose-dependent phenomena.

Adverse drug reactions are pharmacokinetically and pharmacogenetically based. Thus, *a priori* knowledge of anomalous metabolic enzymic deficiencies, excesses, or inductions can permit estimations of proper dosage regimens.

The use of metabolic or pharmacokinetic profiles can give individualized dosage regimens. This should lead to the development of flexible dosage forms that are readily adaptable to unique regimens and are consistent with the known, but ignored, fact—that everyone is different. Delineation of the apparent volumes of distribution, renal insufficiencies, gastrointestinal anomalies, etc., can permit the practicing physician to modify standard dose regimens for the well-being of the individual patient.

The comparison of the pharmacokinetics and metabolisms of a drug in various species may permit the design of molecules that have the desired action without toxicity in man. Certainly, the proper scientific goal is to predict the pharmacokinetics of a new drug species before such studies are made. The pharmacokinetic basis for the pharmacodynamic action of a drug must be impressed on our medicinal chemists so that they cease to merely design molecules that only act effectively when administered directly into the biophase.

REFERENCES

Berman, M., Shahn, E., and Weiss, M. F., 1962, *Biophys. J.* **2**:275.
Dettli, L., 1971, in: *Klinische Pharmakologie und Pharmakotherapie* (H. P. Kuemmerle, E. R. Garrett, and K. H. Spitzy, eds.), Urban und Schwarzenberg Verlag, Munich.
Dost, F. H., 1968, *Grundlagen der Pharmakokinetik*, 2nd ed., Thieme Verlag, Stuttgart.
Garrett, E. R., 1964, *Antibiotica et Chemotherapia, Advances*, Karger Verlag, Basel, Vol. 12, p. 227.
Garrett, E. R., 1969, *Advances in the Biosciences*, Pergamon Press, New York, Vol. 5, p. 7.

Garrett, E. R., 1971, in: *Klinische Pharmakologie und Pharmakotherapie* (H. P. Kuemmerle, E. R. Garrett, and K. H. Spitzy, eds.), Urban and Schwarzenberg Verlag, Munich.
Garrett, E. R., and Alway, C. D., 1964, *Proceedings of the 3rd International Congress on Chemotherapy*, Stuttgart, 1963, Vol. 2.
Garrett, E. R., and Gravenstein, J. S., 1967, *Proceedings of the 5th International Congress on Chemotherapy*, Vienna, 1967, Vol. 4, p. 105.
Garrett, E. R., and Lambert, H. J., 1966, *J. Pharm. Sci.*, **55**:626.
Garrett, E. R., Ågren, A. J., and Lambert, H. J., 1967, *Int. J. Clin. Pharmacol., Therapy, Toxicol.* **1**:1.
Garrett, E. R., Thomas, R. C., Wallach, D. P., and Alway, C. D., 1960, *J. Pharmacol. Exper. Therap.* **130**:106.
Krüger-Thiemer, E., 1964, *Proceedings of the 3rd International Congress on Chemotherapy*, Stuttgart, 1963, Vol. 2, p. 1686.
Krüger-Thiemer, E., 1966, *J. Theoret. Biol.* **13**:212.
Krüger-Thiemer, E., Dettli, L., Spring, P., and Diller, W., 1967, *Proceedings of the 3rd International Congress of Cybernetic Medicine*, Naples, Italy, 1964, p. 249.
Loo, J. C. K., and Riegelman, S., 1968, *J. Pharm. Sci.* **57**:918.
Meyer, M. C., and Guttman, D. E., 1968, *J. Pharm. Sci.* **57**:895.
Nelson, E., 1959, *J. Pharm. Sci.* **48**:489.
Nelson, E., 1960, *J. Pharm. Sci.* **49**:437.
Nelson, E., 1961, *J. Pharm. Sci.* **50**:181.
Röpke, H., and Riemann, J., 1969, *Analog Computer in Chemie und Biologie*, Springer-Verlag, Berlin.
Riegelman, S., Loo, J. C. K., and Rowland, M., 1968, *J. Pharm. Sci.* **57**:117.
Wagner, J., and Nelson, E., 1963, *J. Pharm. Sci.* **52**:610.
Wagner, J., and Nelson, E., 1964, *J. Pharm. Sci.* **53**:1392.

DISCUSSION SUMMARY

Ariens opened the discussion by probing the speaker and the audience for an exact definition of "bioavailability," stating that the literature has applied various meanings to the term. Garrett responded that he felt bioavailability to be a misnomer since the term is not used to mean "available to act" in a pharmacodynamic sense in the body. Instead, bioavailability is usually defined in relation to a measure of the time course of a drug in the general circulation. Although these measurements may be considered a first approximation to the pharmacodynamic availability or to the duration of action of a drug, a more meaningful measure of bioavailability would be the degree and duration of a specific pharmacologic response. Garrett went on to point out that there are many ways in which one can define aspects of bioavailability depending on the methodology employed by the investigator. Ariens thought this definition too general and asked if bioavailability might be defined as the fraction of the administered dose which reaches the general circulation.

Riegelman explicitly defined bioavailability as the extent and rate at which the administered dose reaches the sampling site, usually a peripheral vein. He added that the site of measurement could influence these values. Wagner took a pragmatic approach to the definition: if a tablet or capsule is labeled as containing a certain amount of drug, it is usually assumed that this amount reaches the general circulation. Bioavailability is a measure of the reliability of this assumption in terms of the degree and rate observed relative to a standard dosage form.

Benet returned to the more general approach suggested by Garrett. That is, bioavailability should be a measure of the rate and extent of drug reaching the biophase, the site of drug action. He suggested that the attainment of measurable blood levels for a particular drug may actually be considered one of the basic failures of drug therapy, since measurable blood levels are an indication of the therapist's inability to get the drug directly into the biophase. a number of pharmaceutical companies are developing dosage forms which may be input directly into the biophase or target organ, such as an intrauterine ring impregnated with an anti-fertility compound or a soft plastic lens designed to release drug directly into the eye. For products such as these, measurable levels of drug in the blood would more than likely indicate a toxic dose or a faulty dosage form. Pharmacologic measurements of bioavailabilty would be most appropriate for these products. Benet concluded that, at present, blood level measurements of bioavailability are used as a means of comparing various oral dosage forms, simply because there is not an efficient means of administering the drug directly to its site of action or of measuring its bioavailability at this site.

Sjoqvist responded to the concluding remarks of Garrett's lecture with respect to the fact that most pharmaceutical manufacturers produce drug products as a standard dose, and suggest fixed doses of the drug in various therapeutic situations. He pointed out that the relationship of plasma concentration to pharmacologic effect is known for only about 12 drugs, in comparison to the more than 300 drugs that are used in most hospitals. Optimal drug formulations and individual dosage regimens tailored to the clinical state of the patient can only be realized after clinical studies of the importance of pharmacokinetics and drug response have been carried out. Sjoqvist suggested that information from these types of studies must be fed back to the drug industry and to other clinicians before pharmacokinetics at the bedside can become a reality. Both Garrett and Lemberger suggested that it is the responsibility of the pharmaceutical industry to determine and make available pharmacokinetic data for their drugs and that the responsibility of the clinician is to adjust the dosage of these drugs in a patient. Lemberger added that it is extremely difficult, if not impossible, to determine a pharmacokinetic profile for a drug in every patient, and therefore the clinician falls back on the usual doses suggested by the manufacturer.

Wagner suggested a means of overcoming the inflexible dose problem that tablets or capsules present. His simple concept, especially tailored for use in the hospital where average doses are seldom used, consisted of having a drug formulation extruded in long segments similar to spaghetti. This would allow the pharmacist to cut off a section of the dosage form which would be exactly equal to the milligram dose suggested by the physician.

Returning to the bioavailability problem, Garrett suggested two alternatives which could be employed to overcome the problem of variability in drug products from a number of manufacturers. Either each individual company must take the responsibility of validating the efficacy of their suggested dosage regimen or we must demand that all dosage forms of the same drug must give the same bioavailability when measurements are determined under identical conditions.

Berman pointed out that although the term bioavailability has frequently been used synonymously with the effect of the drug, there may be a considerable gap between the two. A simple example is the use of lithium in the treatment of Graves disease. It has been shown that lithium seems to have an effect in at least two sites related to hydrolysis of thyroglobulin in the thyroid and the disappearance of thyroxin in the periphery. However, the actual clinical effect is a combination of the level of lithium in the thyroid, the degree of abnormality of thyroid hormone synthesis and secretion, the sensitivity of these mechanisms to lithium, and the fact that two sites of action are involved. Thus the blood levels of lithium may not be a consistent therapeutic measure of the clinical effects.

Axelrod stressed the importance of having a measure of bioavailability and that the best reflection of this parameter is measured blood levels, even considering the number of faults found with this measurement. He felt that for patients receiving long-term drug therapy it is crucial to understand how much of the drug is present in the body and how it changes over a period of time. He suggested that with the development of all of our sophisticated medical methodologies, the physician should undertake to determine a half-life for the drug whenever a patient is initially begun on long-term therapy. This half-life value should be checked periodically in light of the possibility of induction or inhibition of drug disposition resulting from the concomitant administration of other drugs or from changes in the pathophysiologic condition of the patient. A knowledge of this value would greatly aid in the rational administration of drug doses. Since the physician undertaking a new patient or course of therapy will routinely screen the patient with a series of laboratory tests, it is logical to include a measurement of drug half-life in this screen.

Garrett closed the discussion by reiterating the point made by Axelrod that all too often dosage regimens are adjusted on the basis of the appearance of toxic symptoms in the patient. Garrett suggested that we have the ability to determine many parameters in addition to half-life, and he reiterated the statements in his formal presentation with respect to the use of subtherapeutic drug cocktails to determine a metabolic pattern in individual patients.

A Modern View of Pharmacokinetics

John G. Wagner

College of Pharmacy and Upjohn Center for Clinical Pharmacology
The University of Michigan
Ann Arbor, Michigan

Publication of the mathematics of accumulation in the one compartment open model by Widmark and Tandberg (1924) and the two papers on the two-compartment open model by the organizer of this conference, Professor Torsten Teorell (1937), were the origins of pharmacokinetics. Many of us who have studied the literature of pharmacokinetics have been amazed at the insight and foresight embodied in Professor Teorell's two papers. The classical one- and two-compartment open linear models have withstood the test of time, achieved accurate assessment of rates of absorption, metabolism, and excretion when applied to certain specific drugs, and been very useful for predictive purposes. Undoubtedly in the future these classical models will continue to be as useful as they have in the past. These classical pharmacokinetics models are based upon systems of linear differential equations, which may conveniently be integrated using Laplace transforms. Kinetic linearity was defined by Krüger-Thiemer (1968a) as direct proportionality of transfer rates to concentrations or concentration differences.

A modern view of pharmacokinetics must include both linear and nonlinear systems. For many years in the linear pharmacokinetic area authors spent a great deal of time and journal space deriving the equations they needed to interpret data. Recently, Benet and Turi (1971) and Benet (1972) made significant contributions in the linear pharmacokinetic area. The Benet method (1972) allows one to write the Laplace transform for the amount of drug in any compartment of a mammillary model and to obtain the inverse Laplace transform (i.e., the final integrated equation) consisting of a sum of exponential terms. The method is highly recommended for those not familiar with the technique. Since Dr. Garrett has reviewed classical pharmacokinetics I will spend most of my time comparing linear and nonlinear pharmacokinetics and discussing nonlinear pharmacokinetics.

HISTORICAL

Evidence of nonlinearities in pharmacokinetics goes back almost as far as the theory of linear pharmacokinetics. Widmark (1933) originated the concept that ethyl alcohol is eliminated at a fixed rate independent of its concentration in the body. After an oral dose of ethyl alcohol, a certain range of alcohol blood concentrations appears to give a straight line when the data are plotted on cartesian coordinate graph paper; but when plotted on semilogarithmic graph paper they give a line with concave decreasing curvature. Although Widmark's concept is still widely accepted and taught, it is really incorrect, as was discussed in a recent paper (Wagner and Patel, 1972).

In searching the literature for this review I was rather amazed to find in my files over 160 articles which contained evidence of nonlinearities in drug absorption, distribution, metabolism, and excretion, and in the pharmacokinetics of drug action. This review is not intended to be an exhaustive search. In the area of pharmacokinetics of drug action only reviews, and not original literature, are cited. Much of the literature has been summarized in a series of tables: Table I lists the evidence of nonlinearities in drug absorption; Table II, the evidence for nonlinearities in drug distribution; Table III, the evidence for nonlinearities in drug metabolism; Table IV, the evidence for nonlinearities in renal excretion of drugs and metabolites; Table V, the evidence of nonlinearities in biliary excretion of drugs; and Table VI, the evidence for nonlinearities in pharmacokinetics of drug action. It may well be that I have missed some significant references, and to the authors of those papers I apologize. However, Tables I through VI summarize the references I could readily find.

COMPARISON OF LINEAR AND NONLINEAR PHARMACOKINETICS

Drug Absorption. In linear pharmacokinetics the process of drug absorption has usually been described mathematically by one or two first order processes. Krüger-Thiemer (1968) stated that deviations from linear drug absorption kinetics may result from low solubility of the drug, from low rate of dissolution, from the many different types of sustained release

TABLE I
Evidence for Nonlinearities in Drug Absorption

Drug	Comments	References
Several	Mathematical description of carrier-mediated transport across a membrane	Wilbrandt and Rosenberg (1961)
Several	Mathematical aspects of effects of drugs on active transport systems	Patlack (1961)
Riboflavin	Saturable absorption process evident in fasted subjects not evident when subjects fed	Levy and Jusko (1966)
^{14}C-Antipyrine	Change in absorption rate with change in intestinal blood flow rate	Ochsenfahrt and Winne (1968)
Griseofulvin	Nonlinear absorption curves in man	Rowland et al. (1968)
Folic acid and 5-methyl-tetrahydrofolate	Absorption obeyed Michaelis–Menten kinetics	Hepner et al. (1968)
	No evidence of saturable absorption process	Strum et al. (1968)
Convallotoxin	In vitro studies indicated active transport mechanism for absorption	Lauterback (1968)
Barbiturates	Absorption rates correlated with binding to mucosal tissue	Kakemi et al. (1969)
Acidic and basic drugs	Theoretical models for drug absorption involving stagnant water layer	Suzuki et al. (1970a)
Sulfaethidole	Change in slope of first order plot for disappearance from intestinal lumen of dog with change in intestinal blood flow rate	Crouthamel et al. (1970)
Several	Kinetics of absorption related to intestinal blood flow rate	Winne (1970)
Several	Kinetics of carrier-mediated ion transport	Langer and Stark (1970)
Guanethidine	Percent of dose absorbed decreased with increasing dose in man	McMartin and Simpson (1971)

TABLE I (continued)

Drug	Comments	References
p-Substituted acetanilides	Hypothesized that tissue binding caused nonlinearity of first order plots in buccal absorption test	Dearden and Tomlinson (1971)
Indomethacin	Drug strongly bound to intestinal tissue during absorption and binding was dependent upon pH	Fuwa et al. (1971)
Pentobarbital	Delay in gastric emptying	Smith et al. (1972)
Acidic and basic drugs	Theoretical models for drug absorption which ignore stagnant water layer	Wagner and Sedman (1972)
Salicylamide	Rate of appearance of glucuronide in plasma, subsequent to intestinal wall metabolism, rate-limited by transport across the basal barrier rather than by metabolism	Barr and Riegelman (1970a,b)

preparations, and from saturable active absorption processes. In addition, one may add: fluctuations and changes in intestinal blood flow rate, as result of the work of Ochsenfahrt and Winne (1968), Crouthamel et al. (1970), and Winne (1970); the change in *p*H of lumenal contents as a basic, acidic, or amphoteric drug moves down the gastrointestinal tract, as the result of the work of Shore et al. (1957), Hogben et al. (1959), and the theoretical papers of Suzuki et al. (1970), and Wagner and Sedman (1972); and the possible effects of binding of drugs to mucosal tissue, as a result of the work of Kakemi et al. (1969), Dearden and Tomlinson (1971), and Fuwa et al. (1971). Delay in gastric emptying, such as caused by food in the stomach, enteric-coated tablets, sustained-release preparations, anticholinergic agents, etc., will also cause nonlinearities in the absorption process. The work of Rowland et al. (1968) with griseofulvin in man illustrates that administration of even a micronized drug powder yields absorption data which cannot be fitted well by simple first-order kinetics.

Metabolism and Active Tubular Secretion in the Kidney. Figure 1 compares linear and nonlinear pharmacokinetics with respect to metabolism and active tubular secretion in the kidney. At the top, a plot of $-dC/dt$

vs. C is linear in conformity with the first-order rate equation $-dC/dt = KC$. At the bottom, a plot of $-dC/dt$ *vs.* C gives a curved line, which approaches an asymptote ($-dC/dt \to V_m$ as $C \to \infty$), in conformity with the equation of Michaelis and Menten (1913), shown inset in the figure. It should be noted that the $K = 2.2$ line at the top is really the tangent line to the $-dC/dt$ *vs.* C plot at the bottom, since $V_m/K_m \to$ a constant (2.2) as $C \to 0$. If Michaelis–Menten kinetics are obeyed the percent saturation of the enzyme is given by Eq. (1).

$$-\frac{dC/dt}{V_m} \times 100 = \frac{C}{K_m + C} \times 100 \qquad (1)$$

It is the relative values of K_m and C which determine whether the Michaelis–Menten equation should be "collapsed" to a zero-order or first-order rate expression. The fundamental assumptions behind linear pharmacokinetics are that (1) saturable rate processes may be "collapsed" to first-order rate equations, and (2) saturable binding processes may be "collapsed" to the equation of a straight line. In actual practice, these both involve the approximation of a segment of a gently curving line by a straight line. The data in Table VII, which were calculated using Eq. (1) and literature values of K_m, suggest that the Michaelis–Menten equation should not be "collapsed" to a zero-order rate expression at least for salicylate, blood alcohol, and diphenylhydantoin. The computer simulation of salicylate urinary excretion data by Levy *et al.* (1972), the computer fitting of whole capillary blood alcohol concentrations by Wagner and Patel (1972), and the plasma diphenylhydantoin concentration data by Gerber and Wagner (1972) support this statement. The estimation of the V_m and K_m of the Michaelis–Menten equation from blood concentration or urinary excretion data is about as easy with a modern computer as the estimation of a first-order rate constant. Since the K_m and V_m values obtained will usually provide an adequate description of the kinetics at *all dose levels*, pharmacokineticists in the future may wish to use this approach rather than report a series of rate constants or half-lives of elimination which vary with the dose administered.

UPTAKE OF DRUG BY TISSUES

Figure 2 compares linear and nonlinear pharmacokinetics with respect to the uptake of drugs by tissues. At the top is the theoretical prediction of the amount of drug in the tissues as a function of dose for the two-compartment open model with rapid intravenous injection. The appropriate equation from which the lines were drawn is shown inset in the figure. The model predicts that the amount of drug in tissues (A_2) will be a linear

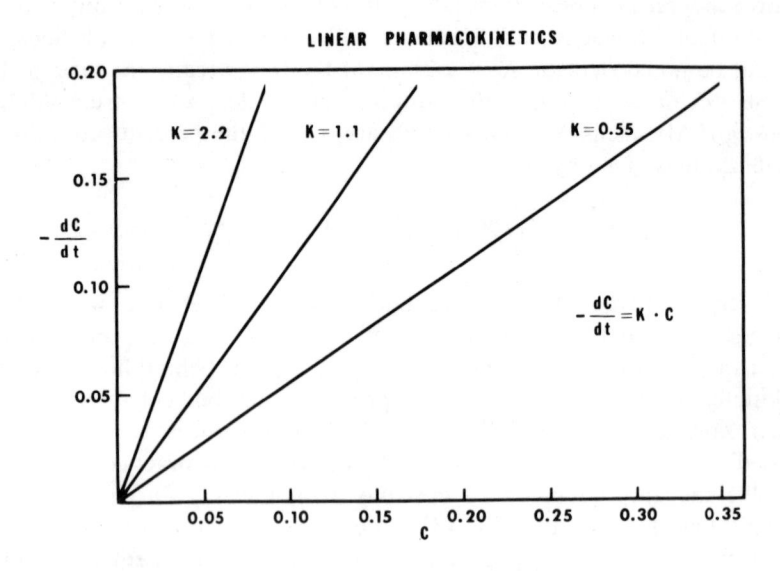

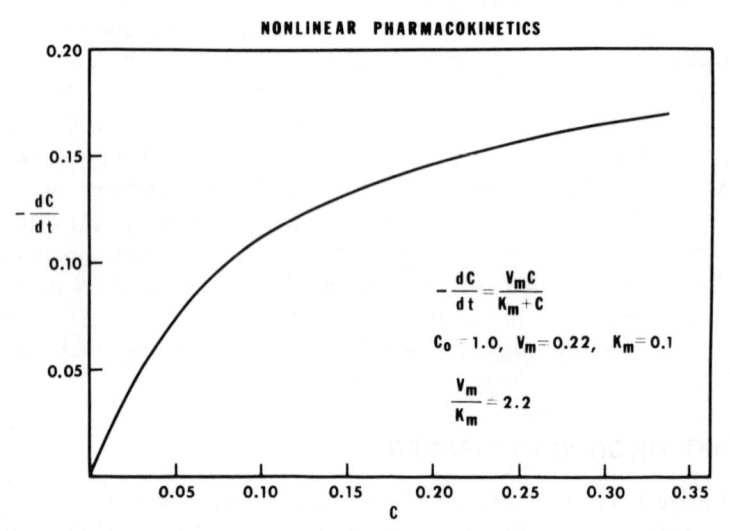

Fig. 1. Comparison of linear and nonlinear pharmacokinetics with respect to metabolism and active tubular secretion. See text for explanation.

function of dose administered, for a fixed value of time t. The type of curves one expects in nonlinear pharmacokinetics is indicated at the bottom of the figure. The asymptotic nature of the curves results from the assumption that there is a limiting amount of drug that can be taken up by the tissues. This appears reasonable since there is obviously only a certain amount of each kind of tissue in the body. The curves shown in Fig. 2 were generated as follows: values of $A = 10$, $B = 1$, and $K = 2.75$ were assigned, and Eq. (2) of Wagner (1971) and DiSanto and Wagner (1972) was numerically integrated for C_0 values of 0.5, 2, 5, 10, 20, and 50, corresponding to doses of 1.917, 4.33, 6.67, 9.55, 14.76, and 29.9 mg/kg, based on an assumed volume of distribution, V, of 0.5 L/kg:

$$\frac{dC}{dt} = \frac{-KC}{1 + AB/(B + C)^2} \quad (2)$$

Hence, the C, t data generated fit the integrated form of Eq. (2), shown as Eq. (3):

$$t = \frac{1}{k}\left\{\left(1 + \frac{A}{B}\right)\ln\left(\frac{C_0}{C}\right) + \frac{A}{B}\ln\left[\frac{B + C}{B + C_0}\right] + A\left[\frac{C - C_0}{(B + C)(B + C_0)}\right]\right\} \quad (3)$$

The amount of drug in the tissue, T', was calculated from a given value of C by means of Eq. (4):

$$T' = \frac{A'C}{B + C} \quad (4)$$

In Eq. (4), the value of A' employed was $A' = AV = (10)(0.5) = 5$ mg/kg. In the simulation, A' represented the maximum amount of drug, with dimensions of milligrams per kilogram of body weight, which could be taken up by tissues.

There is very little literature concerning the measurement of drug in various tissues of the body *as a function of both time and dose*. Recently my co-workers have been generating such data. Figure 3 shows the data of DiSanto and Wagner (1972) on the uptake of methylene blue in four tissues of the rat, presented differently than in the original paper. This is preliminary data since only one rat was studied at each dose. However, nonlinearity is very evident. Dr. Robert N. Smith, while at The Upjohn Center for Clinical Pharmacology, University of Michigan Medical School, administered diphenhydramine in doses of 4, 6, 8, 12, and 16 mg/kg by rapid intravenous injection and killed the rats at 1, 5, 15, 30, 60, 120, 180, and 240 min postinjection. Diphenhydramine was measured by a fluorometric method in brain, lung, heart, spleen, liver, and plasma of four rats at each

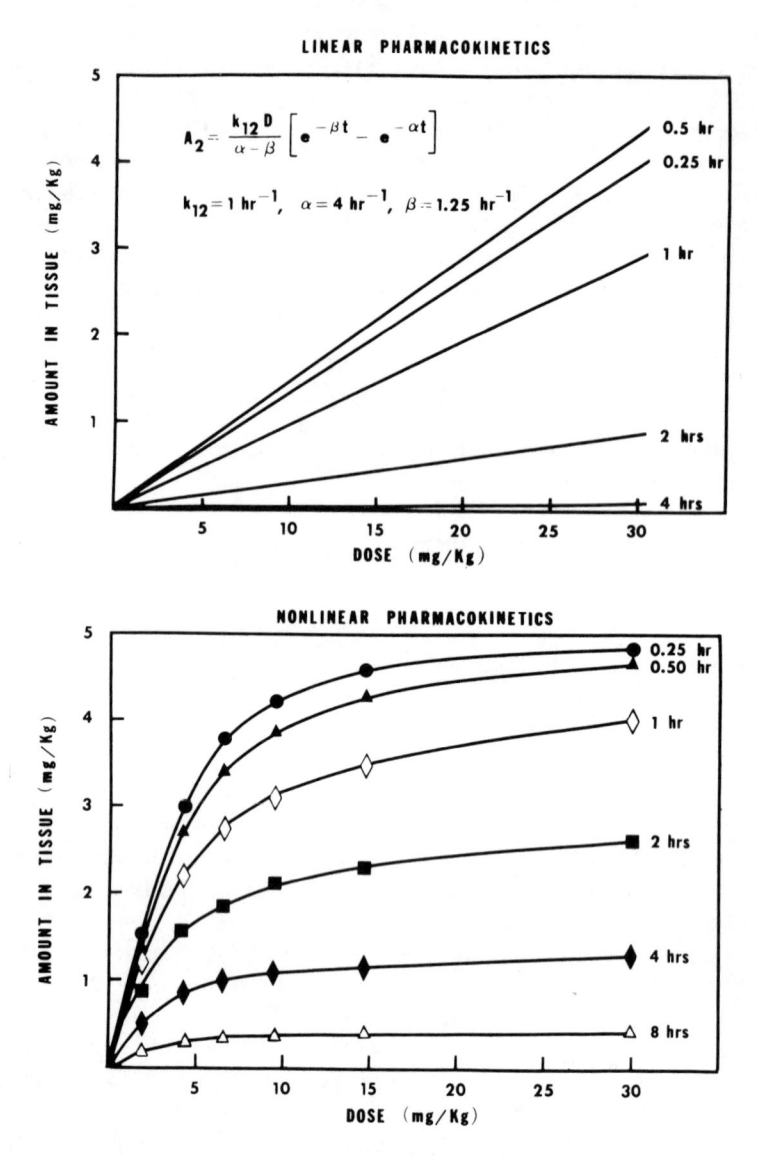

Fig. 2. Comparison of linear and nonlinear pharmacokinetics with respect to uptake of drug by tissues. See text for explanation.

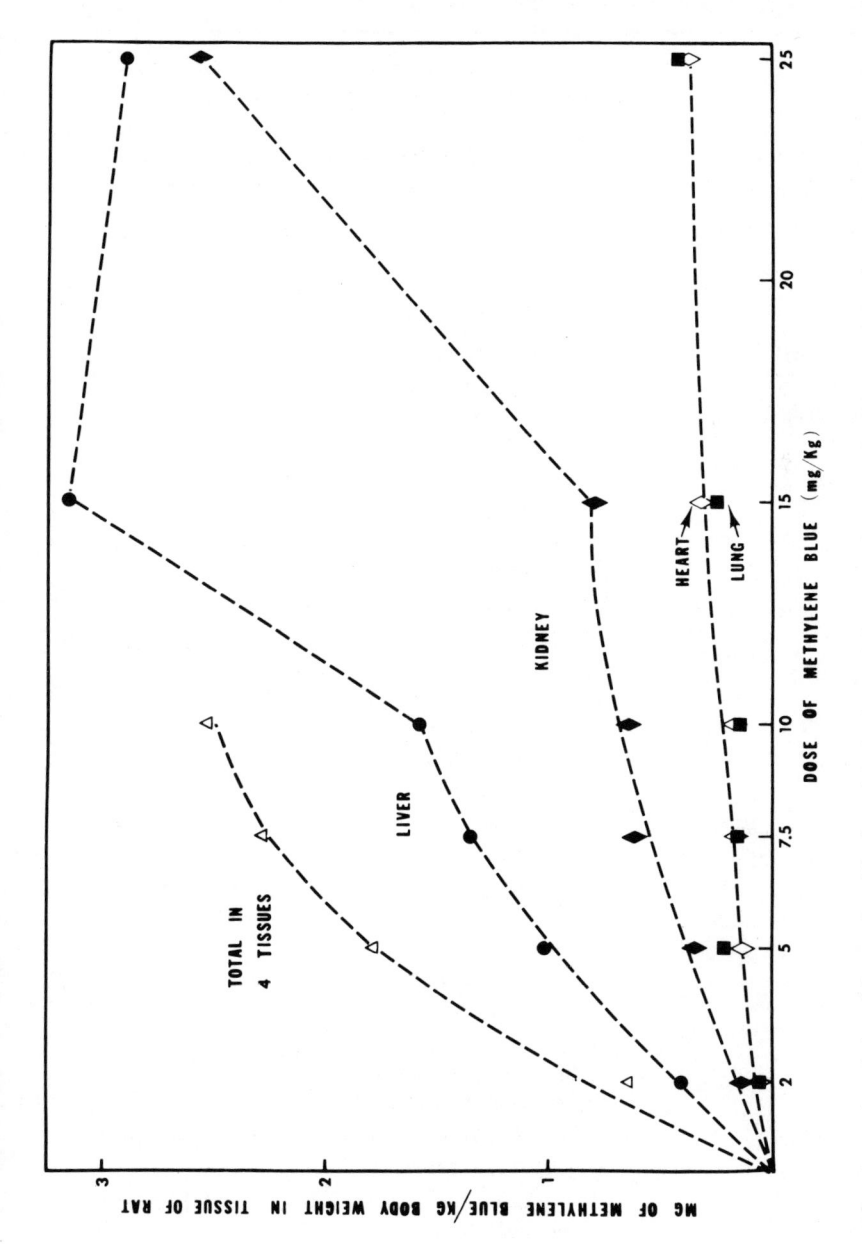

Fig. 3. Plot of mg of methylene blue per kg of body weight in tissue of the rat vs. dose of methylene blue in mg/kg. Data of DiSanto and Wagner (1972d) presented differently than in original paper.

TABLE II
Evidence for Nonlinearities in Drug Distribution

Drug	Comments	References
Several	Mathematical description of drug distribution	Jacquez et al. (1960)
Fat emulsions and chylomicrons	Kinetics of elimination from bloodstream	Carlson and Hallberg (1963); Hallberg (1965a,b)
Sulfobromophthalein	Distribution and rate of uptake by liver	Anderson et al. (1963); Goresky (1964)
	Day to day variation in elimination curves	Winkler and Tygstrup (1964)
Quabain-^{3}H	Distribution in plasma and uptake by heart	Marks et al. (1964)
Guanethidine	Time course in plasma and tissues of rat	Schanker and Morrison (1965)
Methotrexate	Distribution in mice, rats, dogs and monkeys	Henderson et al. (1965)
	Time and dose dependent tissue levels	Zaharko et al. (1970)
	Flow-rate-limited model for distribution in mice	Bischoff et al. (1971)
Kanamycin	Nonlinear kinetics in perilymph from scala vestibuli of guinea pigs	Stupp et al. (1967)
Aspirin	Time courses in plasma and synovial fluid different	Sholkoff et al. (1967)
Bishydroxycoumarin	Unusual interaction with plasma proteins	Nagashima et al. (1968b)
	Liver-plasma distribution affecting rate of metabolism	Nagashima et al. (1968d)
	Three compartment open model	Nagashima et al. (1968c)
	Effect of plasma protein binding on distribution and elimination in rats	Levy and Nagashima (1969)
^{75}Se-Selenite	Dose-dependence of rapid disappearance from blood	Oldendorf (1968)
Thiopental	Flow-rate-limited model for thiopental pharmacokinetics	Bischoff and Dedrick (1968)
Benzylpenicillin	Active transport from CSF to blood	Dixon et al. (1969)

TABLE II (continued)

Drug	Comments	References
Digoxin	Atrial tissue concentrations and plasma concentrations	Hill (1970)
Indocyanine green	Rapid and saturable uptake by liver	Paumgartner et al. (1970)
Diphenhydramine	Very rapid tissue binding in rhesus monkey	Drack et al. (1970)
Benzopyrene	Exponential relationship between tissue concentrations and oral dose	Rees et al. (1971)
Methacycline	Lung tissue and serum concentrations	Timmer et al. (1971)
Methylene blue	Tissue levels in rat as function of dose showed saturation effects	DiSanto and Wagner (1972a and d)
	Blood levels in dog as function of dose showed nonlinearities	DiSanto and Wagner (1972d)
Erythromycin acid erythromycin-2'-propionate ester	Most drug bound to tissues and only about 1 percent bound to plasma proteins	Wiegand and Chun (1972)
Duanomycin	Rapidly taken up and tenaciously held by tissues	Alberts et al. (1971)
Several	Effect of perfusion rate and distribution factors on elimination kinetics in a perfused organ system	Nagashima and Levy (1968)
Salicylate	Decreasing blood pH in rats associated with increasing tissue concentrations	Hill (1970)
Secobarbital	Tissues and blood levels did not obey zero or first order kinetics	Somani et al. (1971)
Griseofulvin	Dose-dependent kinetics in some dogs attributed to changes in tissue distribution	Chiou and Riegelman (1969)
Bupivacaine	Semilogarithmic plasma concentration plots showed continual curvature	Mather et al. (1971)
Methylhydroxycoumarin	Tissue and plasma levels in the rat	Tomura and Akera (1971)

TABLE III
Evidence for Nonlinearities in Drug Metabolism

Drug	Comments	References
Ethyl alcohol	Originated idea of fixed rate of elimination independent of concentration in body	Widmark (1933)
	Showed that apparently linear decline of plasma alcohol concentration (k_0) increased with increase in both dose of alcohol and initial concentration (C_0)	Eggleton (1940)
	Showed that serum alcohol concentration, time data fit the integrated form of the Michaelis–Menten equation.	Lunquist and Wolthers (1958)
	Showed mathematically that $1/k_0$ should be linearly related to $1/C_0$, but V_m and K_m change in same subject from day to day	Wagner and Patel (1972)
Benzoic acid	Conjugation with glycine limited by availability of glycine	Bray et al. (1951)
Salicylic acid	Evidence of saturation effects in formation and active tubular secretion of salicylurate and salicyl phenolic glucoronide following 4-g. oral dose of sodium salicylate in man. Evidence of active tubular secretion of salicylate and salicyl acyl glucuronide	Schachter and Manis (1958)
	Intensive investigation of capacity limited formation of salicylurate	Levy (1965 a,b) Nelson et al. (1966) Levy (1968) Levy and Yaffe (1968) Levy et al. (1969 a,b) Levy and Yamada (1970)
	Capacity limited formation of salicyl phenolic glucuronide	Levy et al. (1966) Levy (1971) Levy et al. (1972)

TABLE III (continued)

Drug	Comments	References
	Competitive inhibition of salicylic acid conjugation with glycine and mutual inhibition in glucuronide formation	Levy and Amsel (1966) Levy and Procknall (1968) Amsel and Levy (1969) Levy and Yamada (1970)
	Complete model to explain salicylate pharmacokinetics	Levy et al. (1972)
Salicylsalicylic acid Aspirin Salicylic acid	Metabolic kinetics	Nordquist et al. (1965)
Salicylamide	Conjugation with sulfate limited by availability of sulfate	Levy and Matsuzawa (1966)
	Pharmacokinetics of elimination in man	Levy and Matsuzawa (1967)
	Effect of capacity-limited metabolism on plasma levels of unchanged drug	Barr and Riegelman (1968)
Salicylic acid and salicylamide	Mutual inhibition in glucuronide formation	Levy and Procknall (1968)
Benzoic acid and salicylic acid	Simultaneous conjugation with glycine	Amsel and Levy (1969)
Acetaminophen and salicylamide or salicylic acid	Biotransformation interaction	Levy and Yamada (1971) Levy and Regardh (1971)
Isoniazid	Inhibition of acetylation by *p*-aminobenzaldehyde	Kakemi et al. (1963)
p-Aminobenzoic acid	Percent acetylation related to dose, rate of administration, and nutritional factors	Drucker et al. (1964)
Diphenylhydantoin Phenylbutazone Biscoumacetate Probenecid	Changes in elimination half-life and apparent volume of distribution with dose	Dayton et al. (1967)
Bishydroxycoumarin	Elimination kinetics in several species	Nagashima et al. (1968a)
Warfarin	Elimination kinetics in several species	Nagashima and Levy (1969)
Novobiocin	Elimination half-life dependent on dose in adults and children	Wagner and Diamiano (1968)

TABLE III (continued)

Drug	Comments	References
2-Pyridinealdoxime methochloride	Log–log relationship between peak plasma concentration and dose	Kondritzer et al. (1968) Sidell et al. (1969)
Heparin	Change in elimination half-life and apparent volume of distribution with dose	Estes et al. (1969)
Tetracycline	Area under serum concentration curve at equilibrium state averaged twice the area from 0 to ∞ after single dose	Wagner (1966)
	Apparent increase in elimination half-life after multiple dosing	Doluisio and Dittert (1969)
Acetanilide	Formation of 4-hydroxyacetanilide shown to obey Michaelis–Menten kinetics	Shibasaki et al. (1968b)
Diphenylhydantoin	Plasma levels following i.v. administration in man.	Glazko et al. (1969)
	I.v. administration in man indicated dose-dependent kinetics did *not* occur	Suzuki et al. (1970b) Blum et al. (1971)
	Oral administration in man indicated dose-dependent kinetics *did* occur	Arnold and Gerber (1970)
	Studies in mice and rats indicated dose-dependent kinetics *did* occur	Gerber and Arnold (1969) Gerber et al. (1971)
	Human and rat data fit with integrated form of Michaelis–Menten equation	Gerber and Wagner (1972)
Several	Properties of the Michaelis–Menten equation and its integrated form which are useful in pharmacokinetics	Wagner (1972)
Amylobarbitane	Influence of dose on distribution and elimination kinetics	Balasubramaniam et al. (1970)

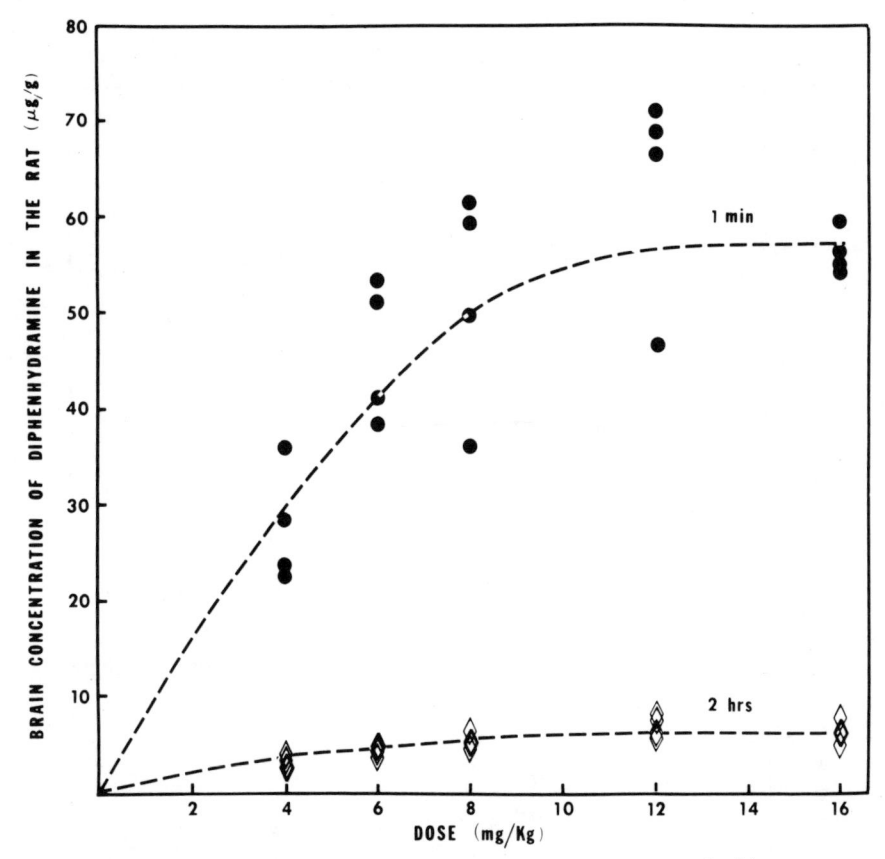

Fig. 4. Plot of brain concentration of diphenhydramine in the rate (μg/g) vs. dose of diphenhydramine in mg/kg administered by rapid intravenous injection. Upper curve 1 min, and lower curve 2 hr, postinjection. Data generated by Dr. Robert N. Smith.

time and each dose level. The tissue concentration and plasma concentration time plots showed marked nonlinearities. The data will be published in the *British Journal of Pharmacology* in the future. Figures 4 and 5 illustrate a small amount of the data collected. In Fig. 4 the brain concentration of diphenhydramine is plotted as a function of dose administered. Each point represents a separate rat. Only the one-minute and two-hour data have been plotted. Figure 5 shows the lung (at the top) and heart (at the bottom) concentration data as a function of dose. It is noteworthy that these data show the nonlinear asymptotic curvature analogous to the curves generated with the simulation example shown in Fig. 2.

Methylene blue is completely ionized at physiological *p*H values and hence anologous to a quarternary ammonium compound. Diphenhydra-

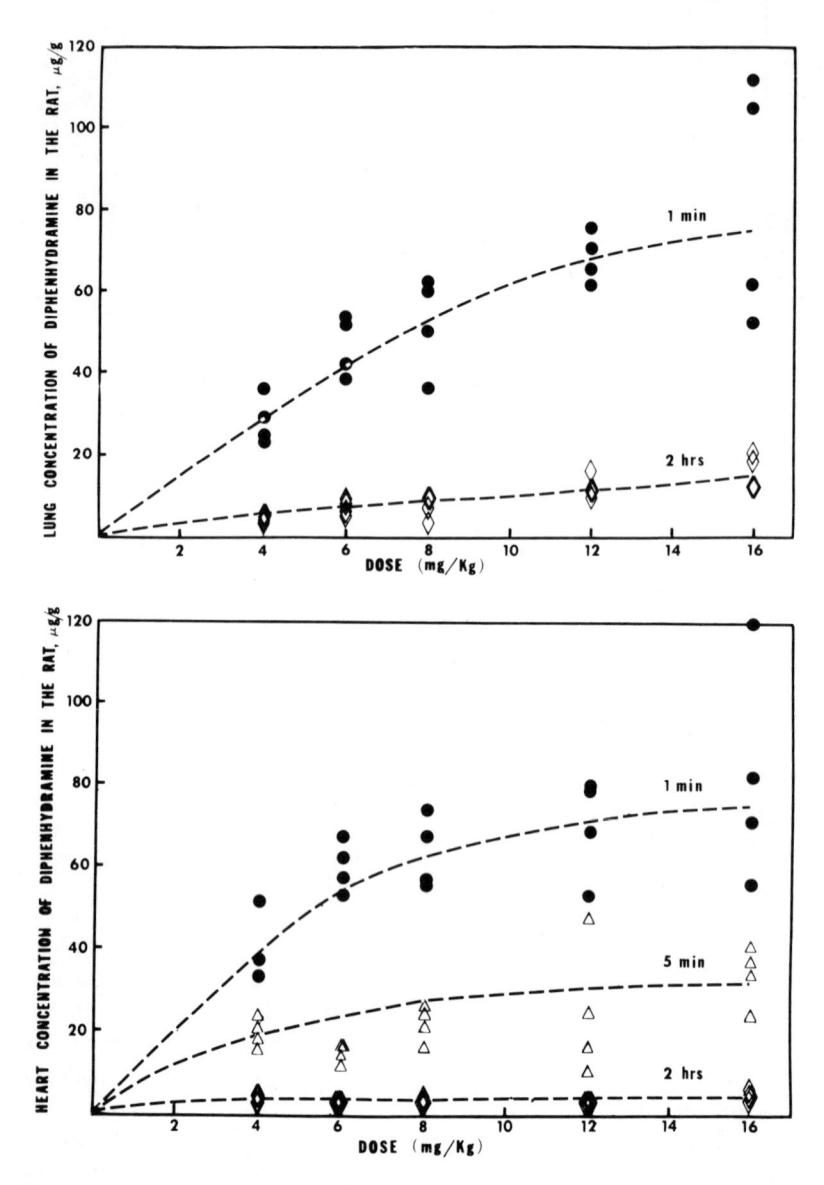

Fig. 5. Plot of lung concentration (upper half) and heart concentration (lower half) of diphenhydramine in the rat (µg/g) vs. dose of diphenhydramine in mg/kg administered by rapid intravenous injection. Data generated by Dr. Robert N. Smith.

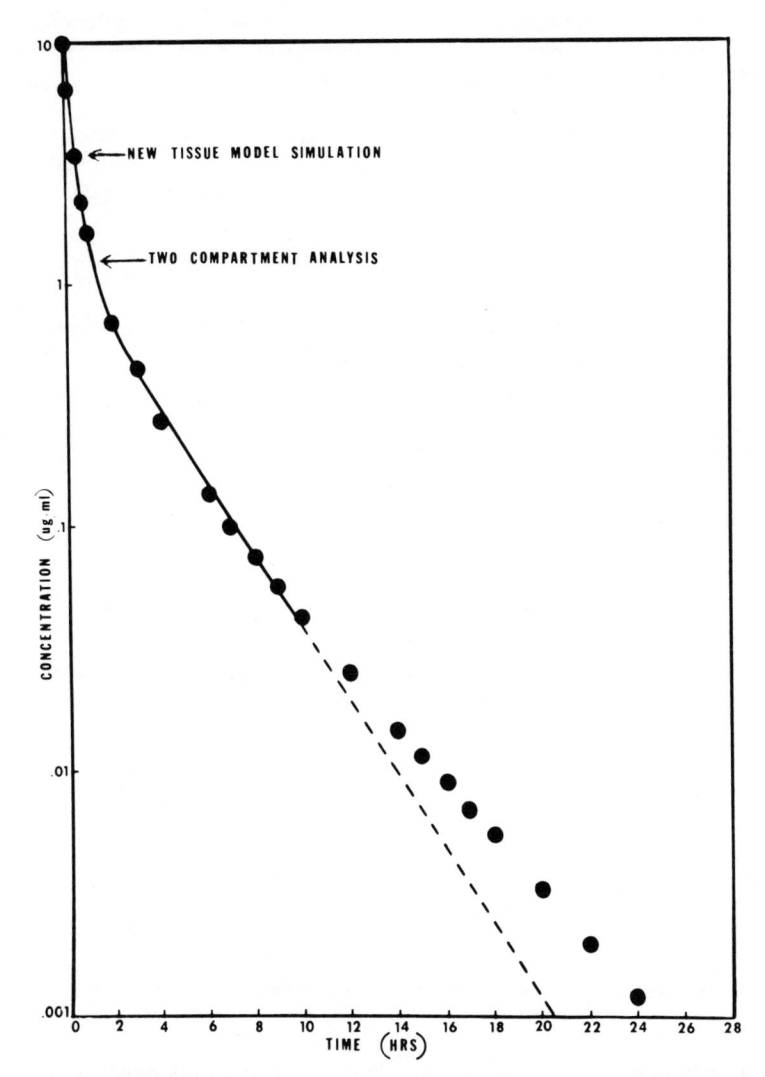

Fig. 6. Solid points are data simulated with Eq. (3). Solid line is from least squares fit of 0 to 9 hr points to Eqs. (5) and (6), based on the two compartment open model. The following values were used in the simulation: $C_0 = 10$, $B = 1.0$, $A = 10$ μg/ml, $K = 2.75$ hr^{-1} and $V = 0.5$ L/kg. Dotted line indicates extrapolation according to the two-compartment analysis. Reprinted from DiSanto and Wagner (1972b) with permission of the Journal of Pharmaceutical Services.

TABLE IV
Evidence for Nonlinearities in Renal Excretion of Drugs and Metabolites

Drug	Comments	References
Several	Renal excretion of weak organic acids and bases	Mudge and Weiner (1963) Weiner and Mudge (1964) Weiner et al. (1964a)
Bile acids	Saturable reabsorptive process	Weiner et al. (1964b)
Amphetamine	Rhythmic urinary excretion due to variable urine pH	Beckett and Rowland (1964)
PAH and other organic acids	Kinetic studies on transport in isolated renal tubules	Huang and Lin (1965)
Riboflavin	Saturable reabsorptive process	Jusko and Levy (1970) Jusko et al. (1970)
Sulfonamides	Diurnal variations in elimination rate	Dettli and Spring (1966)
Basic and acidic drugs	Use of analog computer to predict reabsorption and excretion	Beckett et al. (1968a,b)
Anisotropine methylbromide and propantheline	Periodic excretion peaks	Pfeffer et al. (1969)
Several	Simultaneous chemical reaction and diffusion model for uphill renal transport	Shibasaki et al. (1968a)
Acetaminophen	Formation of metabolite more rapid than excretion of metabolite	Shibasaki et al. (1971)
Methylene blue	Periodic excretion peaks in man	DiSanto and Wagner (1972c)
p-Methyl mandelic acid	Michaelis–Menten kinetics of renal tubular secretion	Nagwekar and Unnikriskan (1971)

mine is a typical weakly basic amine. Both of these drugs were taken up by tissues extremely rapidly; with diphenhydramine the tissue concentration measured one minute after injection was usually the highest concentration observed. With methylene blue an average of 27% of the dose (range 20–32%) was accounted for in only four tissues (liver, kidney, heart, and lung) three minutes after the intravenous dose. Currently Theodore Benya, one of my graduate students, is studying the tissue distribution of warfarin, an acidic drug, in the rat. The same picture is emerging. After intravenous injection the uptake of warfarin in tissues is extremely rapid and the disappearance exceedingly slow. The general picture emerging from these

TABLE V
Evidence for Nonlinearities in Biliary Excretion of Drugs

Drug	Comments	References
Several	Concentrative transfer from blood to bile	Schanker (1962)
Sulfobromophthalein	Transport maximum	Schoenfield et al. (1964)
Several	Influence of enterohepatic circulation on toxicity of drugs	Williams et al. (1965)
Tetracycline	Active transport into bile	Lanman et al. (1970)
Indomethacin	Role of enterohepatic circulation	Yesair et al. (1970)
Methyl orange	Successive demylation and biliary secretion	O'Reilly et al. (1971)
Riboflavin	Two nonlinear processes work in opposite directions. Biliary excretion in rat increases disproportionately with increasing body levels. Tissue binding also nonlinear.	Axelson and Gibaldi (1972)

TABLE VI
Evidence for Nonlinearities in Pharmacokinetics of Drug Action

Subject matter	References
Nonlinear equation for relating response to drug concentration	Wagner (1968b)
Nonlinear equation relating turnover time of goldfish to ethanol concentration in bathing fluid	DiSanto and Wagner (1969)
Dose-dependent decline of pharmacologic effects of drugs with linear pharmacokinetic characteristics	Gibaldi and Levy (1972)
Relationships between drug concentration and response	Wagner (1971)
Pharmacokinetics of drug action	Levy and Gibaldi (1972)
Relationship between dose and plateau levels of drugs eliminated by parallel first-order and capacity-limited kinetics	Tsuchiya and Levy (1972)

studies is that tissue uptake of drug is extremely rapid—much more rapid than one would usually predict from two-compartment analysis, and liberation of the tissue-bound drug is a slow process. Kinetic nonlinearity is very evident. The often repeated statement that highly plasma-protein bound drugs do not get into tissues is apparently incorrect since warfarin is about 97% bound to plasma proteins.

TABLE VII
Calculation of Percent Saturation of "Enzyme System" from Available Literature Values of K_m of the Michaelis–Menten Equation

Dose of salicylate, mg	Percent saturation of "enzyme system," if entire dose were made available to enzyme	
	Salicylurate[b]	Phenolic glucuronide[c]
300	46.9	35.6
600	63.8	52.5
1000	74.6	64.9
2000	85.5	78.7
4000	92.2	88.1

Blood alcohol concentration, mg/ml	Percent saturation of "enzyme system" metabolizing ethyl alcohol[d]
0.1	50.0
0.2	66.7
0.3	75.0
0.4	80.0
0.5	83.3
0.75	88.2
1.0	90.9
1.5	93.75
2.0	95.2
3.0	96.8

Plasma concentration of diphenylhydantoin, µg/ml	Percent saturation of "enzyme system" metabolizing diphenylhydantoin[e]	
50	88.1	} Toxic range
40	85.5	
30	81.6	
20	74.6	} Therapeutic range
10	59.6	
5	42.5	Subtherapeutic

[a] Calculated from Eq. (1) in text.
[b] Based on the K_m value of 340 mg of Levy et al. (1972) for subject A.
[c] Based on the K_m value of 542 mg of Levy et al. (1972) for subject A.
[d] Based on the K_m value of 0.1 mg/ml of Goldstein (1970).
[e] Based on the K_m value of 6.77 µg/ml of Gerber and Wagner (1972).

A CURRENT AND FUTURE PROBLEM IN PHARMACOKINETICS

It is exceedingly difficult, if not impossible, to determine if a *given set* of whole blood, plasma, or serum concentrations of a drug measured after one dose is best described by a classical linear or nonlinear mathematical model. The problem is even more difficult with urinary data. Obtaining data after only one or two doses of a drug is usually insufficient to deduce the appropriate model. It is feasible for known nonlinear data to appear to be linear pharmacokinetic data when only one dose of a drug is studied. This is so even when the drug is administered by rapid intravenous injection. This concept is illustrated by two simulations below.

Example 1

The data points in Fig. 6 obey Eq. (3) and were generated both by numerical integration of Eq. (2) and by use of Eq. (3) and a digital computer. The points in the concentration range 10 to 0.05 µg/ml, and in the time range 0 to 9 hr were fit essentially perfectly by the equations appropriate to the classical two-compartment open model shown as Eqs. (5) and (6):

$$C = \frac{C_0}{\alpha - \beta}[(k_{21} - \beta)e^{-\beta t} - (k_{21} - \alpha)e^{-\alpha t}] \tag{5}$$

$$\alpha, \beta = \tfrac{1}{2}\{(k_{12} + k_{21} + k_{el}) \pm \sqrt{[(k_{12} + k_{21} + k_{el})^2 - 4k_{21}k_{el}]}\} \tag{6}$$

where $\alpha > \beta$.

The solid line through the points in the indicated ranges are the model-predicted concentrations for the two-compartment open model. The dotted line in the figure is the extrapolated two-compartment model prediction. The points deviate from the line beyond 9 hr. However, if this were real data, and if one only had an assay sensitive to 0.05 µg/ml then one could not decide *on the basis of these data only* whether Eqs. (3) or Eqs. (5) and (6) represented the appropriate mathematical model. This example was published by DiSanto and Wagner (1972). If data were available from several simulations with different C_0 values (or real data were available following administration of several different doses) then a distinction between linear and nonlinear pharmacokinetics could be made.

Example 2

The data points for curve A of Fig. 7 are the same as those in Example 1 and Fig. 6. However, in Fig. 7 the least squares log C, t line was drawn through the points in the 5- to 9-hr time region, then was extrapolated

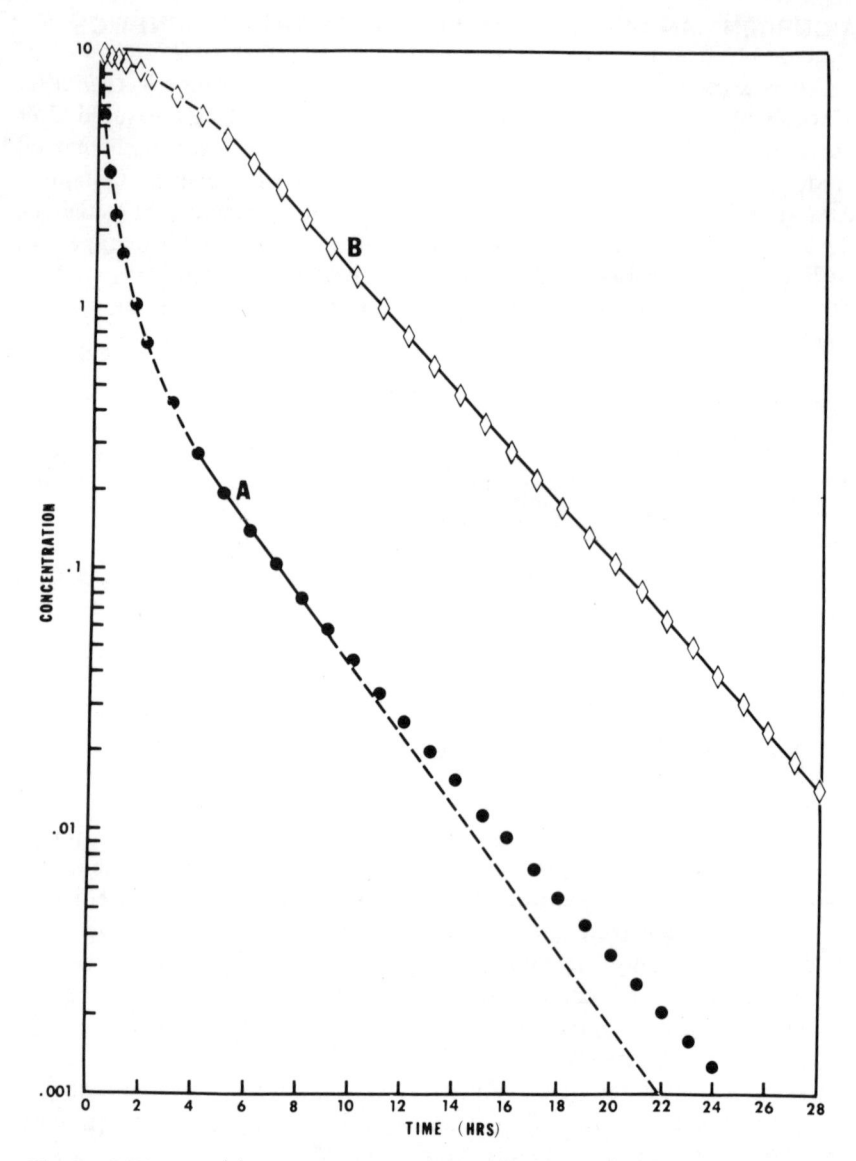

Fig. 7. Solid points (●) are data simulated with Eq. (3) and are same points as in Fig. 6. Solid line is least squares log C, t line based on 5- to 9-hr points and lower dotted line is extrapolation of this line. Open points (◊) were simulated with Eq. (8) using $V_m = 1.375$, $K_m = 0.5$, $A = 10$, $B = 1$, and $C_0 = 10$. Line drawn through the points from 5 to 28 hr is the least squares log C, t line indicating apparent first-order elimination, yet data were really generated from a model involving Michaelis–Menten kinetics and Langmuir-type tissue binding.

(dotted line). Hence, only terminal points, in somewhat less than one log cycle, were linear on the semilogarithmic graph paper. The data points for curve B of Fig. 7 were obtained by numerical integration of Eq. (7), and hence obey the integrated form of Eq. (7), namely, Eq. (8):

$$\frac{dC}{dt} = \frac{-V_m C/(K_m + C)}{1 + AB/(B + C)^2} \qquad (7)$$

$$t = \frac{C_0 - C}{V_m}\left[1 + \frac{A(B - K_m)}{(B + C)(B + C_0)}\right]$$
$$+ \frac{K_m}{V_m}\left[\left(1 + \frac{A}{B}\right)\ln\frac{C_0}{C} + \frac{A}{B}\ln\left(\frac{B + C}{B + C_0}\right)\right] \qquad (8)$$

The line drawn through the data points from 5 to 28 hr is the least squares log C, t line and suggests simple first-order elimination. Yet the equation from which the data points were derived involved a model with Michaelis–Menten elimination kinetics and Langmuir-type binding of drug to tissues. The particular set of parameter values used in the simulation were $V_m = 1.375$, $K_m = 0.5$, $A = 10$, $B = 1$, and $C_0 = 10$. Michaelis–Menten kinetics alone cause concave decreasing curvature when the C, t data are plotted on semilogarithmic graph paper. Langmuir-type tissue binding causes convex decreasing curvature when the C, t data are plotted on semilogarithmic graph paper. A judicious mixture of Michaelis–Menten elimination kinetics and Langmuir-type tissue binding (i.e., the parameters are in a certain "space") yields the result shown as line B in Fig. 7. In a modern view of pharmacokinetics we must be aware that such things can happen and, perhaps, not be as sure as we have in the past that fitting data to a model *proves* that the model is correct.

Three "real world" examples along the same lines will be discussed.

Salicylate

As indicated in Table III, Schachter and Manis (1958) published evidence of saturation effects in the formation and active tubular secretion of salicylurate and salicyl phenolic glucuronide from salicylate following an oral dose of four grams of sodium salicylate in man. They also reported evidence of active tubular secretion of salicylate and salicyl acyl glucuronide. During the period 1965 to 1972, Dr. Levy, who is with us today, intensively studied the aspirin-salicylate problem (*see* citations in Table III under salicylic acid). He has tackled the problem many ways and has certainly shown, at least to my satisfaction, that one must use Michaelis–Menten kinetics to elucidate the formation of salicylurate and salicyl phenolic glucuronide from salicylate. Rowland and Riegelman (1968) and Rowland, et al. (1970) evaluated the pharmacokinetics of *acetyl*salicylic acid in man following intravenous administration by means of the classical two-compartment model for a drug and its metabolite. Wagner (1967) showed that approximately 50% of a metabolite excreted in the urine may be excreted at such rates that the cumulative urinary excretion plot would appear to be nearly linear when the model is a catenary chain with parallel paths involving only first-order rate constants. In a review as late as 1968, Wagner (1968a) supported the first-order elimination kinetics of salicylate. However, currently I agree with Dr. Levy's interpretation. It was undoubtedly Dr. Levy's and Dr. Krüger-Thiemer's papers which first stimulated my interest in nonlinear pharmacokinetics. I'm sure we have all learned a great deal from the saga of salicylate. In case the point is lost, I wish to reiterate that individual sets of nonlinear data can be fit by linear pharmacokinetic equations and therein lies the real problem.

Diphenylhydantoin

Dayton et al. (1967) published data which indicated that the elimination half-life of diphenylhydantoin in the dog apparently increased when the dose was raised from 20 to 50 mg/kg. Analysis of diphenylhydantoin plasma concentration data, obtained following intravenous administration to man, by Suzuki et al. (1970b) and Blum et al. (1971) indicated that dose-dependent kinetics did *not* occur. Plasma concentration data, obtained following oral administration of diphenylhydantoin to man, published by Arnold and Gerber (1969), indicated dose-dependent kinetics *did* occur. Studies in mice (Gerber and Arnold, 1969) and in rats (Gerber et al., 1971) also indicated marked nonlinearity. Recently, Gerber and Wagner (1972) fitted sets of diphenylhydantoin plasma concentration data in man and whole blood diphenylhydantoin concentration data in the rat, to the integrated form of the Michaelis–Menten equation, shown as Eq. (9).

$$C_0 - C + K_m \ln \frac{C_0}{C} = V_m t \tag{9}$$

Although evaluated by the authors according to first-order kinetics, the diphenylhydantoin plasma concentration data of Glazko et al. (1969) exhibit concave decreasing curvature on semilogarithmic graph paper as expected for Michaelis–Menten kinetics. Based on the data published by Suzuki et al. (1970b) and Blum et al. (1971) I, personally, would accept it as conventional two-compartment open model data. However, the data I evaluated with Dr. Gerber, obviously is fitted very well by Eq. (9). I have no further explanation of the discrepancy *in the observed data* at the present time.

Riboflavin in the Rat

Axelson and Gibaldi (1972) discussed an unusual example of nonlinear pharmacokinetics. Estimation of the availability of riboflavin-5'-phosphate after oral administration to the rat is greatly complicated because of the occurrence of a complex and markedly nonlinear, dose-dependent excretion of the vitamin. The elimination of the vitamin involves at least two nonlinear processes occurring simultaneously, and having opposite effects on the dose–total urinary recovery relationship. One process involves biliary excretion which increases disproportionately with increasing body levels of riboflavin. The other process appears to be a binding of the vitamin to tissues, which function kinetically as deep compartments. Apparently, the higher the body level of the vitamin, the smaller the fraction that can be "immobilized" in the compartment and the larger is the fraction that can be detected in the urine. The latter is another way of stating in words what is implied by Eq. (4).

Recognition of Nonlinearities

1. Administer the drug intravenously at several different doses and obtain whole blood or plasma concentrations as a function of time. The entire curve must be defined including samples as early as one and three minutes postinjection. Estimate the C_0 value of each curve by fitting the equation $\ln C = \ln C_0 - Kt$ to only the first two points of each set of data. Calculate the values of the ratios C/C_0 and plot vs. time. Put all sets for all doses on the same piece of semilogarithmic graph paper. If each set forms its own curve and the data are not superimposible, then some type of nonlinearity exists. If the curves are superimposible then the data are linear.

2. Fit each set of data (one dose per set) to the equations appropriate to the two-compartment open model, i.e., Eqs. (5) and (6). If the estimated parameters change in a uniform manner with dose then this is strong evidence of a nonlinear system.

3. If drug is administered orally or intramuscularly, then divide each plasma concentration by the dose, or the normalized dose, and plot the ratios vs. time. If the curves are not superimposible then some type of nonlinearity exists.

4. Measure tissue concentrations of unchanged drug as a function of both time and dose. If one obtains curves, such as shown at the bottom of Fig. 2, and in Figs. 3 and 5, then nonlinear tissue binding exists.

5. Administer a metabolizable drug in a readily available form such as an aqueous solution at several dose levels. Collect the urine until essentially all of the metabolite(s) is (are) excreted. Plot the amount of each metabolite excreted as a percentage of the total urinary excretion against

the dose. If the percentage decreases uniformly as the dose increases, then Michaelis–Menten kinetics should be suspected.

6. Administer the drug on a multiple dose regimen at several dose levels, establish an equilibrium state, then measure the metabolite concentration in the whole blood or, plasma in a dosage interval at the equilibrium state. If the area under the metabolite concentration curves at the equilibrium state are not a linear function of dose, but rather a curvilinear function of dose, then this is excellent evidence for the operation of Michaelis–Menten kinetics in the formation of the metabolite. One must be careful to ensure that excretion is rate-limited by formation of the metabolite, and that one is not dealing with a case such as acetaminophen where the formation step of conjugation proceeds much more rapidly then the subsequent excretion step (Shibasaki *et al.*, 1971).

NONLINEAR MODELS AND THE FITTING OF DATA

Plasma Protein Binding

The effects of plasma protein binding of drugs on drug distribution and elimination is still controversial. One type of deviation from first-order elimination kinetics from the human body is characterized by a diminishing steepness of the slope of the total plasma concentration, time curve on semilogarithmic graph paper (i.e., convex decreasing curvature). This type of deviation exists for some sulfonamides which show a high degree of binding to plasma proteins and was discussed and referenced by Krüger-Thiemer (1968a). The higher the affinity for protein binding, the greater will be the bending of the log-concentration–time curve. This is just the opposite behavior to that Martin (1965) predicted from a judgment of the same problem. Krüger-Thiemer (1968a) published a mathematical model which could explain such deviations. In the conclusion of a review on the binding of drugs by plasma proteins, Meyer and Guttman (1968) stated: "An impression, gained from the literature, is that there appears to be a tendency to overemphasize the general importance of the binding phenomenon in the behavior of drugs in the body. Evidence exists that only in the case of highly bound agents will binding be important in a practical sense. Many workers, in attempting to extrapolate *in vitro* data to *in vivo* expectations tend to lose sight of the fact that the plasma comprises a relatively small fraction of the total volume available for drug distribution and that protein-drug complexes of rather extraordinary stability must be formed to substantially reduce the amount of drug that exists in the body in the active, diffusible, unbound form. A number of important drugs do, however, fall in the category of 'strongly bound' and these serve as examples which emphasize the need to at least consider protein binding as a necessary parameter in the characterization of drug behavior." Coffey et al. (1971) described numerical methods for the solution of differential equations arising from nonlinear binding of drugs to plasma proteins, assuming one- and two-compartment pharmacokinetic models. The results suggested that binding of drugs to plasma proteins should cause detectable nonlinearity in the log C vs. t plot only if doses are sufficiently high to approach saturation of binding sites, or if the number of binding sites in plasma is small. The effect of competition for binding sites in plasma was also studied by the same authors. They reported: "It appears that unless the tissue distribution volume is quite small competition for binding sites would not be expected to have a large effect." Curry (1970) also studied this problem but his results are discussed under tissue-binding.

During his lifetime Dr. E. Krüger-Thiemer contributed a great deal to pharmacokinetics. Only a few of his many papers are cited in this review (Krüger-Thiemer, 1966, 1968a,b,c), but the cited papers contain many references to his work. He was mainly concerned with the problem of accumulation of drugs, the pharmacokinetics of suitable dosage requirements for individual patients, and the establishment of sufficient plasma concentration of free (unbound) drug once the parameters of binding of the specific drug to plasma proteins were known. He developed and applied many mathematical models to reach these objectives. He developed many digital computer programs to allow the fitting of observed data to a specific mathematical model.

For a 70-kg man, total plasma albumin is about 120 g, and total interstitial albumin is about 156 g (Reeve, 1964). Hence total body albumin is about 0.276 kg, or about 0.4% of body weight. If total body water is taken as 60% of body weight, the "total tissue" expressed as dry weight is 28 kg, or 40% of body weight. Thus the ratio of total dry tissue mass to total albumin mass is about 100/1. Since there are about 70 cardiac passes of blood per minute, and the dissociation of plasma protein–drug complexes, where they have been measured, is an exceedingly rapid process, with a half-life of the order of 20 msec (Thorp, 1964), it is not difficult to see that in most cases the binding of drugs to tissues will be kinetically much more important than the binding of drugs to albumin. This was pointed out also by Gillette (1971). It is perhaps fortuitous but Wiegand and Chun (1972), after studying the serum protein and tissue binding of erythromycin and erythromycin 2'-propionate ester, calculated that drug bound to serum proteins is only about 1% of the dose, and that most of the drugs are bound to tissues.

Tissue Binding

In light of the discussion above, it is amazing that so little experimental investigation has been conducted on the measurement of tissue concentrations of drug *as a function of both time and dose*. Most "distribution" data of specific drugs in animals and man have resulted from measurement of tissue concentrations at only one or two times postadministration and usually following only one specific dose of drug. Such data give no insight into the kinetics of drug distribution. Recently, some investigators have measured tissue and plasma or whole blood concentrations as a function of time and dose. Drs. Bischoff and Dedrick, who are reviewers of other topics during this conference, have reported such data and developed pharmacokinetic models to explain such data. Dedrick and Bischoff (1968) discussed pharmacokinetics in application to the artificial kidney; Bischoff and Dedrick (1968) described thiopental pharmacokinetics; Zaharko et al. (1970) reported on time and dose-dependent tissue concentrations of methotrexate; and Bischoff et al. (1970, 1971) described methotrexate pharmacokinetics. Dr. Bischoff won the 1972 Ebert Prize for his 1971 article on *Methotrexate Pharmacokinetics* which was published in the *Journal of Pharmaceutical Sciences*. The flow rate-limited model, described in that paper, incorporated compartments for the gastrointestinal tract, the liver and enterohepatic circulation, plasma, kidney, and muscle. Three compartments-in-series were used to simulate bile formation and secretion time in the liver. Transit of drug down the gastrointestinal tract was handled similarly, except that provision was made for transport through the intestinal wall. Tissue binding was assumed to be the sum of a linear nonspecific binding and a strong binding, presumed to be associated with dihydrofolate reductase, in conformity with Eq. (10):

$$C_{\text{tissue}} = RC_p + \frac{aC_p}{\varepsilon + C_p} \quad (10)$$

The model predicted the time courses of methotrexate in lumenal contents of small intestine, liver, kidney, muscle, and plasma of mice, rats, and dogs with reasonable accuracy. As part of the model for thiopental pharmacokinetics, Bischoff and Dedrick (1968) used two-term equations, such as Eq. (11), to estimate the bound concentration x, of thiopental in tissues and in plasma:

$$x = \frac{B_1 K_1 C}{1 + K_1 C} + \frac{B_2 K_2 C}{1 + K_2 C} \quad (11)$$

where C represents the free (unbound) concentration of drug.

Curry (1970) reported that concentrations of chlorpromazine fluctuate in the plasma of dogs and man after intravenous doses. He examined the possibility that the fluctuations could arise from movement of the drug between tissue and plasma stores by performing simulations. His calculations showed that small changes in protein binding of drugs in plasma and tissues could cause redistribution of highly bound drugs between tissues and plasma. Also, redistribution would be greatest after changes in tissue binding of highly bound drugs. He hypothesized that fluctuations in chlorpromazine plasma concentrations could be caused this way.

A generalized nonlinear pharmacokinetic model was elaborated by DiSanto (1971) and Wagner (1971a). The model takes into account the nonlinear tissue binding of drug to one or more tissues associated with one or more fluid compartments. Dose-dependent metabolism or urinary excretion may be incorporated into the generalized model by replacing the first-order elimination constant by an expression of the Michaelis–Menten type. Several specific applications of the general theory were discussed. The chapter (Wagner, 1971) contains 126 equations, hence is too extensive to be reviewed here. Equations (2) and (3), above, result from the simplest specific application of the generalized model, and were employed by DiSanto and Wagner (1972b) in simulations, and by DiSanto and Wagner (1972d) in interpreting whole-blood concentrations obtained following rapid intravenous injection of five different doses of methylene blue in a dog. Figure 8 shows the results of a simultaneous fit of the whole blood concentration data, obtained following the five different doses of methylene blue, to Eq. (3) above; only one value of each of the parameters A, B, and K and five different C_0 values were estimated during the digital computer fitting with Dr. Metzler's program NONLIN, modified by addition of a rootfinder subroutine. It is feasible that such an approach, with the same or alternate mathematical models, may yield valuable information for studies in comparative pharmacology. In such a case the number of parameters estimated in small, and comparison of the values obtained from one species of animal to another with those estimated from human data may be a useful clue as to the appropriate species of animal for long-term toxicologic studies.

Metabolism

Lundquist and Wolthers (1958) were the first to use the intergrated form of the Michaelis–Menten equation, shown as Eq. (9) above, to explain blood concentration data. They fitted terminal serum concentrations of ethyl alcohol in man to the equation. The parameters, K_m, V_m, and C_0 for the fitting were obtained by graphical methods. The differential form, that

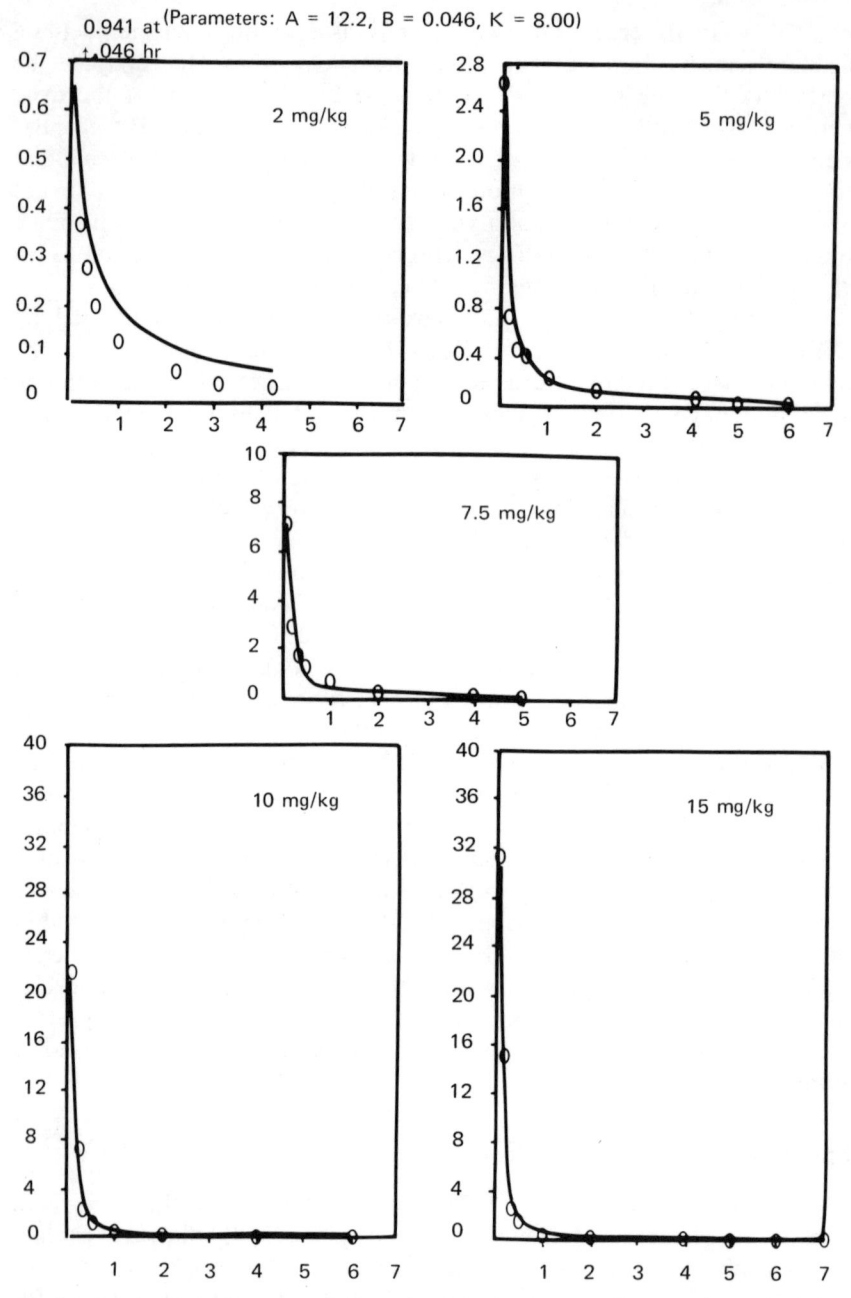

Fig. 8. Results of simultaneous nonlinear least squares fitting of five sets of methylene blue whole blood concentrations to Eq. (3). Data from DiSanto and Wagner (1972d).

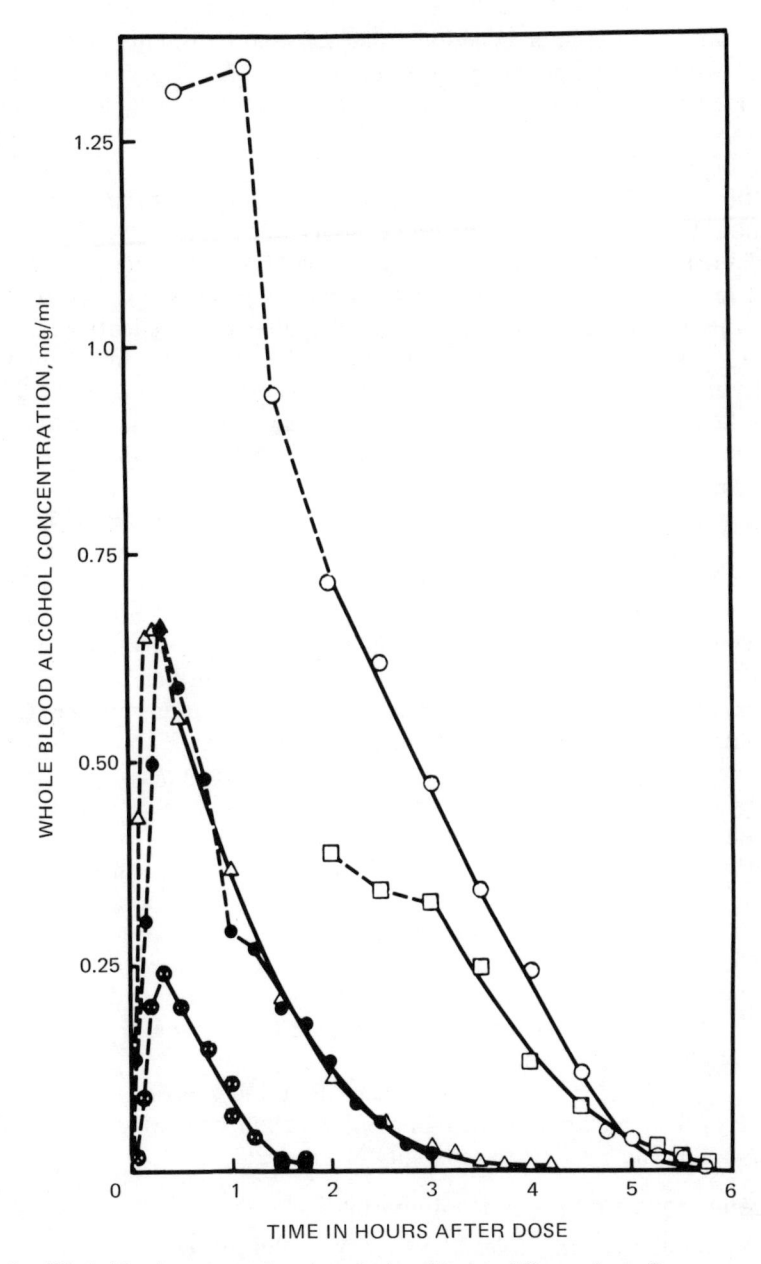

Fig. 9. Whole blood concentrations in a single subject at different times. Doses were 15 ml (⊗), 30 ml (△ and ●), and 60 ml (○ and □) of 95% ethanol. Solid lines are least squares fits of terminal concentrations to Eq. (9). From Wagner and Patel (1972). Reprinted from *Research Communications in Chemical Pathology and Pharmacology* **4:** 61 (1972) with permission of PJD Publications Ltd., 10 Oakdale Drive, Westbury, N. Y. 11590.

is, the Michaelis–Menten equation itself, was used by Bischoff and Dedrick (1968) in their thiopental pharmacokinetic model. Levy *et al.* (1972) simulated the time courses of the urinary excretion rate of total salicylic acid and metabolites, salicyluric acid, salicyl acyl glucuronide, salicyl phenolic glucuronide, gentisic acid, and salicylic acid in four subjects following a 3-g oral dose of salicylic acid as sodium salicylate in aqueous solution. In order to do this, it was necessary to determine the values of 14 individually determined constants (Levy, 1971). The formidable technical effort required an average of over 400 analyses per dose per subject. The constants estimated following the 3-g dose allowed excellent predictions following 1- and 0.19-g doses. The model equations employed involved Michaelis–Menten equations for the formation of salicylururate and salicyl phenolic glucuronide and first-order equations for formation of salicyl acyl glucuronide, gentisic acid and for excretion of unchanged salicylic acid and its absorption from the gut.

Figure 9 is taken from the paper of Wagner and Patel (1972). The points are whole capillary blood ethanol concentrations measured in the same subject at different times. Two of the curves resulted from 60-ml, two of the curves resulted from 30-ml, and one curve resulted from 15-ml oral doses of 95% ethyl alcohol. The solid lines drawn through the terminal points are the model-predicted values, based on fitting to Eq. (9) by numerically integrating the Michaelis–Menten equation on the digital computer, and the assignment of equal weights. It was found in this study that the absorption rate of ethanol and the values of K_m and V_m varied widely in the same subject and apparently in a random manner not related to dose or time of administration.

Figure 10 is taken from the paper of Gerber and Wagner (1972). It shows the fit of plasma concentrations of diphenylhydantoin in a human subject to Eq. (9). The data were collected starting 12 hrs after the last dose when doses of 2.3, 4.7, and 7.9 mg/kg of sodium diphenylhydantoin (as Dilantin®) were administered daily for three days during different time periods. The V_m value estimated was 0.253 μg/(ml × hr) and the K_m value estimated was 6.77 μg/ml.

Krüger-Thiemer and Levine (1968c) discussed several non-first-order models of drug metabolism including one which incorporated both capacity-limitation and restricted availability of substrate.

Miscellaneous Causes of Nonlinearities

As summarized in Tables I, IV, and V nonlinearities can occur in drug absorption, in active tubular secretion and reabsorption in the kidney and in biliary excretion of drugs and their metabolites. Circadian rhythm in hepatic drug metabolizing enzyme activity, as discussed by Civen *et al.*

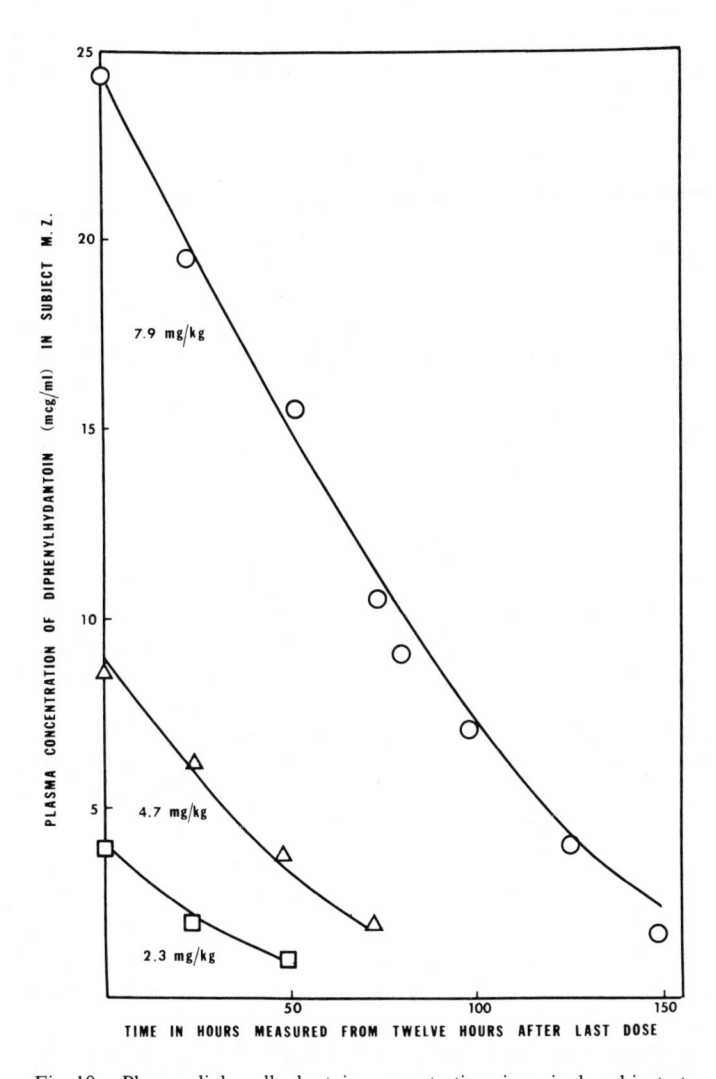

Fig. 10. Plasma diphenylhydantoin concentrations in a single subject at different times fitted to Eq. (9). "Zero time" is 12 hr after the last of multiple doses of 2.3, 4.7, and 7.9 mg/kg of sodium diphenylhydantoin. From Gerber and Wagner (1972); reprinted from *Research Communications in Chemical Pathology and Pharmacology* **3:** 455 (1972) with permission from PJD Publications Ltd., 10 Oakdale Drive, Westbury, N.Y. 11590.

(1967) and Radzialowski and Bousquet (1967), will undoubtedly cause nonlinearities even though we may not be able to "see" them readily. Enzyme stimulation and inhibition (Burns and Conney, 1968) may also cause nonlinearities.

Data Fitting Aids

The fitting shown in Fig. 10 was achieved by successive trials of numerical integration of the Michaelis–Menten equation by the Runge–Kutta method using a simple electronic calculator. This is analogous to the use of an analog computer, and suffers from the fact that no standard deviations of the estimated parameters, or other mathematical and statistical information, is obtained along with the fitting. Usually one uses a high-speed digital computer with a suitable nonlinear least squares estimation program. Dr. Berman's SAAM program, Dr. Metzler's NONLIN, and Control Data's MIMIC are examples of successful programs which have been used widely for data fitting and simulation purposes. Recently, Atkins (1971) described a new versatile digital computer program for nonlinear regression analysis. The iteration procedure used in this program possesses two important advantages over those used in the past, namely, that second partial derivatives need not be calculated and convergence is guaranteed. Quasilinearization, discussed by Buel and Kulaba (1968), may prove to be an aid in fitting of nonlinear models to experimental data.

Pooling of Parallel Paths

If there are parallel first-order paths in classical linear pharmacokinetics one can simply add the first-order rate constants to obtain the overall elimination rate constant. But can we pool parallel Michaelis–Menten paths and parallel Langmuir-type tissue binding equations justifiably? About a year ago I gave this problem to one of my graduate students, Allen J. Sedman, and at the meeting of the A.Ph.A. Academy of Pharmaceutical Sciences in April, 1972, we presented a paper entitled: "Quantitative Pooling of Both Parallel Michaelis–Menten Formation Equations and Langmuir-type Equations for Binding of Drugs to Tissues" (Sedman and Wagner, 1972). In the paper we answered the above question with a qualified "yes." Sedman developed equations which allowed calculation of the pooled parameters, V_{mp} and K_{mp}, from the microscopic parameters V_{m1}, V_{m2}, K_{m1}, and K_{m2} for parallel Michaelis–Menten paths and also for the Langmuir-type equations. The simulated data could always be fit essentially exactly using the calculated pooled parameters. When the parameters have a certain relationship to each other there is no problem in the sense that the pooled parameters need not change with change in dose. In certain cases, which are usually predictable, the pooled parameters will change with change in dose. The simulations suggested the appropriate experimentation with a given drug. One should study as low a dose as one can measure adequately, and as high a dose as one may give safely, and see if the nonlinear parameters appear to change with dose. If they do not, then one is reasonably safe with the pooling concept within that dose range with that drug. In this rapidly moving field one is never alone. When we returned from the Houston meeting we found papers by Spears et al. (1971) and Neal (1972) which treated the same problem, but in a different way.

SOME COMMENTS ABOUT MICHAELIS–MENTEN KINETICS

In Wagner (1972) and Wagner and Patel (1972) the properties of the Michaelis–Menten equation and its integrated form are discussed extensively. We do not have space here to delve deeply into those papers. However, one or two points are worthy of special consideration. As one can see in Figs. 9 and 10 when Eq. (9) is obeyed (solid lines), there is initially an apparently linear segment then a sharp break in the curve—the whole curve taking on a "hockey stick" shape. The apparently linear segment has often been assumed to be linear because the assumption has been made that the enzyme is saturated. But this is a poor assumption because independent of the initial C_0 value, the integrated form of the Michaelis–Menten equation always gives a pseudolinear portion over about two-thirds of the range or more. It is only pseudolinear since the derivative changes when the concentration changes, as evidenced by looking at the Michaelis–Menten equation itself. If one does assume that this pseudolinear segment is linear, and we symbolize the slope by k_0 then one can derive Eq. (12):

$$\frac{1}{k_0} = \frac{1}{V_m} + \frac{K_m}{0.632 V_m} \times \frac{1}{C_0} \qquad (12)$$

Equation (12) indicates that if V_m and K_m remain constant then a plot of the reciprocal of the slope of the pseudolinear portion will be linearly related to the reciprocal of the initial concentration or C_0 value. This shows why the classical concept of ethanol metabolism in man and animals is really incorrect. The apparently linear decline of alcohol blood levels will vary with the dose administered even if K_m and V_m remain constant, and the slope will also be a function of the volume of distribution and sometimes of the absorption rate. However, as stated formerly, when I took five doses of ethanol at different times, the values of K_m, V_m, and k_0 varied widely. Hence, the classical concept that alcohol in a given individual is eliminated at a fixed rate independent of its concentration in the body was not supported by our studies. Also, once the value of K_m for the particular system is known, one can use Eq. (1) to calculate the percent saturation of the "enzyme system" at different C values of interest.

A CHECK LIST FOR POSSIBLE FUTURE PHARMACOKINETIC STUDIES

From my reading and experimental investigations certain guidelines have emerged. For those present at this meeting the listing of these would be unnecessary. But in presenting the following list I am thinking of the many readers of the publication to result from this conference.

1. Preferably do intensive sampling after intravenous administration of several (preferably five or six) doses in at least one species of animal. The data from such studies provide much more information when only one or two rats or dogs are used per dose then when five to ten rats or dogs are dosed with only one or two doses of a drug.

2. After rapid intravenous injection take initial samples very early after injection such as 1, 3, and 5 min, etc. Continue sampling until assay sensitivity is reached *following all doses*. Much of the apparent dose-dependent "first-order" kinetics in the literature was caused by estimating the first-order rate constant in a different concentration region after each dose. Also, extremely rapid uptake of many drugs by tissues has been "missed" since the first tissue samples were taken at one or two hours postinjection.

3. Measure tissue levels as a function of both time and dose in at least one species of animal such as the rat. The rapid intravenous route of administration is preferred and sampling should be as discussed above.

4. After oral administration of many rapidly absorbed drugs, blood samples should be taken as early as 10 to 20 min postadministration in order to obtain data on the "up part" of the plasma or blood concentration curve. *Some drugs are absorbed by passive diffusion extremely rapidly in fasting subjects.* We have a distorted view since in most human studies the first blood sample has been taken one hour or later after administration. Recently, we found that the first blood sample, taken 20 min after oral administration of sodium p-aminosalicylate in an aqueous solution to a fasting human subject, gave the highest plasma concentration of PAS.

5. To check quickly for tissue saturation effects, by measuring only plasma levels, perform a "loading dose" experiment. Give, say, 5 mg/kg of drug by rapid intravenous injection and measure plasma concentrations of unchanged drug at 1, 5, and 10 min. Then, give 10 mg/kg, and 1 hr later give 5 mg/kg, and measure the plasma concentration again at 1, 5, and 10 min after the 5 mg/kg dose. If the plasma levels are appreciably higher in the loading dose experiment this constitutes good evidence of some saturation phenomenon and usually it will be saturable tissue binding. With some drugs the cited doses obviously would have to be drastically altered.

6. Be sure the analytical method used is specific for the unchanged drug and one or more metabolites, and that the method has good sensitivity and reproductibility. After intravenous administration it is preferable to be able to measure drug concentrations through at least two and preferably three or more log cycles on semilogarithmic graph paper. After oral administration the assay method should be sensitive enough to follow the drug levels down to at least one-tenth or one-twentieth of the peak concentration. Samples should be collected so that this criterion can be met after each treatment if possible. The literature is replete with erroneous half-lives of drugs since plasma levels were not measured for a long enough period of time. In drug availability studies the calculation of "bioavailability" from measurement of the area under only one-half or two-thirds of the plasma concentration curve is just plain misleading.

7. Estimate elimination half-lives after different doses are administered to the same subject or animal in the *same concentration range*, not necessarily in the *same time range*.

REFERENCES

Alberts, D. S., Bachur, M. R., and Holtzman, J. L., 1971, *Clin. Pharmacol. Therap.* **12**: 96.
Amsel, L. P., and Levy, G., 1969, *J. Pharm. Sci.* **58**: 321.
Anderson, E., Norberg, B., and Teger-Nilsson, A. C., 1963, *Scand. J. Clin. Lab. Invest.* **15**: 577.
Arnold, K., and Gerber, N., 1970, *Clin. Pharmacol. Therap.* **11**: 121.
Atkins, G. L., 1971a, *Biochim. Biophys. Acta* **248**: 405.
Atkins, G. L., 1971b, *Biochim. Biophys. Acta* **248**: 421.
Axelson, J. E., and Gibaldi, M., 1972, *J. Pharm. Sci.* **61**: 404.
Balasubramaniam, K., Mawer, G. E., and Simons, P. J., 1970, *Brit. J. Pharmacol.* **40**: 578.
Barr, W. H., and Riegelman, S., 1968, "Effect of Capacity Limited Metabolism on Plasma Levels of Free Salicylamide in Man." Presented to A.Ph.A. Academy of Pharmaceutical Sciences, Miami Beach, Florida, May 6, 1968.
Barr, W. H., and Riegelman, S., 1970a, *J. Pharm. Sci.* **59**: 154.
Barr, W. H., and Riegelman, S., 1970b, *J. Pharm. Sci.* **59**: 164.
Beckett, A. H., and Rowland, M., 1964, *Nature* **204**: 1203.
Beckett, A. H., Boyes, R. N., and Tucker, G. T., 1968a, *J. Pharm. Pharmacol.* **20**: 269.
Beckett, A. H., Boyes, R. N., and Tucker, G. T., 1968b, *J. Pharm. Pharmacol.* **20**: 277.
Benet, L. Z., 1972, *J. Pharm. Sci.* **61**: 536.
Benet, L. Z., and Turi, J. S., 1971, *J. Pharm. Sci.* **60**: 1593.
Binnion, P. F., Morgan, L. M., Stevenson, H. M., and Fletcher, E., 1969, *Brit. Heart J.* **31**: 636.
Bischoff, K. B., and Dedrick, R. L., 1968, *J. Pharm. Sci.* **57**: 1347.
Bischoff, K. B., Dedrick, R. L., and Zaharko, D. S., 1970, *J. Pharm. Sci.* **59**: 149.
Bischoff, K. G., Dedrick, R. L., Zaharko, D. S., and Longstreth, J. A., 1971, *J. Pharm. Sci.* **60**: 1128.
Blum, M., McGilvery, I., Becker, C., and Riegelman, S., 1971, *Clin. Res.* **19**: 121, abstract.
Bray, H. G., Thorpe, W. V., and White, K., 1951, *Biochem. J.* **48**: 88.
Buell, J., and Kalaba, R., 1968, Technical Report USCEE-312, Electronic Sciences Laboratory, University of Southern California, Los Angeles, California.

Burns, J. J., and Conney, A. H., 1965, *Proc. Roy. Soc. Med.* **58:** 955.
Carlson, L. A., and Hallberg, D., 1963, *Acta Physiol. Scand.* **59:** 52.
Chiou, W. L., and Riegelman, S., 1969, *J. Pharm. Sci.* **58:** 1500.
Civen, M., Ulrich, R., Trimmer, B. M., and Brown, C. B., 1967, *Science* **157:** 1563.
Coffey, J. J., Bullock, F. J., and Schoenemann, P. T., 1971, *J. Pharm. Sci.* **60:** 1623.
Crouthamel, W., Doluisio, J. T., Johnson, R. E., and Diamond, L., 1970, *J. Pharm. Sci.* **59:** 878.
Curry, S. H., 1970, *J. Pharm. Pharmacol.* **22:** 753.
Dayton, P. G., Cucinell, S. A., Weiss, M., and Perel, J. M., 1967, *J. Pharmacol. Exp. Therap.* **158:** 305.
Dearden, J. C., and Tomilson, E., 1971, *J. Pharm. Pharmacol.* **23:** 685, Suppl.
Dedrick, R. L., and Bischoff, K. B., 1968, *Chem. Engr. Prog. Symp. Ser.* **64:** 32.
Dettli, L., and Spring, P., 1966, *Helv. Med. Acta* **33:** 291.
DiSanto, A. R., and Wagner, J. G., 1969, *J. Pharm. Sci.* **58:** 1077.
DiSanto, A. R., 1971, "A New Nonlinear Pharmacokinetic Model with Specific Application to Methylene Blue." A dissertation submitted in partial fulfillment of the requirements for the degree of Doctor of Philosophy (Pharmacy) at the University of Michigan.
DiSanto, A. R., and Wagner, J. G., 1972a, *J. Pharm. Sci.* **61:** 598.
DiSanto, A. R., and Wagner, J. G., 1972b, *J. Pharm. Sci.* **61:** 552.
DiSanto, A. R., and Wagner, J. G., 1972c, *J. Pharm. Sci.* **61:** 1086.
DiSanto, A. R., and Wagner, J. G., 1972d, *J. Pharm. Sci.* **61:** 1090.
Dixson, R. L., Owens, E. S., and Rall, D. P., 1969, *J. Pharm. Sci.* **58:** 1106.
Doluisio, J. T., and Dittert, L. W., 1969, *Clin. Pharmacol. Therap.* **10:** 690.
Drach, J. C., Howell, J. P., Borondy, P. E., and Glazko, A. J., 1970, *Proc. Soc. Exp. Biol. Med.* **135:** 849.
Drucker, M. M., Blondheim, S. H., and Wislicki, L., 1964, *Clin. Sci.* **27:** 133.
Eggleton, M. G., 1940, *J. Physiol. (London)* **98:** 239.
Estes, J. W., Pelikan, E. W., and Krüger-Thiemer, E., 1969, *Clin. Pharmacol. Therap.* **10:** 329.
Fuwa, T., Iga, T., Hanano, M., Nogami, H., and Kashima, K., 1971, *J. Pharm. Soc. Japan* **91:** 1223.
Gerber, N., and Arnold, K., 1969, *J. Pharmacol. Exp. Therap.* **167:** 77
Gerber, N., and Wagner, J. G., 1972, *Res. Comm. Chem. Pathol. Pharmacol.* **3:** 455.
Gerber, N., Welles, W. L., Lynn, R., Rangno, R. E., Sweetman, B. J., and Bush, M. T., 1971, *J. Pharmacol. Exp. Therap.* **178:** 567.
Gibaldi, M., and Levy, G., 1972, *J. Pharm. Sci.* **61:** 567.
Gillette, J. R., 1971, *Ann. N. Y. Acad. Sci.* **179:** 43.
Glazko, A. J., Chang, T., Bankema, J., Dill, W. A., Gaulet, J. R., and Buckanan, R. A., 1969, *Clin. Pharmacol. Therap.* **10:** 498.
Goresky, C. A., 1964, *Am. J. Physiol.* **207:** 13.
Hallberg, D., 1965a, *Acta Physiol. Scand.* **64:** 299.
Hallberg, D., 1965b, *Acta Physiol. Scand.* **64:** 306.
Henderson, E. S., Adamson, R. H., Denham, C., and Oliverio, V. T., 1965, *Cancer Res.* **25:** 1008.
Hepner, G. W., Booth, C. C., Cowan, J., Hoffbrand, A. V., and Mollin, D. L., 1968, *Lancet* Aug. **10:** 302.
Hill, J. B., 1970, *Federation Proc.* **29:** 934, abstract.
Hogben, C. A. M., Tocco, D. J., Brodie, B. B., and Schanker, L. S., 1959, *J. Pharmacol. Exp. Therap.* **125:** 275.
Huang, K. C., and Lin, D. S. T., 1965, *Am. J. Physiol.* **208:** 391.
Jacquez, J. A., Bellman, R., and Kalaba, R., 1960, *Bull. Math. Biophys.* **22:** 309.

Jusko, W. J., and Levy, G., 1970, *J. Pharm. Sci.* **59:** 722.
Jusko, W. J., Levy, G., Yaffe, S. Y., and Gorodescher, R., 1970, *J. Pharm. Sci.* **59:** 473.
Kakemi, K., Arita, T., Sezaki, H., and Hanano, M., 1963, *J. Pharm. Soc. Japan* **83:** 260.
Kakemi, K., Arita, T., Hori, R., Koniski, R., and Nishimura, K., 1969, *Chem. Pharm. Bull. (Tokyo)* **17:** 248.
Kondritzer, A. A., Zvirblis, P., Goodman, A., and Paplanas, S. H., 1968, *J. Pharm. Sci.* **57:** 1142.
Krüger-Thiemer, E., Diller, W., and Bünger, P., 1966, *Antimicrobiol Agents Chemother.* **1965:** 183.
Krüger-Thiemer, E., 1968a, *Farmaco (Pavia) Ed. Sci.* **23:** 717.
Krüger-Thiemer, E., 1968b, "Pharmacokinetics and Dose-Concentration Relationships," in: Proceedings of the Third International Pharmacological Meeting, July 24-30, 1966, Vol. 7., *Physico-Chemical Aspects of Drug Actions*, Pergamon Press, New York. Vol. 7, p. 63.
Krüger-Thiemer, E., and Levine, R., 1968c, *Arzneim. Forsch.* **18:** 1575.
Lanman, C., Muranishi, S., and Schanker, L. S., 1970, *Pharmacologist* **12:** 293, abstract.
Lauger, P., and Stark, G., 1970, *Biochem. Biophys. Acta* **211:** 458.
Lauterback, F., 1968, *Biochem. Biophys. Acta* **150:** 146.
Levy, G., 1965a, *J. Pharm. Sci.* **54:** 496.
Levy, G., 1965b, *J. Pharm. Sci.* **54:** 959.
Levy, G., 1968, "Dose-Dependent Effects in Pharmacokinetics," in: *Importance of Fundamental Principles in Drug Evaluation* (Tedeschi, D. H. and Tedeschi, R. E.,eds.),Raven Press, New York.
Levy, G., 1971, *Chem. Biol. Interactions* **3:** 291.
Levy, G., and Amsel, L. P., 1966, *Biochem. Pharmacol.* **15:** 1033.
Levy, G., Amsel, L. P., and Elliott, H. C., 1969b, *J. Pharm. Sci.* **58:** 827.
Levy, G., and Gibaldi, M., 1972, *Ann. Rev. Pharmacol.* **12:** 85.
Levy, G., and Jusko, W. J., 1966, *J. Pharm. Sci.* **55:** 285.
Levy, G., and Matsuzawa, T., 1966, *J. Pharm. Sci.* **55:** 222.
Levy, G., and Matsuzawa, T., 1967, *J. Pharmacol. Exp. Therap.* **156:** 285.
Levy, G., and Nagashima, R., 1969, *J. Pharm. Sci.* **58:** 1001.
Levy, G., and Procknal, J. A., 1968, *J. Pharm. Sci.* **57:** 1330.
Levy, G., and Regardh, C. G., 1971, *J. Pharm. Sci.* **60:** 608.
Levy, G., Tsuchuja, T., and Amsel, L. P., 1972, *Clin. Pharmacol. Therap.* **13:** 258.
Levy, G., Vogel, A. W., and Amsel, L. P., 1969c, *J. Pharm. Sci.* **58:** 503.
Levy, G., Weintraub, L., Matsuzawa, T., and Oles, S. R., 1966, *J. Pharm. Sci.* **55:** 1319.
Levy, G., and Yamada, H., 1970, *J. Pharm. Pharmacol.* **22:** 964.
Levy, G., and Yamada, H., 1971, *J. Pharm. Sci.* **60:** 215.
Levy, G., and Yaffe, S. J., 1968, *Clin. Toxicol.* **1:** 409.
Lundquist, F. and Wolthers, H., 1958, *Acta Pharmacol. Toxicol.* **14:** 265.
Mackey, M. C., 1971a, *Biophys. J.* **11:** 75.
Mackey, M. C., 1971b, *Biophys. J.* **11:** 91.
Marks, B. H., Dutta, S., Gauthier, J., and Elliott, D., 1964, *J. Pharmacol. Therap.* **145:** 351.
Martin, B. K., 1965, *Nature* **207:** 274.
Mather, L. E., Long, G. J., and Thomas, J. T., 1971, *Clin. Pharmacol. Therap.* **12:** 935.
McMartin, C., and Simpson, P., 1971, *Clin. Pharmacol. Therap.* **12:** 73.
Meyer, M. C., and Guttman, D. E., 1968, *J. Pharm. Sci.* **57:** 895.
Michaelis, L., and Menten, M. L., 1913, *Biochem. Z.* **49:** 333.
Mudge, G. H., and Weiner, I. M., 1963, "Renal Excretion of Weak Organic Acids and Bases," in: *Drugs and Membranes*, Vol. IV (Hogben, C. A. M., ed.), The Macmillan Company, New York, p. 157.

Nagashima, R., and Levy, G., 1969, *J. Pharm. Sci.* **58**: 845.
Nagashima, R., and Levy, G., 1968, *J. Pharm. Sci.* **57**: 1991.
Nagashima, R., Levy, G., and Back, N., 1968a, *J. Pharm. Sci.* **57**: 68.
Nagashima, R., Levy, G., and Nelson, E., 1968b, *J. Pharm. Sci.* **57**: 58.
Nagashima, R., Levy, G., and O'Reilly, R. A., 1968c, *J. Pharm. Sci.* **57**: 1888.
Nagashima, R., Levy, G., and Sarcione, E. J., 1968d, *J. Pharm. Sci.* **57**: 1881.
Nagwekar, J. B., and Unnikrishnan, A., 1971, *J. Pharm. Sci.* **60**: 375.
Neal, J. L., 1972, *J. Theoret. Biol.* **35**: 113.
Nelson, E., Hanano, M., and Levy, G., 1966, *J. Pharmacol. Exp. Therap.* **153**: 159.
Nordquist, P., Harthorn, J. G., and Karlson, R., 1965, *Nord. Med.* **74**: 1024.
Ochsenfahrt, H., and Winne, D., 1968, *Life Sci.* **7**: 493.
Oldendorf, W. H., 1968, *Intern. J. Appl. Radiation Isotopes* **19**: 411.
O'Reilly, W. J., Pitt, P. A., and Ryan, A. J., 1971, *Brit. J. Pharmacol.* **43**: 167.
Patlak, C. S., 1961, *Bull, Math. Biophys.* **23**: 173.
Paumgartner, G., Probst, P., Kraines, R., and Leevy, C. M., 1970, *Ann. N. Y. Acad. Sci.* **170**: 134.
Pfeffer, M., Schor, J. M., Bolton, S., and Jacobson, R., 1968, *J. Pharm. Sci.* **57**: 1375.
Radzialowski, F. M., and Bousquet, W. F., 1967, *Life Sci.* **6**: 2545.
Rees, E. D., Mandelstram, P., Lowry, J. A., and Lipscomb, H., 1971, *Biochem. Biophys. Acta* **225**: 96.
Reeve, E. R., 1964, "The Plasma Albumin System. A First Attempt at a Kinetic Description in Dynamic Clinical Studies with Radioisotopes." Proceedings of a Symposium held at the Oak Ridge Institute of Nuclear Studies, October 21-25, 1963. U.S. Department of Commerce, TID 7678, Office of Technical Services, U.S. Dept. of Commerce, Washington, D.C., p. 445.
Rowland, M., Benet, L. Z., and Riegelman, S., 1970, *J. Pharm. Sci.* **59**: 364.
Rowland, M., and Riegelman, S., 1968, *J. Pharm. Sci.* **57**: 1313.
Rowland, M., Riegelman, S., and Epstein, W. L., 1968, *J. Pharm. Sci.* **57**: 984.
Schachter, D., and Manis, J. G., 1958. *J. Clin. Invest.* **37**: 800.
Schanker, L. S., 1962, *Biochem. Pharmacol.* **11**: 253.
Schanker, L. S., and Morrison, A. S., 1965, *Intern J. Nevropharmacol.* **4**: 27.
Schoenfield, L. J., McGill, D. B., and Foulk, W. T., 1964, *J. Clin. Invest.* **43**: 1424.
Sedman, A. J., and Wagner, J. G., 1972, "Quantitative Pooling of Both Parallel Michaelis–Menten Formation Equations and Langmuir-type Equations for Binding of Drugs to Tissues." Abstracts of Symposia and Contributed Papers Presented to the A.Ph.A. Academy of Pharmaceutical Sciences at the 119th Annual Meeting of the American Pharmaceutical Association, Houston, Texas, April 22-28, 1972, Vol. 2, No. 1, p. 61, abstract 16.
Shibasaki, J., Koizumi, T., and Higuchi, W., 1968a, *Chem. Pharm. Bull.* (*Tokyo*) **16**: 2273.
Shibasaki, J., Koizumi, T., and Tanaka, T., 1968b, *Chem. Pharm. Bull.* (*Tokyo*) **16**: 1661.
Shibasaki, J., Konishi, R., Takeda, Y., and Koizumi, T., 1971, *Chem. Pharm. Bull.* (*Tokyo*) **19**: 1800.
Sholkoff, S. D., Eyering, E. J., Rowland, M., and Riegelman, S., 1967, *Arthritis Rheumatism* **10**: 348.
Shore, P. A., Brodie, B. B., and Hogben, C. A. M., 1957, *J. Pharmacol. Exp. Therap.* **119**: 361.
Sidell, F. R., Groff, W. A., and Ellin, R. I., 1969, *J. Pharm. Sci.* **58**: 1093.
Smith, R. B., Dittert, L. W., Griffin, W. D., Jr., and Doluisio, J. T., 1973, *J: Pharmacokinetics and Biopharmaceutics* **1**: 5.
Somani, S. M., Schumacher, D., Thompson, R., and McDonald, R. H., Jr., 1971, *Fed. Proc.* **30**: 1335, abstract.
Spears, G., Sneyd, J. G. T., and Loten, E. G., 1971, *Biochem. J.* **125**: 1149.

Strum, W. B., Nixon, P. F., Binden, H. J., and Bertino, J. R., 1970, *Clin. Res.* **18**: 389, abstract.
Stupp, H., Rouch, S., Sous, H., Brun, J. P., and Lagler, F., 1967, *Arch. Otolaryngol.* **86**: 63.
Suzuki, A., Higuchi, W. I., and Ho, N. F. H., 1970a, *J. Pharm. Sci.* **59**: 644.
Suzuki, A., Higuchi, W. I., and Ho, N. F. H., 1970a, *J. Pharm. Sci.* **59**: 651.
Suzuki, T., Saitoh, Y., and Nishihara, K., 1970b, *Chem. Pharm. Bull. (Tokyo)* **18**: 405.
Teorell, T., 1937, *Arch. Inter. Pharmacodyn.* **57**: 205 and 226.
Thorp, J. M., 1964, "The Influence of Plasma Proteins on the Action of Drugs," in: *Absorption and Distribution of Drugs*, p. 64 (Binns, T. B., ed.), The Williams and Wilkins Company, Baltimore.
Timmes, J. J., Demos, N. J., and Chong, S. I., 1971. *Clin. Pharmacol. Therap.* **12**: 920.
Tomura, M., and Akera, T., 1971, *Jap. J. Pharmacol.* **21**: 682.
Tsuchuja, T., and Levy, G., 1972, *J. Pharm. Sci.* **61**: 541.
Wagner, J. G., 1966, *Can. J. Pharm. Sci.* **1**: 55.
Wagner, J. G., 1967, *J. Pharm. Sci.* **56**: 586.
Wagner, J. G., 1968a, *Ann. Rev. Pharmacol.* **8**: 67.
Wagner, J. G., 1968b, *J. Theoret. Biol.* **20**: 173.
Wagner, J. G., 1971a, *Biopharmaceutics and Relevant Pharmacokinetics*, Chapter 40, p. 302, Drug Intelligence Publications, Hamilton, Illinois.
Wagner, J. G., 1971b, *J. Mondial de Pharmacie* **14**: 279.
Wagner, J. G., 1973, "Properties of the Michaelis–Menten Equation and Its Integrated Form Which Are Useful in Pharmacokinetics," *J. Pharmacokinetics & Biopharmaceutics*, **1**: 103.
Wagner, J. G. aud Damiano, R. E., 1968, *J. Clin. Pharmacol. J. New Drugs* **8**: 102.
Wagner, J. G., and Patel, J. A., 1972, "Variations in Absorption and Elimination Rates of Ethyl Alcohol in a Single Subject," *Res. Com. Chem. Pathol. Pharmacol.* **4**: 61.
Wagner, J. G., and Sedman, A. J., 1973, "Quantitation of Rate of Gastrointestinal and Buccal Absorption of Acidic and Basic Drugs Based on Extraction Theory," *J. Pharmacokinetics & Biopharmaceutics*, **1**: 23.
Weiner, I. M., and Mudge, G. H., 1964, *Am. J. Med. Sci.* **36**: 743.
Weiner, I. M., Blanchard, L. C., and Mudge, G. H., 1964a, *Am. J. Physiol.* **207**: 953.
Weiner, I. M., Glasser, J. E., and Lach, L., 1964b, *Am. J. Physiol.* **207**: 964.
Widmark, E. M. P., 1933, *Biochem. Z.* **267**: 128.
Widmark, E. M. P., 1933, *Biochem. Z.* **267**: 135.
Widmark, E., and Tandberg, J., 1924, *Biochem. Z.* **147**: 358.
Wiegand, R. G., and Chun, A. H. C., 1972, *J. Pharm. Sci.* **61**: 425.
Wilbrandt, W., and Rosenberg, P., 1961, *Pharmacol. Rev.* **13**: 109.
Williams, R. T., Milburn, P., and Smith, R. L., 1965, *Ann. N. Y. Acad. Sci.* **123**: 110.
Winkler, K. and Tygstrup, H., 1964, *J. Clin. Lab. Invest.* **16**: 481.
Winne, D., 1970, *J. Theroret. Biol.* **27**: 1.
Yesair, D. W., Callahan, M., Remington, L., and Hensler, C. J., 1970, *Biochem. Pharmacol.* **19**: 1579.
Zaharko, D. S., Dedrick, R. L., and Oliverio, V. T., 1970, *Fed. Proc.* **29**: 932, abstract.

DISCUSSION SUMMARY

Teorell expressed surprise that linear kinetic models, such as the model he had introduced in 1937, did such an adequate job of describing the pharmacokinetics of drugs in the body. He reviewed the forces in the body related to membrane transport processes and suggested that future workers would one day combine pharmacokinetics with a complete force analysis. At that time electropotential measurements as well as pressure gradient measurements would necessitate the use of nonlinear models which are not monotonic in the time phase.

Lemberger asked whether the pharmacologic effect of a drug may result in the nonlinear kinetics seen following its administration. For example, high doses of diphenhydramine affect the intraventricular conducting system and could cause a possible asystole. He suggested that in asystole less of the drug would get into the brain, resulting in the nonlinearity of kinetics as described by Wagner.

Wagner agreed that pharmacologic action could not be disregarded. However, he felt that every drug would show tissue binding saturation at high dose levels regardless of any specific pharmacologic effect. There is only so much tissue in the body, and if the dose is raised to a sufficiently high level, this tissue will be saturated just like plasma proteins.

Garrett felt that much of the data could be analyzed in a manner consistent with an hypothesized multicompartment linear model containing a deep compartment, as well as by the nonlinear methods of Wagner. Wagner agreed that in a limited dose range a linear compartment model could describe the data and would be a useful adjunct in making therapeutic decisions. For example, this would be true for lincomycin in the 250 mg to 1-g-per-day dose range. However, when this drug is given at a dosage level of 10 g per day, the blood concentration can no longer be described by the linear model.

Levy reminded the audience that it took pharmacokineticists a number of years to realize that the first-order kinetics observed for many drugs may only be the limiting case for a process described by Michaelis–Menten kinetics. However, now that this possibility is recognized, it is important to also realize that pharmacokinetic processes may be subject to substrate and produce inhibition. For example, O'Reilly's studies with dicumerol yield half-life changes with increasing dose even when plasma concentrations are measured in the same range for all doses. This data cannot be rationalized by simple Michaelis–Menten kinetics or by simple binding models. Rather, a more complex model such as product inhibition must be invoked. The inhibition of diphenylhydantoin and phenylbutazone metabolism following the administration of the hydroxy metabolites of these compounds are further examples of possible product inhibition. Levy also pointed out that the pharmacokinetic parameters and product inhibition potential determined following an *i.v.* administered metabolite might not necessarily reflect the kinetics observed when the metabolite is formed endogenously in contrast to being administered exogenously, even though the peripheral blood levels in the two studies may be comparable.

Riegelman agreed that although nonlinearity is a very interesting aspect of pharmacokinetics, nonlinear treatments are usually not necessary at normal dose levels or in the clinical situation. He pointed out that the greatest application of pharmacokinetics in the clinical situation has been by workers such as Dettli and in these cases the simplistic one-compartment model is often sufficiently accurate.

Translation of Pharmacokinetics to Clinical Medicine*

L. Dettli

Department of Internal Medicine
University of Basel, Buergerspital
Basel, Switzerland

More than four hundred years ago the famous natural scientist and physician Theophrastus Paracelsus said: "Alle Dinge sind Gift und nichts ist ohne Gift. Nur die Dosis macht's, dass ein Ding kein Gift sei." These words for the first time clearly stated that the biological effect (E) of a substance depends quantitatively on the dose (D) administered, i.e.,

$$E = f(D) \qquad (1)$$

It took several centuries for pharmacologists to confirm Paracelsus' discovery in a somewhat modified way by the fundamental statement that the bioactivity of a substance depends on its concentration (c) at the site of action and on its "intrinsic activity" (α). A further refinement was brought about by the development of the receptor theory. Based on the law of mass action the terms "binding affinity" and "binding capacity" were introduced and characterized by appropriate constants (K_i, β_i). By means of these constants, the binding characteristics of drug molecules of both pharmacologically active and inactive (e.g., plasma albumin) macromolecules of the organism can be described (Ariens, 1964). Furthermore, we know today that in an open system such as the organism, the concentration at the site of action depends on many factors such as the absorbed fraction (F) of the dose, the time interval between the doses (τ), the rate constants of

---

* Aided by Schweizerischer Nationalfonds zur Foerderung der wissenschaftlichen Forschung.

absorption, distribution, metabolism, and excretion (k_i), and on the distribution volumes (V_i) of the drug. As a consequence, the assumption of Paracelsus as symbolized in Eq. (1) may be transformed in the following way:

$$E = f(c, \alpha) = f(D, \tau, F, V_i, k_i, \beta_i, K_i, \alpha) \qquad (2)$$

Pharmacokinetics is defined as the mathematical description of concentration changes of drugs within the organism. The symbols on the right side of Eq. (2) demonstrate in principle the importance of this discipline in pharmacotherapeutics: F, V_i, and K_i are obviously pharmacokinetic factors, whereby factor F may be influenced to some extent by biopharmaceutical procedures, e.g., modifications of the dosage form; V_i and k_i, however, are constants which are usually beyond the control of the physician. The same is true for β_i, K_i, and α. The factors β_i and K_i are either of a pharmacokinetic nature (when they describe "silent" receptors such as plasma albumin) or of a pharmacodynamic nature (when they refer to pharmacologically active receptors). On the other hand, α characterizes the pharmacodynamic or chemotherapeutic properties of the drug. Consequently, in the light of Eq. (2), the translation of pharmacokinetics to clinical medicine means answering the following question: *When the pharmacodynamic or chemotherapeutic activity (α) of a drug is known, how must its dosage regimen (D, τ) be adapted to its pharmacokinetic characteristics in order to reach and maintain the desired therapeutic effect (E)?*

It is the purpose of the following presentation to discuss some examples of pharmacokinetic analysis which influenced the practice or the principles of practical therapeutics. First of all, it should be stressed that pharmacokinetic reasoning has opened up a new way of thinking in clinical medicine. Physicians always intuitively appreciated the basic importance of *pharmacodynamics* because they are primarily interested in the action of a drug on the patient. In pharmacokinetics we consider the fact that there is not only a unidirectional action but rather a mutual *interaction* between drug and organism (Dettli, 1968). The action of the organism on the drug may be summarized by the terms "absorption," "distribution," and "elimination" (metabolism and excretion). According to Eq. (2), these three processes which are the object of pharmacokinetics control the concentration of the drug at the site of action and consequently its pharmacological effect. As a consequence, a growing number of physicians are recognizing that pharmacokinetics is a basic clinical problem just as much as is pharmacodynamics. As a result, several reviews and monographs emphasizing the clinical significance of pharmacokinetics have been published (Dominguez, 1950; Krueger-Thiemer, 1960, 1961; Nelson, 1961; Freerksen *et al.* 1964; Dettli and Spring, 1968; Dost, 1953, 1968; Wagner, 1971).

DEFINING THE TERM "DRUG" IN THE LIGHT OF PHARMACOKINETICS

A World Health Organization Scientific Group (1966) adopted the following definition: "A drug is any substance or product that is used or intended to be used to modify or explore physiological systems or pathological states for the benefit of the recipient." Evidently the term "drug" is here used in the sense of a "preparation" as it is administered to the patient, and not in the sense of a "bioactive substance" as used by the pharmacologist, because a bioactive substance is completely defined by its molecular structure and its biological activity whether or not it is used for the benefit of patients. My first proposal is to delete the word "substance" from the above definition because a drug, in the sense of "drug preparation," is never a substance but always a "product" which *contains* one or more bioactive substances. Numerous bioavailability studies using pharmacokinetic-methodology have shown beyond doubt that two drugs containing identical amounts of identical bioactive substances may be of totally different therapeutic efficacy on account of differences in the dosage form. The fact that the importance of bioavailability was brought to the attention of the physician is one of the most fundamental contributions of pharmacokinetics to practical medicine. Furthermore, there are obviously many other "products" that are used to modify pathological states for the benefit of the "recipient," e.g., artificial teeth or other protheses. The basic difference between an artificial tooth and a bioactive substance is the fact that the latter acts in *molecular dispersion*: absorption, distribution, metabolism, excretion, and binding to biological macromolecules; in other words, the whole pharmacokinetic and pharmacodynamic behavior of a bioactive substance depends on molecular dispersion! Therefore, this fundamental fact should be incorporated in the definition of the terms "drug" and "bioactive substance."

DRUG ACCUMULATION

In practical medicine, drug accumulation is a serious problem. Curiously enough, a definition of the term seems to be lacking in the textbooks of therapeutics and pharmacology. As a qualitative definition we may adopt the following simple statement (Dettli, 1971): "The amount of drug in the organism after repeated administration of a dose is higher than that after the administration of one dose." In order to gain real insight into the nature of the process, a quantitative definition is needed which elucidates the factors responsible for drug accumulation. Of course, there would be no difficulty in formulating such a definition based on the well-known equations describing multiple dose elimination kinetics (Dost, 1953; Wagner, 1971). However, any translation of pharmacokinetics to practical medicine must meet one condition of utmost importance: the condition of *simplicity*. Any definition must be adapted to the mathematical background of the physician even if this means the risk of a certain amount of error. Our starting point is the well-known equation introduced into pharmacokinetics by Teorell (1937) which describes the amount of drug in the organism, m, after the paravascular administration of one dose, D. In many cases of practical importance the speed of absorption, compared to the speed of elimination, is so great that the short absorption process may be neglected without introducing a considerable error. Under these conditions, Teorell's equation is transformed into an equation of pure exponential elimination. As a consequence, the drug amount in the organism, $m_{0,1}$, at the beginning of the first dosage interval, τ, will be (Dettli, 1970):

$$m_{0,1} = D \tag{3}$$

and at the end of the dosage interval

$$m_{\tau,1} = D \cdot e^{-k_e \cdot \tau/t_{1/2}} = D \cdot e^{-\ln 2 \cdot \tau/t_{1/2}} \tag{4}$$

where $t_{\frac{1}{2}}$ is the biological half-life and $k_e = \ln 2/t_{\frac{1}{2}}$ is the "overall" elimination rate constant of the drug. After the administration of an "infinite" number of doses, the amount of drug in the organism approaches its maximum or steady-state level, $m_{0,\infty}$, which is described by

$$m_{0,\infty} = \frac{D}{1 - e^{-\ln 2 \cdot \tau/t_{1/2}}} \tag{5}$$

Introducing the relative dosage interval $\varepsilon = \tau/t_{\frac{1}{2}}$ according to Krueger-Thiemer (1960) and dividing Eq. (5) by Eq. (3) results in the expression

$$R = \frac{m_{0,\infty}}{D} = \frac{1}{1 - 2^{-\varepsilon}} \tag{6}$$

R is called *accumulation factor*. According to Eq. (6), R describes the amount of drug in the organism ($m_{0,\infty}$) after reaching the steady-state of accumulation as a multiple of the dose: $m_{0,\infty} = R \cdot D$. Equation (6) quantitatively defines, therefore, the *extent* of drug accumulation. Furthermore, the following conclusions of practical importance can be drawn from Eq. (6) (Dettli, 1970): The extent of drug accumulation is entirely defined by the relative dosage interval, ε, i.e., by the relationship between the dosage interval, τ, and the biological half-life, $t_{1/2}$, of the drug. Consequently, accumulation is not a quality of the drug itself but rather a property of the dosage regimen. The common view that there are "accumulating" and "nonaccumulating" drugs is therefore a misconception. Since the value of ε can be freely chosen, it is the physician rather than the drug who decides on the extent of accumulation: The lower the value of ε chosen the more pronounced is the tendency of accumulation, and vice-versa.

Table I shows some values of R as a function of ε. It should be noted that the accumulation factor R is numerically identical with the "dose ratio" $R^* = D^*/D$ according to Krueger-Thiemer (1960) which describes the correct quantitative relationship between the loading dose, D^*, and the maintenance dose, D. When a loading dose $D^* = R \cdot D$ is administered, the steady-state level of the drug in the organism is already reached after the first dose. We have shown elsewhere (Dettli, 1970; 1971) that the time course of drug accumulation is also completely defined by the relative dosage interval: The smaller the value of ε chosen the longer the accumulation process will last, and vice versa.

TABLE I

The Accumulation Factor R as a Function of the Relative Dosage Interval $\varepsilon = \tau/t_{1/2}$ [a]

$\epsilon = \tau/t_{1/2}$	0.01	0.05	0.1	0.2	0.3	0.4	0.5	0.6	0.7	0.8	0.9	1.0	2.0	3.0	4.0	5.0
$R = m_{0,\infty}/D$	145	29.4	14.9	7.7	5.3	4.1	3.4	2.9	2.6	2.3	2.15	2.00	1.33	1.14	1.07	1.03

[a] Calculated according to eq. (6) (for explanations see text).

KRUEGER-THIEMER'S DOSAGE THEORY OF BACTERIOSTATIC AGENTS

It is evident that any theory relating pharmacokinetic data to therapeutic effects is of general clinical significance (Levy, 1964; 1966; Levy and Nelson, 1965). Krueger-Thiemer's theory on the dosage regimen of bacteriostatic agents is one of the most beautiful translations of pharmacokinetic reasoning to clinical pharmacology (Krueger-Thiemer, 1960; 1961). The starting point of the theory is the simple assumption that the drug concentration in the plasma water, c, which produces the desired therapeutic effect is proportional to the concentration μ which produces an identical effect in the *in vitro* experiment:

$$c = \sigma \cdot \mu \tag{7}$$

Since this effect is a reversible one (e.g., bacteriostasis), Krueger-Thiemer postulates that c should be maintained during the whole period of therapy.

When this is accomplished by continuous infusion of the drug, the following steady-state concentration, c, is reached and maintained in the plasma water:

$$c = c' \cdot f = \frac{f \cdot D/t}{k_e \cdot V'} \tag{8}$$

where c is the steady-state concentration in the plasma water; c' is the total steady-state concentration in the plasma; $f = c/c'$ is the fraction of molecules not bound to the plasma proteins; D/t is the dose per hour; and V' is the distribution volume of the drug. The factor f considers the fact that the *in vitro* experiment is usually performed in a protein-free medium, whereas in the organism the drug is partly bound to the plasma proteins. Introducing Eq. (8) into Eq. (7) and solving for D/t results in

$$\frac{D}{t} = \sigma \cdot \left(\frac{\mu \cdot k_e V'}{f}\right) \tag{9}$$

In order to reach the steady-state concentration immediately, the following loading dose D^* has to be administered:

$$D^* = \frac{D/t}{k_e} \tag{10}$$

It should be noted that all parameters between parentheses in Eq. (9) can be determined *in vitro* (μ, f) or in the pharmacokinetic experiment *in vivo* (k_e, V'). Consequently, there remains the proportionality constant, σ, as the only unknown to be determined in the therapeutic experiment. This is accomplished by varying σ until the optimum therapeutic result is reached. All other time-consuming "trial and error" procedures can then be avoided. Thus, the fundamental importance of Krueger-Thiemer's equations is the fact that the therapeutic efficacy of two compounds can be compared based on a true quantitative null hypothesis (Krueger-Thiemer, 1962; Dettli, 1966).

To work out the principles clearly, we restricted our discussion to the case of continuous infusion and introduced some simplifications. For example, in Krueger-Thiemer's original theory, f is a function of the plasma concentration according to the law of mass action:

$$f = \frac{c}{c'} = \frac{1}{1 + (\beta \cdot p)/(K + c)} \tag{11}$$

where β is the apparent maximum binding capacity; K is the dissociation constant of the drug–albumin complex; and p is the concentration of the binding proteins. The relevant biological constants of Eqs. (9) and (11) have been determined for all commonly used sulfonamides (Krueger-Thiemer,

1961; Scholtan, 1961; 1962; Spring, 1966; Dettli and Spring, 1966; 1968) and for several experimental compounds (Krueger-Thiemer et al., 1966; 1969). Several sulfonamides have been evaluated in therapeutic trials according to Krueger-Thiemer's principles (Buenger et al., 1961; Buenger, 1963). A value of $\sigma \cong 10$ was found for all sulfonamides studied so far, when the minimum bacteriostatic concentration μ in vitro was compared with the minimal chemotherapeutically effective concentration in the plasma water of the patients. The dosage regimens for intermittent administration listed in Table II are calculated based on this result and compared with the dosage regimens presently recommended by the manufacturers.

PHARMACOKINETICS AND THE INDIVIDUAL PATIENT

Since physicians have to treat individual patients, the question "How variable are pharmacokinetic constants in a sample of patients or in one individual patient at different times?" is of practical significance. As far as gastrointestinal drug absorption is concerned, it appears that drug formulation and food constituents in the gastrointestinal tract play a greater role than intraindividual and interindividual differences in the strict sense (Heizer et al., 1971; Wagner, 1971). In contrast, increasing evidence has accumulated that many internal and external factors may profoundly influence drug metabolism and excretion (Dettli and Spring, 1968a). The elimination rates and consequently the steady-state levels after repeated administration of a drug may vary by more than an order of magnitude (Brodie et al., 1959). Interindividual differences may be partly explained by induction or inhibition of the drug metabolizing enzymes caused by prior or concomitant administration of other substances. There is no doubt, however, that many of these differences are genetically determined (Evans, 1962). Pharmacogenetics—a special branch of pharmacokinetics—will possibly develop into a powerful tool for genetic research in man (Kalow, 1962).

In all these instances it is hardly possible to recognize which one of the patients is kinetically abnormal and to what extent. As a consequence, a safe and effective drug therapy is often possible only when the drug concentration in the patient can be determined. The development of laboratories suitable for this purpose is one of the most important problems of present-day therapeutics. The contribution of pharmacokinetics consists mainly in predicting from a one-dose experiment the steady-state drug levels in chronically treated patients.

On the other hand, there are several well-defined factors, discussed below, which influence drug kinetics and may be recognized or at least suspected in the individual patient.

TABLE II
Dosage Regimens of Sulfonamides According to Krueger-Thiemer (1960)[a]

| Compound | Pharmacokinetic parameters ||||||| Dosage regimens |||||
| | μ (mg/L) | Δ' (L/kg) | K (μmol/L) | β (μmol/g) | f | k_e (hr^{-1}) | Calculated ||| Conventional ||
							τ (hr)	D (mg)	D^*/D	τ (hr)	D (mg)	D^*/D
Sulfadiazine	0.250	0.31	1193	31,50	0.501	0.058	12	111	1.9	4–6	1000	2
Sulfamethoxy-pyrazine	0.448	0.25	341	29,75	0.233	0.011	24	102	4.3	24	200	4
Sulfamethoxy-pyridazine	0.336	0.20	70	29,75	0.065	0.019	24	418	2.7	24	500	2
Sulfamethoxy-diazine	0.364	0.25	105	29,75	0.091	0.019	24	404	2.7	24	500	2
Sulfadimethoxine	0.279	0.15	11,5	31,50	0.016	0.019	24	1058	2.7	24	500	2

[a] Pharmacokinetic parameters (left) and calculated and conventional dosage regimens (right) of five sulfonamide compounds μ: minimum inhibitory concentration *in vitro* against mycobacterium smegmatis in a medium free of protein and antagonists; G: body weight of the patient; $\Delta' = V^c/G$: relative distribution volume; K: dissociation constant of the sulfonamide-albumin complex in human plasma at 27°C; β: apparent maximum binding capacity of human plasma albumin for the sulfonamide; f: the fraction of sulfonamide in human plasma not bound to albumin when $c = 10 \cdot \mu$; k_e: overall elimination rate constant; D: maintenance dose; D^*: loading dose; τ: dosage interval. These dosage regimens for intermittent administration have been calculated based on the following standard values: $G = 70$ kg; concentration of albumin in the plasma $p = 40$ g/liter; $\sigma = 10$.

Age of the Patient

It is well known that pediatricians are reluctant to administer sulfonamides to newborn children. In contrast, the generally accepted doses related to body weight in older children are several times higher than that in the adult. It has been shown that these empirically established rules of sulfonamide dosage are in accordance with pharmacokinetic facts: The elimination of sulfonamides in newborn children is much slower than in adults. During the first years of life however, the elimination rate increases sharply up to sevenfold and then decreases slowly with increasing age until the "normal" value of the adult is reached at about 20 years (Krauer et al., 1968; Krauer, 1972). A further decrease of the elimination rate during adult life has been reported for sulfamethoxazole (Otaya, 1971). On the other hand, the distribution volume decreases steadily and slightly in parallel with the decreasing extracellular space during the same time period (Rindt and Gladtke, 1964; Krauer, 1972).

pH of Body Fluids and State of Wakefulness

According to the theory of nonionic diffusion (Milne et al., 1958) the permeation of acidic and basic drugs through cellular membranes is practically restricted to the neutral moiety and should depend therefore on the pH of the biological fluids. As a consequence, it can be expected that the pharmacokinetic characteristics of acidic drugs are influenced in the following way by the pH of the body fluids (the opposite effects may be expected with basic drugs): Tubular reabsorption decreases with increasing urine pH, resulting in an increased renal elimination rate. Furthermore, the distribution volume of the drug should decrease with increasing pH values of the extracellular fluid, and vice versa. These expectations have been verified experimentally (Kostenbauder et al., 1962; Dettli and Spring, 1964; Rowland et al., 1965; Dettli et al., 1967). Since sleep induces a slight acidosis (Birchfield et al., 1959) we put forward the working hypothesis that the biological half-life and the distribution volume of acidic drugs such as sulfonamides will increase during sleep, resulting in a bicyclic diurnal elimination pattern. These hypotheses have also been verified experimentally (Dettli and Spring, 1966a; Spring et al., 1967). Interestingly enough, the diurnal periodicity of elimination is absent in the newborn child and develops during the first year of life (Krauer, 1969; 1970; 1972) in parallel with the transition of the sleeping behavior from a polycyclic to a bicyclic behavior (Kleitmann, 1963). Whereas the influence of the pH on the distribution volume is small, it can be seen from Table III that sleep or differences in the urine pH may change the elimination rate constant of some sulfonamides by several hundred percent and that the differences are more pronounced with compounds of a low pKa'. The influence of disturbances of the acid–base equilibrium on pharmacokinetics may well be of clinical significance because many disease states influence the pH of the body fluids much more than sleep.

TABLE III

The Influence of the Urine pH and of Sleep on the Elimination Rate of Sulfonamides[a]

Compound	pKa'	Q_{pH}	$Q_{n/d}$
Sulfisoxazole	4.9	2.0	–
Sulfaethidole	5.1	2.7	–
Sulfasymazine	5.5	2.4	2.9
Sulfamethoxazole	5.7	1.5	1.6
Sulfadimethoxine	5.9	–	1.5
Sulfamethoxypyrazine	6.1	–	2.3
Sulfadiazine	6.4	–	1.4
Sulfamethoxine	6.5	–	3.6
2-Sulfa-5-ethylpyrimidine	6.9	–	2.5
Sulfadimethyloxazole	7.2	1.2	–
Sulfisomidine	7.4	1.2	1.4
Sulfanilamide	10.5	1.0	1.1

[a] In a first series of experiments the urine of the patients was maintained at $pH < 5.5$, or $pH > 7.8$, by the continuous infusion of ammonium chloride or sodium bicarbonate, respectively. The mean elimination rates of the drugs at low urinary pH were lower by the factor Q_{pH}.

In a second series of experiments the elimination rates of the sulfonamides were measured during day and during night. The mean elimination rates during night were lower by the factor $Q_{n/d}$ (Dettli and Spring, 1968).

Saturation Phenomena

When speaking of linear or first-order elimination kinetics it is wise to add the term "apparent." This is especially true in the case of metabolic disposition of a drug because it must be assumed *a priori* that enzymatic processes do not follow first-order kinetics, i.e., $-dc/dt = k_e \cdot c$, but rather Michaelis–Menten kinetics, i.e.,

$$\frac{-dc}{dt} = \frac{v_{\max}}{V} \cdot \frac{c}{K + c} \qquad (12)$$

where K and $v_{\max}$ are the dissociation constant of the drug-enzyme complex and the maximum reaction rate, respectively. First-order kinetics will only prevail when $c \ll K$. This condition is apparently fulfilled in most pharmacokinetic experiments published so far. It should be emphasized, however, that the predictive value of such experiments is strictly limited to the dose range studied. Higher doses could result in saturation kinetics because the condition $c \ll K$ no longer holds. As a consequence, after repeated administration of the drug much higher steady-state levels than predicted by Eq. (5) and a correspondingly increased risk of toxicity will result. The clinician (and the drug addict) should interpret Levy's remarkable analysis of salicylate kinetics as a serious warning against this possibility (Levy, 1968; Levy et al., 1972). In addition, when several drugs are administered concomitantly, mutual competitive inhibition of drug metabolism is a problem of increasing clinical importance (Levy, 1971).

Similar problems arise in connection with the binding of drugs to plasma proteins. Several authors demonstrated in *in vitro* experiments an increase of the unbound drug fraction $f = c/c'$ in the plasma [see Eq. (11)] caused by genetic factors, disease states (e.g., uremia) or by the presence of other drugs (Silverman et al., 1956; Anton, 1960; Reidenberg, 1971). Under the assumption that an increase in f will result in a proportional increase in c, it must be postulated that the risk of toxicity is increased even when the total plasma concentration (c') remains unaltered, because it is the concentration of unbound molecules which determines the pharmacological effect (Dettli, 1961; Krueger-Thiemer, 1965). When discussed in the light of our knowledge of drug distribution, it can be shown that this assumption is usually not correct:

In the plasma space (V_p) and in the interstitial space (V_i), the total drug concentration $(c'_p = c_p/f_p$ and $c'_i = c_i/f_i$, respectively) consists of protein-bound molecules and of a certain fraction of freely dissolved molecules (f_p and f_i, respectively). Under equilibrium conditions we will have $c_i = c_p$. With anionic or cationic drugs, the concentration c_c of unbound drug in the intracellular water space (V_c) must be corrected for the pH difference between intracellular and extracellular water: Under equilibrium conditions, the concentrations of neutral molecules are identical in both spaces $(c_p \cdot \psi_i = c_c \cdot \psi_c)$. However, the pH-dependent fractions of neutral molecules (ψ_i and ψ_c, respectively) and consequently the total concentrations, are different, whereby

$$\psi_a = \frac{1}{1 + 10^{p\text{H}-p\text{K}}}$$

and (13)

$$\psi_b = \frac{1}{1 + 10^{p\text{K}-p\text{H}}}$$

for the neutral fractions of acidic (ψ_a) and basic (ψ_b) drugs, respectively. Furthermore, a specialized intracellular space (V_m) must be assumed where only a fraction (f_m) of the total concentration $(c'_m = c_m/f_m)$ is freely dissolved. The rest is bound to macromolecules (e.g., metabolizing enzymes, etc.). Finally, the neutral drug molecules will penetrate into the lipid space (V_j) according to the lipid–water partition coefficient (γ) of the drug. These facts may be described by the following equation (Dettli and Spring, 1973):

$$D = V' \cdot c' = \frac{c}{f_p}\left[V_p + V_i\left(\frac{f_p}{f_i}\right) + (V_c - V_m)\left(\frac{f_p \cdot \psi_i}{\psi_c}\right) + V_m\left(\frac{f_p \cdot \psi_i}{\psi_c \cdot f_m}\right) + V_j(f_p \cdot \psi_i \cdot \gamma)\right]$$

(14)

Based on Eq. (14) which describes the relationship between the formal distribution volume (V') as used in pharmacokinetics and the "real" fluid-compartments of the organism, the factors influencing the free drug concentration (c) can be discussed. As mentioned above, changes in the water or fat content of the organism, disturbances of the acid–base equilibrium in the extracellular space, or any factor influencing macromolecular drug binding will influence drug distribution. However, as indicated in Eq. (14), macromolecular binding is not restricted to the intravascular space. In fact, Levy has shown that the influence of intracellular macromolecules on the distribution of dicoumarols is much more pronounced than the influence of plasma albumin (Levy, 1970). Furthermore, when the fraction f_p of unbound drug increases in the plasma it should be realized that this will result in a redistribution of the drug in the organism. As a consequence, in most cases, the increase in c_p will be much less than the increase in f_p. Based on Eq. (14), we have shown elsewhere (Dettli and Spring, 1973) that under the following conditions, the increase of c_p as a consequence of drug displacement from serum albumin, can probably be neglected: When the drug is normally less than about 90% bound ($f_p > 0.1$), a high distribution volume, marked extravascular macromolecular binding, cationic dissociation, or pronounced lipophilic properties of the drug (see also Gillette, 1968). In contrast, serious side effects of highly albumin-bound substances such as bilirubin (Silverman *et al.*, 1956) and tolbutamide (Kristensen and Christensen, 1969) are reported in the literature.

It should be noted that any factor influencing the distribution volume will also influence drug elimination because the overall elimination rate constant of a drug (k_e) is not only proportional to its overall clearance ($\dot{V}'$) but also inversely proportional to its distribution volume (V'):

$$k_e = \frac{\dot{V}'}{V'} \qquad (15)$$

Kidney Disease

One of the sessions of the last International Congress on Pharmacology was devoted to the modifying effects of physiological variables and disease upon pharmacokinetics. In summarizing these discussions we may say that the influence of several disease states upon pharmacokinetics is now firmly established and should be recognized by the practicing physician (Okita and Acheson, 1972). However, in most instances, these modifying effects are relatively small and cannot be quantitatively analyzed in daily practice to such an extent that well-defined dosage modifications can

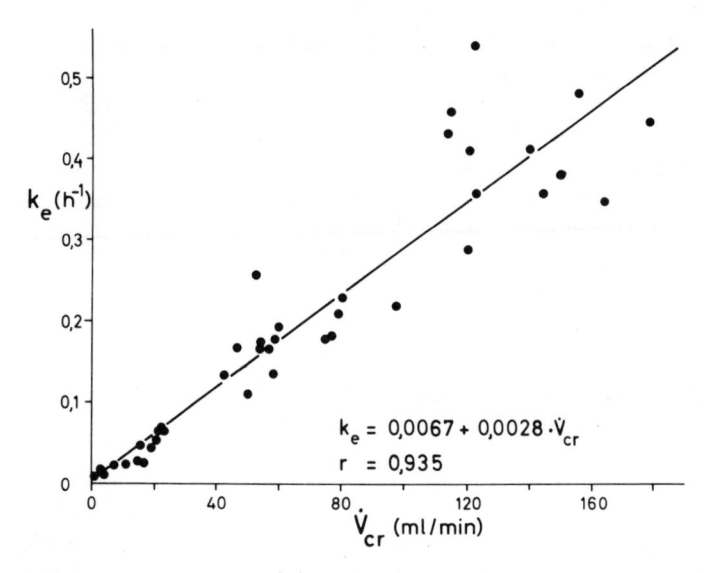

Fig. 1. Elimination rate constants (k_e) of gentamicin as a function of the endogenous creatinine clearance ($\dot{V}'_{cr}$) in 12 healthy volunteers and in 28 patients with kidney disease. The regression line corresponds to the following numerical solution of Eq. (16): $k_e = 0.0067 + 0.0022 \cdot \dot{V}'_{cr}$, indicating that the mean elimination rate of gentamicin in anuric patients is about 50 times smaller than that in patients with normal kidney function (Spring and Buergi, 1973).

be proposed. Renal failure is an exception to this rule. After the pioneer work of Kunin et al. (Kunin and Finland, 1959; Kunin, 1967; 1968), on the relationship between the biological half-life of drugs and the endogenous creatinine clearance of patients with renal disease, several authors (Jelliffe, 1967; Dettli, 1969; Dettli et al., 1970; 1971, 1971a; 1972; Spring et al., 1973; Wagner, 1971) demonstrated a linear relationship between the overall elimination rate constant (k_e) and the endogenous creatinine clearance ($\dot{V}'_{cr}$):

$$k_e = k_{nr} + \delta \cdot \dot{V}'_{cr} \qquad (16)$$

where k_{nr} is the mean extrarenal elimination rate constant in anuric patients and δ is a constant relating $\dot{V}'_{cr}$ to the renal elimination rate constant (k_r) of the drug. The assumptions underlying the theory have been discussed elsewhere. At present, Eq. (16) can be used for about forty drugs. Furthermore, simple nomographic methods have been devised which allow the estimation of the rate of drug elimination in the individual patient with kidney disease from his value of $\dot{V}'_{cr}$ (Dettli et al., 1971; Wagner, 1971). Based on the estimated individual elimination rate constant, a modified dosage regimen may be calculated according to pharmacokinetic principles. For the problems connected with dosage adjustment, the reader is referred to the literature (Dettli et al., 1971; Wagner, 1971). Such methods of individual dosage modification based on pharmacokinetic analysis are now used widely in clinical practice throughout the world. The practical importance of the problem is due to the fact that the elimination rate of drugs predominantly excreted by the kidneys may be reduced fiftyfold or more in patients with severe renal impairment (see Fig. 1). On the other hand, modern therapeutic techniques help keep such patients alive for years.

TRANSLATION OF PHARMACOKINETICS TO CLINICAL MEDICINE: A DIDACTIC PROBLEM

Mathematics may be defined as the science describing relationships among elements. Mathematical language must be used by the clinician when the relationships among clinical elements are too complex to be described intuitively and by means of colloquial language. The relationship between drug dosage on one hand and drug effects on the other is a beautiful illustration for such a complex situation. The introduction of pharmacokinetic techniques is the answer to the problem. However, even the most correct pharmacokinetic analysis is useless in clinical practice unless it can be adapted to the physician's educational background in mathematics. Therefore, the urgent need for promoting mathematical thinking in medical education should be emphasized. It is not necessary that we, as clinicians, solve our pharmacokinetic problems by ourselves. However, we should be able to discuss our problems in a quantitative, unequivocal language with the professional pharmacokineticist. In most cases relatively rough kinetic approximations will suffice for clinical purposes. Furthermore, a clear insight into the limitations of a pharmacokinetic model is often more important than mathematical sophistication (Wagner, 1971). The conventional types of analog and digital computers proved to be powerful tools in the kinetic analysis of highly complex pharmacokinetic problems. In our experience however a simulator, i.e., the simplest form of an analog computer, is much better suited for educational purposes (Dettli and Spring, 1970).

REFERENCES

Anton, A. H., 1960, *J. Pharmacol. Exp. Ther.* **129**: 282.
Ariens, E. J., 1964, *Molecular Pharmacology*, Vol. 1, Academic Press, New York.
Birchfield, R. I., Sieker, H. O., and Heyman, A., 1959, *J. Lab. Clin. Med.* **54**: 216.
Brodie, B. B., Burns, J. J., and Weiner, M., 1959, *Med. Exp.* **1**: 290.

Buenger, P., 1963, *Chemotherapia (Basel)* **6:** 237.
Buenger, P., Diller, W., Fuehr, J., and Krueger-Thiemer, G., 1961, *Arzneimittelforsch.* **11:** 247.
Dettli, L., 1966, in: *Pathogenesis and Treatment of Thromboembolic Diseases,* F. Koller, ed. Schattauer, Stuttgart.
Dettli, L., 1961, *Arzneimittel-Forsch.* **11:** 861.
Dettli, L., 1969, in: *Advances in the Biosciences, Vol. 5.* p. 39, (G. Raspé, ed., Pergamon Press, Oxford and Vieweg.
Dettli, L., 1971, in: *Klinische Pharmakologie und Pharmakotherapie,* H. P. Kuemmerle, E. R. Garrett, and K. H. Spitzy, eds., Urban and Schwarzenberg, Munich.
Dettli, L., 1972, *Abstract 119th Annual Meeting of the American Pharmaceutical Association* Houston.
Dettli, L., Spring, P., 1964, *Proc. 3rd Int. Congr. Chemother.* **1:** 641, Thieme, Stuttgart.
Dettli, L., Spring, P., 1966, *Regensburg. Jb. Aerztl. Fortbild.* **14:** 17.
Dettli, L., Spring, P., 1966a, *Helv. Med. Acta* **33:** 291.
Dettli, L., Spring, P., 1968, *Proc. 3rd. Int. Congr. Pharmacol.,* Vol. **7,** p. 5., Pergamon Press, Oxford.
Dettli, L., Spring, P., 1968a, *Farmaco (Ed. Sci.)* **23:** 795.
Dettli, L., Spring, P., 1970, *Proc. 4th Int. Congr. Pharmacol.* **1:** 227, Basel and Stuttgart.
Dettli, L., Spring, P., 1972, *Proc. 5th Int. Congr. Pharmacol.* **3,** Karger, Basel (in press).
Dettli, L., Spring, P., and Raeber, I., 1967, *Int. J. Clin. Pharmacol.* **1:** 130.
Dettli, L., Spring, P., and Habersang, R., 1970, *Postgrad. Med. J. Suppl.* **46:** 32.
Dettli, L., Spring, P., and Ryter, S., 1971, *Acta Pharmacol.* **29:** 3, 211.
Dettli, L., Spring, P., and Ryter, S., 1971, in: *Medikamentoese Therapie bei Nierenerkrankungen* (R. Kluthe, ed.), Thieme, Stuttgart.
Dominguez, R., 1950, *Medical Physics* Vol. 2, p. 476 (O. Glasser, ed.), The Year Book Publishers, Chicago.
Dost, F. H., 1953, *Der Blutspiegel,* Thieme, Leipzig.
Dost, F. H., 1968, *Grundlagen der Pharmakokinetik.* Thieme, Stuttgart.
Evans, P. D. A., 1962, *Méd. Hyg.* **20:** 905.
Freerksen, E., Dettli, L., Krueger-Thiemer, E., and Nelson, E., 1964, *Antibiotica et Chemotherapia,* Vol. 14, Karger, Basel.
Gillette, J. R., 1968, in: *Importance of Fundamental Principles in Drug Evaluation* (D. H. Tedeschi and Tedeschi R. E., eds.), Raven Press, New York.
Heizer, W. D., Smith, T. W., and Goldfinger, S. E., 1971, *New Engl. J. Med.* **285:** 257.
Jelliffe, R. W. A., 1967, *Math. Biosci.* **1:** 305.
Kalow, W., 1972, *Pharmacogenetics,* Saunders, Philadelphia.
Kleitman, N., 1963, *Sleep and Wakefulness,* University of Chicago Press, Chicago.
Kostenbauder, H. B., Portnoff, J. B., and Swintosky, J. V., 1962, *J. Pharm. Sci.* **51:** 1084.
Krauer, B., 1970, *Z. Kinderheilk.* **108:** 231.
Krauer, B., 1972. Unpublished observations.
Krauer B., and Dettli, L., 1969, *Chemotherapy* **14:** 1.
Krauer, B., Spring, P., and Dettli, L., 1968, *Pharmacol. Clin.* **1:** 47.
Kristensen, M., and Christensen, L. K., 1968, *Acta Diabetol. Lat.* **6:** 116.
Krueger-Thiemer, E., 1960, *J. Am. Pharm. Assoc. (Sci. ed.)* **49:** 311.
Krueger-Thiemer, E., 1961, in: *Handbuch der Haut- und Geschlechtskrankheiten,* Supplement, Vol 1, p. 962 (J. Kimmig, ed.), Springer, Berlin.
Krueger-Thiemer, E., 1962, *Klin. Wschr.* **40:** 153.
Krueger-Thiemer, E., Wempe, E., and Toepfer, M., 1965, *Arzneimittelforsch.* **15:** 1309.
Krueger-Thiemer, E., Buenger, P., Dettli, L., Spring, P., and, Wempe, E., 1966, *Chemotherapia* **10:** 325.

Krueger-Thiemer, E., Berlin, H., Brante, P., Buenger, P., Dettli, L., Spring, P., and Wempe, Ellen, 1969, *Chemotherapy* **14**: 273.
Kunin, C. M., 1967, *Ann. Internal. Med.* **67**: 151.
Kunin, C. M., 1968, *Ann. Internal Med.* **69**: 397.
Kunin, C. M., and Finland, M., 1959, *Arch. Internal Med.* **104**: 204.
Levy, G., 1964, *J. Pharm. Sci.* **53**: 342.
Levy, G., 1966, *Clin. Pharmacol. Therap.* **7**: 362.
Levy, G., 1968, in: *Importance of Fundamental Principles in Drug Evaluation* (D. H. Tedeschi and R. E. Tedeschi, eds.), Raven Press, New York.
Levy, G., 1971, *Ann. N. Y. Acad. Sci.* **179**: 32.
Levy, G., 1969, *Proc. 4th Int. Congr. Pharmacol.*, Vol. 4, p. 150, Schwabe, Basel.
Levy, G., and Nelson, E., 1965, *J. Pharm. Sci.*, **54**: 812.
Levy, G., Tsuchiya, I., and Amsel, L. P., 1972, *Clin. Pharmacol. Therap.* **13**: 681.
Milne, M. D., Scribner, B. H., and Crawford, M. A., 1958, *Am. J. Med.* **24**: 709.
Nelson, E., 1961, *J. Pharm. Sci.* **50**: 181.
Okita, G. T., and Acheson, G. H., eds. 1973, *Proc. 5th Int. Congr. Pharmacology*, Vol. 3, p. 165 Karger, Basel.
Otaya H., 1971, *Personal communication*.
Reidenberg, M. M., 1971, *Renal Function and Drug Action*, Saunders, Philadelphia.
Rind, H., and Gladtke, E., 1964, *Mschr. Kinderheilk.* **112**: 239.
Rowland, M., Becket, A. H., and Turner, P., 1965, *Lancet* **I**: 303.
Scholtan, W., 1961, *Arzneimittelforsch.* **11**: 707.
Scholtan, W., 1962, *Makromol. Chem.* **54**: 24.
Silverman, W. A., Andersen, D. H., Blanc, W. A., and Crozier, D. M., 1956, *Pediatrics* **18**: 614.
Spring, P., 1966, *Arzneimittelforsch.* **16**: 346.
Spring, P., Dettli, L., and Raeber, I., 1967, *Proc. 5th Int. Congr. Chemother.* Vol. 4, p. 161.
Spring, R., Buergi, M., Dettli, L., and Reber, H., 1973, *Praxis* (in press).
Teorell, T., 1937, *Arch. Int. Pharmacodyn.* **57**: 205.
Wagner, J. G., 1971, *"Biopharmaceutics and Relevant Pharmacokinetics,"* Hamilton Press, Hamilton.
World Health Organization Technical Report, Ser. 341, 1967, World Health Organization.

DISCUSSION SUMMARY

Teorell questioned Dettli with respect to the bedside application of pharmacokinetics and as to how the average hospital patient may benefit from its use. Dettli responded that the most successful applications have been in the administration of drugs to patients with kidney disease. This is due to the fact that, for many drugs, a linear relationship exists between the endogenous creatinine clearance and the elimination constant for the drug. He cited a number of drugs, such as digoxin, gentamycin, and kanamycin, where nomographs have been developed which relate the drug dosage to the creatinine clearance.

Wagner asked if it might not be appropriate for the National Institutes of Health to provide funds for the establishment of Biopharmaceutic-Pharmacokinetic laboratories in a number of hospitals. Thus it would be possible to obtain individual measurements of half-life, clearance, and volume of distribution (as suggested by Axelrod in an earlier discussion) and to demonstrate the benefit of these measurements in the clinical management of the patient. Sjoqvist told the audience that all regional hospitals in Sweden now have monitoring services for determining the plasma levels of diphenylhydantoin. It is felt that these assays are necessary for appropriate neurological treatment due to the overlapping range of effective and

Translation of Pharmacokinetics to Clinical Medicine

toxic doses for this drug as well as the good correlation found between blood levels attained and efficacy of the drug. However, he pointed out that the limitation of the application of pharmacokinetics at the bedside may often be related to changes in the pattern of patient compliance.

Melmon reminded the conference that the application of almost any basic science information to the actual practice of medicine lags far behind the development of the basic science. For example, Dettli has shown that there may be a relationship between the basic science aspects of pharmacokinetics and the practical decision processes in medicine. However, so far, applications have only been utilized with respect to the simplest model and only in the simplest situation where the major drug is given in a well defined and reasonably stable disease state, specifically, where the major factor in body clearance is glomerular filtration. Melmon pointed out that simple one-compartment pharmacokinetic analysis has been useful in determining the proper dosing of digoxin, and that the utility of this model may be greatly improved when the clinician is provided blood levels after the first, second, or third dose. These blood levels provide information which may be utilized in a feedback loop and may be useful in correcting the one-compartment model so that the error rate of the model itself decreases without the necessity of introducing a more complicated and cumbersome model capable of describing the drug in all situations. That is, there is an individualization of the pharmacokinetic model to the particular patient being treated with digoxin.

Azarnoff stated that drug blood levels for certain drugs are being determined in his hospital and pointed out three specific areas of concern. First, measuring blood levels usually requires the development of new methodology for analysis and standardization. These new methods serve as an internal control since many of the routine drug analyses performed by the clinical laboratories will not yield measurements of sufficient accuracy so that the reported drug levels may be used in a predictive sense in a pharmacokinetic model. Second, it is extremely important to know when the blood sample is obtained. Drug blood levels are not like serum potassium or other clinical values which remain fairly constant throughout the day, and it is often difficult to get the house staff to record the time that the sample is obtained. Obviously, if a drug level is going to be used in a predictive sense, it is important to know when the drug level is obtained as compared to when the drug is administered. Third, it is important for the clinician using a pharmacokinetic model and the investigator developing that model to realize that the dosage regimens suggested must realistically conform to the practices prevalent in the hospital. For example, in most hospitals, if a physician orders a drug three times a day, the drug will most likely be administered at 9:00 a.m., 5:00 p.m., and 9:00 p.m., not every eight hours, even though that is what the physician ordered. Similarly, many patients may be taking up to 10 or more drugs a day. If the dosage schedule for each is different, the actual dosing of the drug by the patient, with the assistance of the hospital staff, would be most impractical.

Effect of Route of Administration on Drug Disposition[*]

S. Riegelman and M. Rowland

Department of Pharmacy
University of California
San Francisco, California

An increasing body of information tends to support the hypothesis that drug effect, therapeutic or toxic, is more closely correlated with plasma concentration than dose (Levy, 1968). Absorption is one important determinant of drug plasma levels. Distribution and elimination are others. Most drugs are administered as drug products, not drug entities. The biologic performance of a drug product can be affected by its bioavailability (defined as a measure of the rate and extent to which a drug reaches a sampling site (usually a peripheral vein) or its site of action). Biophasic availability is generally reserved for situations where pharmacologic data are used to assess biologic performance (Smolen, 1971). This paper discusses the various factors that can influence the bioavailability of drug products. Major emphasis is placed on preparations intended for oral administration.

Most oral dosage forms are solids. To be absorbed, the drug must first dissolve. Dissolution is usually complete for most drug substances, but may cause variation in its rate of release from the product. Occasionally dissolution, especially of sparingly soluble drugs, is sufficiently protracted that absorption is incomplete with a commensurate appearance of intact drug in feces. Figure 1 illustrates possible factors that can influence bioavailability. During the manufacture of solid dosage forms (e.g., cap-

[*] The work reported here was supported in part by Grant NIGMS 16496-05.

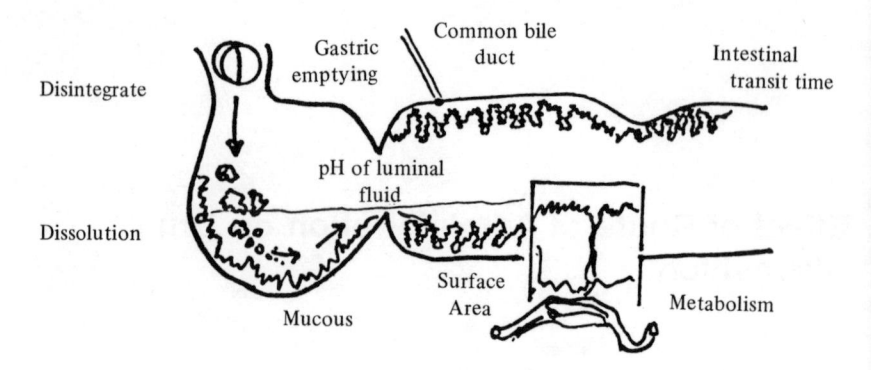

Fig. 1. Schematic of the stomach and intestines indicating some of the physiological factors that can influence the rate and extent of bioavailability. A drug product must disintegrate and dissolve prior to drug absorption. The manufacturing process, physiochemical properties of the drug, its chemical stability, gastrointestinal environment and mobility can all influence the bioavailability profile.

sules and tablets), many factors can cause marked changes in the rate of disintegration and dispersion of the granules into individual particles of drug substance by affecting the physical characteristics. These changes thereby alter the rate at which the surface becomes available for dissolution. Also, the direct contact of the solid with either mucous or food may reduce both the rate of water transfer and the diffusion of drug molecules away from the solid surface. The gastrointestinal fluids, including bile, can interact with the drug molecules, in some cases solubilizing the drug and in others causing precipitation on the surface of a slowly dissolving complex (Riegelman, 1969). Drug absorption often appears to be somewhat limited to certain segments of the upper intestinal tract. Accordingly, the rate of dissolution and absorption may be modified by G.I. transit time and the intensity of peristalsis.

Even when completely dissolved, many factors can influence the bioavailability of a drug product. Enzymes within the gastrointestinal fluids, microflora and mucosa, liver and lung encountered by the orally administered drug are all capable of drug metabolism to a greater or lesser extent. Loss at any site reduces the availability of the drug. Table I lists some of the dosage form and physiologic factors which can modify bioavailability. Sometimes these physiologic factors may be the overriding consideration affecting drug availability. Acetylsalicylic acid (Rowland et al., 1972), salicylamide (Barr and Riegelman, 1969), lidocaine (Boyes, 1970), and propranolol (Dollery et al., 1970) all pass rapidly across the gastrointestinal mucosa but systemically are still poorly available. The major

TABLE I
Physiological and Dosage Form Factors that Modify Bioavailability

Physiological factors

Properties of luminal fluids
   Hydrogen ion concentration
   Mucous interaction
   Complexing components
   Surface activity
   Bile interaction

Factors affecting G.I. transit
   Gastric emptying
   Food effects
   Bed rest
   Motility
   Enterohepatic cycling

Factors at site of absorption
   Surface area
   Permeability of barrier
   Specialized transport
   Local blood flow
   Intestinal metabolism

Metabolic aspects
   Hepatic metabolism
     Enzyme levels
     Hepatic portal blood flow
     Drug binding proteins
   Extrahepatic metabolism
     Saturation phenomena
   Gut wall metabolism
   Kidney metabolism

Distribution effects
   Plasma protein levels
   Obesity

Disease states
   Achlorhydria
   Thyrotoxicosis
   Biliary atresia
   Congestive heart failure

Pharmacological effects of drugs
   Modification of blood flow
   Parasympatholytic activity

Dosage form factors

Physical properties of drug
   Water solubility
   Lipid solubility
   Partition coefficient
   pK_a

Properties of dosage form
   Disintegration time
   Dissolution rate
     Surface area of particles
     Crystal size
     Polymorphic form
     Solvates
     Salt form
     Excipients

Manufacturing variables
   Granulating process
   Lubricant concentration
   Compression pressure
   Tablet coatings

contributory factors are either gut wall metabolism and/or high hepatic extraction, as all absorbed drug must pass through the liver before reaching the general circulation. Recently Dollery (1970) attributed the ratio of the intravenous to oral chromotropic potency of isoproteronol in man of 1000/1 to the formation of an inactive ethereal sulfate during the transfer across the gut wall and passage through the liver. Diczfalusy and Levitz (1970) and Scheidl (1968) also emphasized the distinction between oral absorption and physiologic availability of some steroids which are extensively metabolized within the gut wall and liver.

Saturable drug metabolizing enzymes existing within the intestinal secretions, flora (Sheline, 1968), and epithelium (Barr and Riegelman, 1970) can influence the kinetics of the presentation of the drug to the liver. Therefore, dose-dependent absorption kinetics, as measured from the hepatic portal or peripheral vein can be anticipated. In the absence of gut or gut wall metabolism, loss from the gastrointestinal tract is matched by appearance of drug in the portal circulation. When a metabolic process occurs and the intestinal drug concentration is well below the capacity of the enzyme system, gut metabolism is maximal and the rate of presentation of drug to the liver is less than the disappearance from the intestinal lumen. At concentrations below the capacity of the enzyme system, gut metabolism is first order and disappearance from the luminal contents (sum of gut metabolism and absorption) is maximal. Absorption, as viewed from a peripheral vein, may appear first order but the fraction appearing systemically intact is small relative to the total dose administered. At higher concentrations in the intestinal fluids, enzyme saturation may occur for part of the absorption process and the fraction of the dose undergoing gut metabolism will be reduced while the kinetics of appearance of drug at the liver will be more complex. At still higher concentrations, saturation of the gut enzymes occurs during the majority of the absorption process and the percent of loss by metabolism during the absorption process will be the smallest. If it is negligible, appearance of drug in the portal vein will again approximate the loss of drug from the luminal contents. Even this fairly complex picture will be further complicated by the continually changing environment along the entire gastrointestinal tract.

L-Dopa is an example of a compound showing dosage form modified and physiological modified bioavailability arising from both nonenzymatic and enzymatic metabolism in the gastrointestinal lumen as well as metabolism to the ethereal sulfate and other inactive forms upon passage through the gastrointestinal mucosa. The result is a highly unpredictable bioavailability, making it difficult to define a dosage of this drug and to achieve a desired response. Nonspecific esterases exist along the entire gastrointestinal tract (at varying concentrations) and these enzymes cause variable hydrolysis of orally administered aspirin and possibly other esters (Rowland, 1972). Para-aminobenzoic acid and isoniazid are partly acetylated during passage through the gastrointestinal mucosa. Intestinal glucuronidation and sulfate formation also occurs. Intestinal amide hydrolysis of p-aminohippuric acid has been suggested recently (Boxenbaum and Riegelman, 1973).

The rate of release of the drug substance from the dosage form at the absorption site will influence the degree and rate of bioavailability of most drugs, and has a large effect on drugs undergoing gut and/or hepatic metabolism. Indeed, decreasing the release rate of the dose of salicylamide, which is glucuronidated and sulfated in the intestinal mucosa (Barr, 1969) diminishes its availability in man (Fig. 2). Increasing doses of the drug

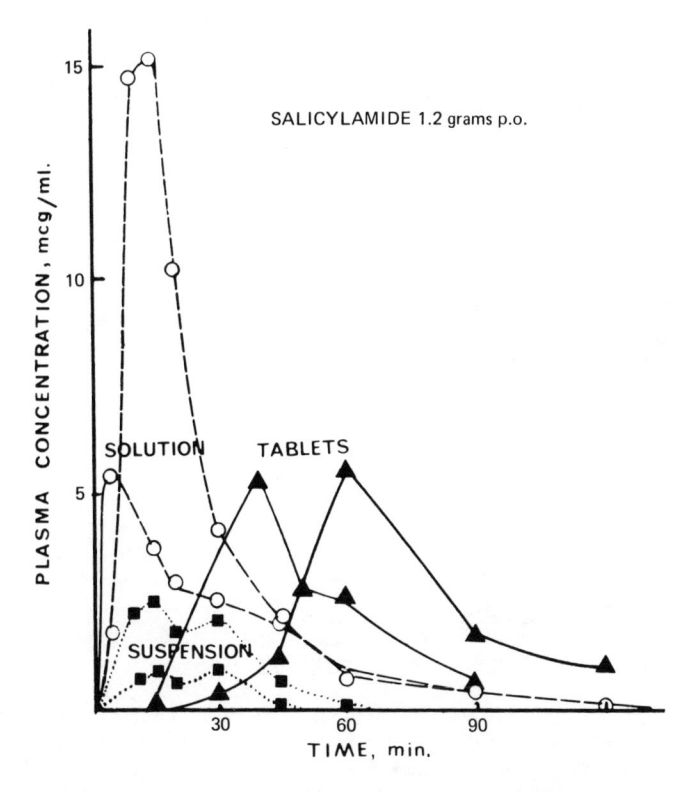

Fig. 2. Difference in systemic availability following a 1.2 g orally administered dose of salicylamide in solution, a commercial tablet suspension and a commercial tablet. Interestingly, the suspension, which is usually thought to be a good dosage form, has poorer availability than the tablet.

administered in solution to man resulted in a disproportionate increase in the area under the blood curve (Fig. 3). Yet, when the drug was administered orally and compared with the same intravenous dose the data shown in Fig. 4 resulted, indicating that drug was being absorbed but metabolized during the absorption process. To distinguish between intestinal and hepatic metabolism, a drug must be introduced in a manner which bypasses the gastrointestinal tract, either by direct infusion into the hepatic portal vein or perhaps by intraperitoneal administration (Lucas, 1971). At this moment, however, intraperitoneal administration must be viewed with caution. Most of the data has been obtained from rats and might not be

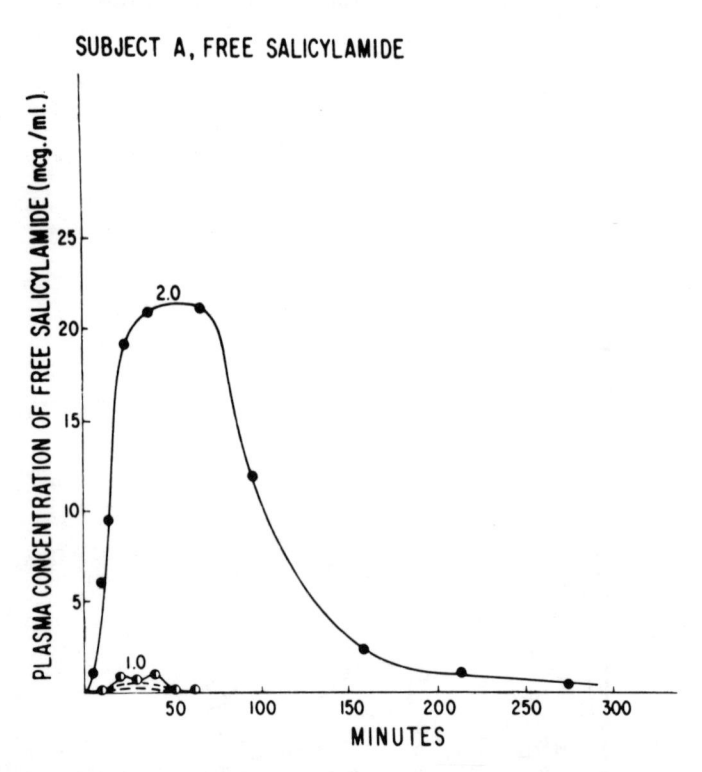

Fig. 3. Comparison of the plasma concentrations of the intact salicylamide when given as a 1-g and as a 2-g dose in solution to the same subject. Dotted lines show the plasma concentrations resulting from a 0.5-g dose and a 0.3-g dose. Note the enormous increase in area upon going from 1 to 2 g. This is due in part to an increase in availability and in part to saturation of the hepatic enzymes during the elimination of the systematically available drug following the 2-g dose.

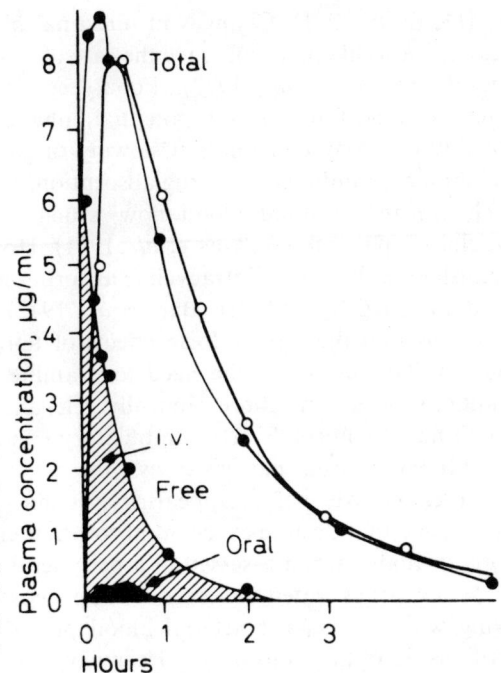

Fig. 4. Plasma concentrations of intact salicylamide (shaded area) and total drug (by acid hydrolysis) following 300 mg given *i.v.* or orally as a solution. Although great differences in the concentrations of intact drug are observed, there are no differences in the plasma concentrations of the total drug.

extrapolated to other animals. Further, the rates of drug presentation to the liver following intraperitoneal administration may be different than when drugs are given orally.

Drugs are primarily removed from the gastrointestinal site by blood flow. Lymphatic uptake is minor, as lymph flows 500 to 700 times more slowly than blood. Changes in intestinal blood flow may alter the rate of absorption in several ways. A reduced flow may diminish the rate of removal of the drug absorbed by passive diffusion or by reducing the supply of oxygen below a certain level, impairing the active transport system. The absorption of other, more polar molecules, is limited not by perfusion, but more by permeability (diffusion) through the intestinal membrane and hence will be flow independent. For example, Barr and Riegelman (1970) found that salicylamide, a lipid soluble drug, showed perfusion-limited absorption while its polar glucuronide, formed within the epithelial cells, did not. Winne and coworkers (1971) have shown blood flow dependency of tritiated water and the flow independency of absorption of the polar ribitol. Other workers have shown perfusion-limited absorption for aniline antipyrine, salicylic acid (Crouthamel *et al.*, 1970), and sulfaethylthiadiazole (Doluisio, 1971). Changes in intestinal blood flow, brought about by stress, are also likely to influence the rate of absorption of perfusion-limited drugs (Rowland *et al.*, 1973). Food, especially protein (Brandt, 1955), increases blood flow but any potential enhancement of drug absorption is probably offset by concomitant slowing of gastric emptying. Bed rest can have a marked influence on drug absorption. Some of this, of course, is due to change in intestinal blood flow which is greater in supine than in ambulatory patients (Wilkins *et al.*, 1951). However, intestinal mobility is diminished by bed rest. Tetracycline absorption from varying dosage forms was diminished by bed rest (Barr *et al.*, 1972). Indeed, it was under these conditions that the dosage form effects of tetracycline seemed to be most manifest. This points to the need to examine the availability of drugs in conditions simulating more clinically relevant circumstances, rather than only in healthy normals in an ambulatory condition.

Whatever drug passes across the gastrointestinal tract must still encounter the liver before appearing systemically. Hepatic removal can be so extensive that despite excellent absorption characteristics, a drug can be poorly available when assessed in a peripheral drug vessel.

When drugs enter the liver via the hepatic portal vein, intermittent mixing with the hepatic arterial blood probably takes place before drug partitions into the sinosoids (Greenway and Stark, 1971). The hepatic extraction ratio is a fraction of the drug entering the liver which is cleared by elimination processes. Only the remainder, F_L, or one minus the extraction ratio, is available to the circulation. If the extraction ratio is expressed in terms of the hepatic clearance and blood flow to the liver, the value of F_L is the fraction available through the liver, as given by

$$F_L = 1 - \frac{\text{Hepatic clearance}}{\text{Hepatic flow}} \qquad (1)$$

One needs to know in any animal or subject the hepatic clearance of the drug and hepatic flow. The hepatic clearance can be estimated from intravenous data. Total clearance is the sum of metabolic and renal clearance and, provided it is constant, is determined by dividing the intravenous dose by the total area under the blood concentration time curve. Knowing the fraction of available drug excreted unchanged, one can readily assess this extrarenal clearance. Hepatic clearance is the difference between total and renal clearance, if one assumes this extrarenal clearance is hepatically eliminated. For drugs totally available prior to encountering the liver, Eq. (1) offers a simple means of estimating the bioavailability of an oral dose. For example, the average hepatic extraction ratio of a local anesthetic, lidocaine, has been calculated from clearance data (Rowland,

1972) and experimentally determined to be approximately 0.7 (Stenson, 1971) in man. Theory also predicts that the oral availability of lidocaine, being readily cleared by the liver, should be sensitive to minor changes in the hepatic extraction ratio. Such minor differences between subjects probably explains the large intersubject variation of the oral availability of lidocaine (Boyes *et al.*, 1971; Prescott and Nimmo, 1971), propranolol (Shand *et al.*, 1972), and perhaps other hepatically cleared drugs (Rowland, 1973).

A high clearance should not be equated only with a short half-life. Clearance is the measure of the functional ability of a substance to be removed by the eliminating organs. The half-life, determined from the terminal log linear portion of an intravenous blood curve $(t_{1/2})$ depends upon clearance and volume of distribution (Riegelman *et al.*, 1968).

$$\text{Total body clearance} = \frac{0.693}{t_{1/2}}(V_d)_{\text{area}} \qquad (2)$$

In a multicompartmental body model, clearance is also given by the product $k_{10} V_1$, where k_{10} is the rate constant associated with the loss of drug from the central compartment of volume V_1 (Riegelman *et al.*, 1968). For a given clearance, which normally cannot exceed organ blood flow, $t_{1/2}$ is usually thought to be inversely related to the volume of distribution. Thus, the total body clearance of lidocaine (Boyes *et al.*, 1971) is slightly greater than aspirin (Rowland and Riegelman, 1968), even though the half-life of

TABLE II

Drugs in Which Luminal and/or Mucosal Metabolism is Suspected

Ester hydrolysis	*Conjugation*
Acetylsalicylic acid	Estrogens
Organic nitrates	Salicylamide
Propoxyphene	L-Dopa
Meperidine	α-Methyldopa
Methadone	
Pentazocine	
Dexamethasone phosphate	
N-Acetylation	*Reduction*
p-Amino benzoic acid	Hydrocortisone
Certain sulfonamides	Cortisone
Amide hydrolysis	Aldosterone
	Progesterone
p-Amino hippuric acid	Testosterone
Hippuric acid	

TABLE III
Drugs in Which First Pass Hepatic Metabolism Is Suspected[a]

Propranolol	Tryptophan
Lidocaine	Dopamine
Alprenolol	Serotonin
Desmethylimipramine	Pheniprazine
Nortriptyline	
Oxyphenbutazone	
Reserpine	

[a] All drugs in Table II suspected of G.I. metabolism

the former ($t_{1/2} = 100$ min) is much longer than the latter ($t_{1/2} = 13$ min). This is explained by lidocaine having a much larger volume of distribution (1.4 L/kg) than aspirin (0.18 L/kg). In fact, those amines including propoxyphene, nortriptyline, propranolol, and pentazocine, which are highly cleared by the liver, have, commensurate with a large volume of distribution, relatively long half-lives. The apparent volume of distribution of some amines can be 500–1000 L in man. These large apparent volumes of distribution are more than enough to compensate for the small elimination rate constant yielding a large overall total body clearance. This has been reported by Sjoqvist *et al.* (1971) on the drug nortriptyline. It is likely that similar events will take place with other polycyclic amines such as the phenothiazines. Table III is a compilation of some of the compounds which appear to show the first pass effect. The list is by no means complete. The dose and the rate at which these drugs become available for absorption through the intestinal mucosa and the liver during the first pass will markedly affect the disposition of the compound and probably control its therapeutic activity within the body as a whole.

To predict oral availability from intravenous data using Eq. (1) assumes clearance is constant. Then, availability should be independent of dose or rate of administration. For many drugs, insufficient data exist to know whether that condition holds over the therapeutic dose range or doses given to animals. At least for salicylamide (Barr, 1969) and propranolol (Shand *et al.*, 1970), it does not. In each case availability appears to increase with dose. One possible explanation is the existence of saturation processes within the gut wall or liver. Figure 5 is a plot of the area *vs.* dose for the same subject as shown in Fig. 3. As the oral dose is increased beyond 1.0 g, the area increases enormously. Just by doubling the dose to 2 g, the area increases severalfold. The dose at which this sudden break occurs was referred to by Barr and Riegelman as the "breakthrough" dose and corresponds to about 1.5 g dose of salicylamide. Probably in this region of

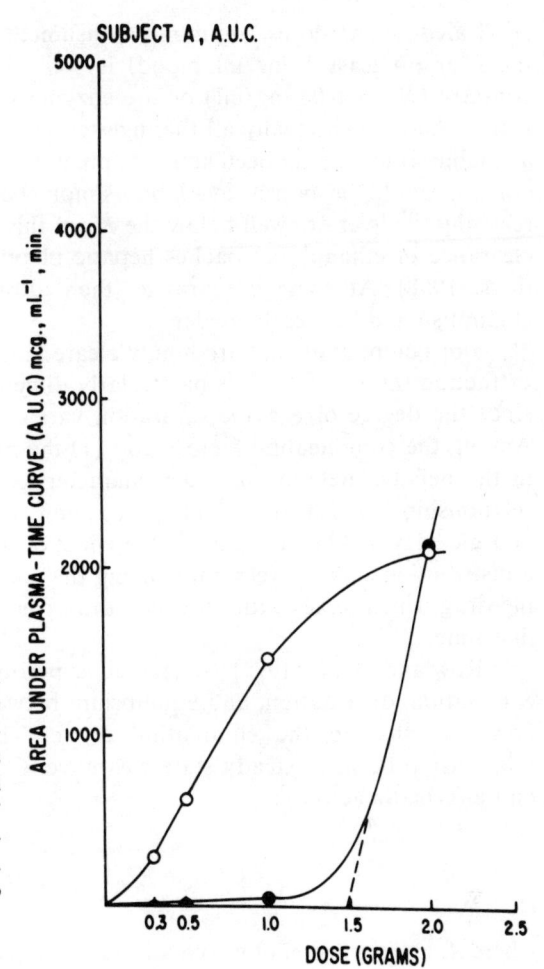

Fig. 5. Areas under the plasma concentration time curve (AUC) for intact salicylamide and glucuronide in the same subject as shown in Fig. 3. The extrapolated line shows the "breakthrough" dose necessary to saturate the metabolic processes following an $i.v.$ dose. With increase of the dose to 2 g, the areas increase severalfold.

dose, the glucuronidases and sulfatases within the gastrointestinal mucosa have become saturated and a concentration entering the liver may be sufficient to approach V_m of the hepatic enzymes. This is possible since the drug is in solution and is apparently rapidly available to the liver. In contrast, solid dosage forms of salicylamide yield a slower rate of hepatic availability and probably do not result in hepatic portal concentrations sufficient to involve Michaelis–Menten kinetics. For propranolol, gut wall metabolism appears absent. The availability was complete for propranolol in a subject with portalcaval anastomosis (Shand and Rango, 1972).

Saturation of hepatic enzymes by therapeutic dose of some drugs or dosage regimens is well established (Levy, 1968). A classical example is ethyl alcohol. At doses commonly consumed, the concentration reaching the liver (at least 1 mg/ml blood) is well above the Michaelis–Menten constant ($K_m = 0.08$ mg/ml) of the enzyme system (Lundquist and Wolthers, 1958), and virtually all the ingested ethanol is probably systemically available. Had ethanol been active at much lower doses, it is likely that oral ethanol would be poorly available, simply because when concentrations reaching the liver are well below the K_m of this enzyme system, the hepatic clearance of ethanol approaches hepatic blood flow (Lundquist and Wolthers, 1958). At some dose range, then, dose-dependent availability of ethanol should be clearly evident.

For compounds that are highly cleared at low concentrations (hepatic extraction ratio > 0.5), it is particularly difficult to predict bioavailability, since the degree of enzyme saturation varies with the rate of absorption. Among the complicating factors are: (1) the number of enzymes involved in the hepatic metabolism, each characterized by a K_m and V_{max}; (2) the relationship between the hepatic extraction ratio, organ blood flow (Q_B), and the enzyme kinetics; and (3) the effect of the rest of the body acting as a distribution sink, thereby influencing the concentration of the recirculating drug which mixes with absorbed drug passing through the liver for the first time.

Rowland et al. (1972) considered a perfusion model with first-order elimination, distribution, and equilibrium between drug in emergent blood flow and that in the eliminating organ. They derived the following relationship between steady state clearance, CL_{SS}, organ blood flow (Q_B), and enzymatic activity:

$$CL_{SS} = Q_B\left(\frac{A}{Q_B + A}\right) \quad (3)$$

where A, an expression of enzymatic activity, may be regarded as the steady state clearance of the drug if there were no flow limitation, i.e., $Q_B \gg A$. The term in parentheses is the extraction ratio of the drug by the organ. This expression holds even when the drug exhibits dose-dependent elimination kinetics, except that A and hence clearance will change with differing incoming concentrations of drug. In contrast, both terms, A and clearance, are independent of concentration when elimination is a first-order process. Of moment, if under conditions of nonsaturation, the extraction ratio is 0.9 ($A = 9Q_B$), a diminution in the enzymatic activity by one-half, e.g., 50% saturation ($A = 4.5Q_B$), will only reduce the extraction ratio to 0.82. This small change in the extraction ratio (and hence clearance) may go unnoticed when drug is given intravenously. However, availability, given by one minus the extraction ratio, would increase from 10% to 18%, a significant and noticeable increase. Thus, the oral availability of a drug, which apparently displays drug independent intravenous kinetics, might be sensitive to dose and rapidity of absorption (Fig. 6). Interestingly, propranolol, which has a large volume of distribution, displays many of these facets (Shand and Rangno, 1972).

Unless there is the development of specific hepato-portal bypasses, all absorbed drug must pass through the liver before entering the general circulation. The hepato-portal concentration of drug resulting directly from

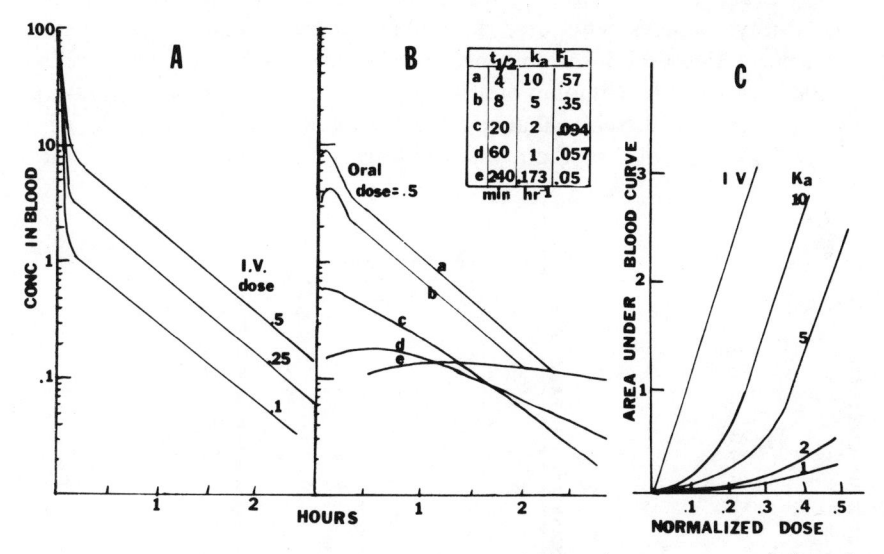

Fig. 6. Influence of route of administration, dose and absorption rate constant (k_A) on the availability and disposition kinetics of a drug with a volume of distribution of 42 L. The data were generated using the CSMP digitial computer program (IBM) assuming a perfusion model with blood flow (volume 5 L, output 6 L/min) to a noneliminating tissue (volume 34 L, flow 4.5 L/min) and the liver (volume 3 L, flow 1.5 L/min) containing a single saturable metabolic enzyme system. The partition of drug between tissue and emergent venous blood was set at unity, corresponding to a volume of distribution of 42 L. The hepatic extraction ratio at concentrations well below the K_m of the enzyme system was fixed at 0.95. Administered dose was normalized to a fraction of the maximum velocity (V_{max}) of the enzyme system. Figure 6A indicates that over a fivefold intravenous dose range (0.1–0.5 units), the disposition kinetics appear dose-independent, even though calculation showed that appreciable enzyme saturation had occurred during the distribution and part of the elimination phase. In contrast, Fig. 6B indicates that decreasing the absorption half-life of an oral dose (0.5 units) not only decreases the time for and increases the peak blood concentration but also dramatically increases the availability (f_L). Also, because area under the intravenous blood concentration time curve is proportional to dose, oral availability is given by the ratio of the oral dose to intravenous doses which gives the same area. Thus, as seen in Fig. 6C, the intravenous dose corresponding to the same area obtained following an oral dose of 0.4 units, $K_A = 5$ hr^{-1} is 0.1 dose units, i.e., oral availability is 0.25.

absorbed drug is a function of the absorption rate (dose, absorption half-life, and time) and blood flow. Any systemically available drug thus distributes to the tissues and only a portion recirculates to the liver. The recirculating drug may be regarded as a competitive inhibitor to the drug passing for the first time through the liver. For drugs with volumes of distribution exceeding 100 L, the contribution of systemically available drug to the hepatic concentration can safely be ignored. The smaller the volume of distribution, the more significant the contribution of the recirculating drug to the hepatic concentration and the more dramatically availability changes with oral dose (Fig. 7). It is conceivable that at sufficiently high oral doses, this inhibitory effect may be so pronounced as to decrease the actual amount of absorbed drug removed in the first passage through the liver, thereby enhancing the availability still further. Also, since a significant fraction of the available drug is now undergoing nonlinear

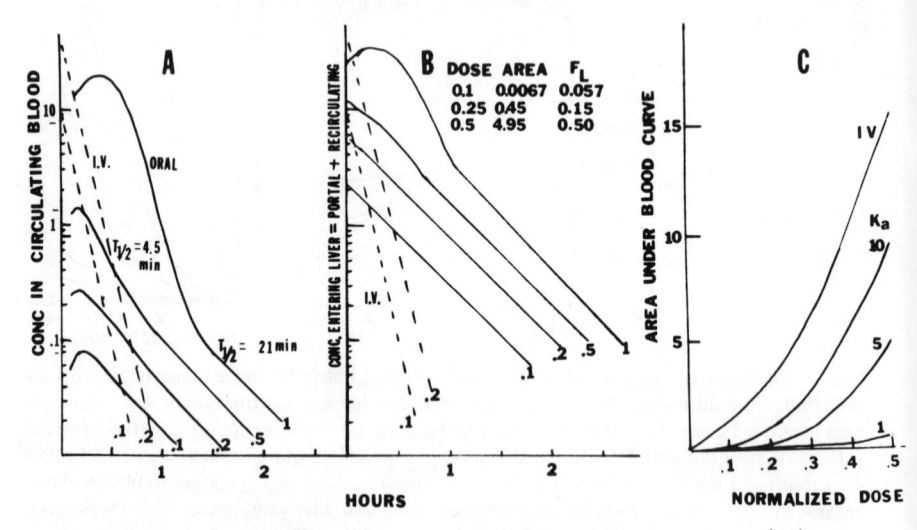

Fig. 7. Influence of route of administration, dose and absorption rate constant (K_A) on the availability and disposition kinetics of a drug with a volume of distribution of 8.7 L. The model is the same as that discussed in the legend for Fig. 6 except that the partition of drug between tissue and emergent venous blood was set at 0.1. In Fig. 7A, below 0.2 dose units the intravenous disposition kinetics appear dose-independent (half-life 4.5 min) but above this dose frank dose dependency is noted, as seen from the area–dose relationships (Fig. 7C). As the oral dose increases, while the absorption rate constant is maintained at 2.0 hr^{-1} ($t_{1/2}$ = 21 min), availability increases (Fig. 7B) and the contribution of recirculating drug to the portal concentration becomes more evident. Also, area increases even more dramatically than the availability. Thus, while doubling the oral dose from 0.25 to 0.5 units increases the availability threefold (0.146 to 0.50), area increases almost elevenfold (0.45 to 4.95). Since absorption is the rate limiting step, the terminal part of the blood concentration time curve declines with a half-life of 21 min, not 4.5 min.

elimination, the area increases even more rapidly than availability (Fig. 7C). The dose-dependent intravenous elimination kinetics make it extremely difficult to assess oral availability from blood concentration–time curves. Similar events may partially explain the enormous increase in the area of salicylamide with increasing oral dose (Fig. 5). The area under the metabolite blood curve seen after giving fully available drugs should be independent of the route of drug administration. For drugs highly cleared by the liver, the low oral availability should be associated with a rapid rise in metabolite levels. Support for this idea can be seen with the weak analgesic, propoxyphene. Even though the elimination half-life is approximately 7 hr, high and maximal plasma concentrations of the more stable metabolite norpropoxyphene (half-life approximately 18 hr, McMahon *et al.*, 1971) are seen within a few hours of propoxyphene ingestion (Wagner *et al.*, 1971). Also, doses as large as 500 mg of lidocaine are sometimes needed to produce therapeutic concentrations, usually achieved with a 100 mg *i.v.* bolus (Boyes *et al.*, 1971). The dizziness reported with the large oral dose of lidocaine is probably caused by the rapid appearance of high concentrations of metabolites produced by the first pass effect. With salicylamide (Barr and Riegelman, 1971) and isoproteronol (Dollery *et al.*, 1971), the metabolites are inactive, although appearing in high concentration following oral doses.

The design of therapeutic agents is fraught with many difficulties. For those intended for oral administration, the bioavailability of the drug product is an additional concern. When a drug product exhibits poor bioavailability in animal testing or in man, it is important to distinguish between dosage form and physiologically modified bioavailability. The former often has a solution through suitable changes in formulation or manufacture. Unfortunately, solutions for the latter, if required, are more traumatic. Generally a new agent or appropriate analog must be synthesized. An optimal choice, with a minimum trial and error, will only come with a greater understanding of the influence of structure on the physicochemical properties, pharmacokinetics, pharmacological and toxicological activity of the potential drug substances (Ariens, 1968).

REFERENCES

Ariens, E. J., 1968, *Il Farmaco. Sci. Ed.* **24:** 1.
Barr, W. H., 1969, *Drug Information Bulletin, Jan./June,* **27**.
Barr, W. H., Gerblach, L. A., Letcher, K., Plant, M., and Strahl, N., 1972, *Clin. Pharmacol. and Therap.* **13:** 97.
Barr, W. H., and Riegelman, S., 1970, *J. Pharm. Sci.* **59:** 164.

Bischoff, K. B., and Dedrick, R. L., 1968, *J. Pharm. Sci.* **57:** 1346.
Boyes, R. N., 1970, *J. Pharmacol. and Exp. Therap.* **174:** 1.
Boyes, R. N., Scott, D. B., Jebson, P. J., Godman, M. J., and Julian, D. G., 1971, *Clin. Pharmacol. Therap.* **12:** 105.
Boxenbaum, H., and Riegelman, S. (unpublished results).
Brandt, J. L., Castelman, L., Rushkin, H. P., Greenwald, J., Kelly, J. J., Jr., and Jones, A., 1955, *J. Clin. Invest.* **34:** 1017.
Crouthamel, W. G., Doluisio, J. T., Johnson, R. E., and Diamord, L. J., 1970, *J. Pharm. Sci.* **59:** 878.
Davies, D. S., Morg, C. D., Connolly, M. E., Paterson, J. W., Sardler, M., and Dollery, C. T., 1970, *Fed. Proc.* **28:** 797.
Diczfalusy, E., and Levitz, M., 1970, in: *Chemical and Biological Aspects of Steroid Conjugation* (Bernstein, S. and Solomon, S., ed.), Springer-Verlag, Berlin.
Dollery, C. T., Davies, D. S., and Connolly, M. E., 1971, *Ann. N. Y. Acad. Sci.* **179:** 108.
Eger, F. I., 1962, in: *Uptake and Distribution of Anesthetic Agents* (E. M. Papper and R. J. Katz, ed.), McGraw-Hill Book Co., Inc., New York.
Greenway, C. V., and Stark, R. D., 1971, *Physiol. Rev.* **51:** 1.
Kety, S. S., 1951, *Pharmacol. Rev.* **3:** 1.
Levy, G. 1968, in: *Importance of Fundamental Principles in Drug Evaluation*, p. 41 (D. H. Tedeschi and R. E. Tedeschi, eds.), Raven Press, New York.
Lucas, G., Bridle, S. D., and Greengard, P., 1971, *J. Pharmacol. and Exp. Therap.* **178:** 562.
Lundquist, F., and Wolthers, M., 1958, *Acta Pharmacol. Toxicol.* **14:** 267.
McMahon, R. E., Ridolfo, A. S., Culp, H. W., Wolen, R. L., and Marshall, W. F., 1971, *Toxicol. Appl. Pharmacol.* **19:** 427.
Perl, W., Rackow, H., Salantre, E., Wolf, G. L., and Epstein, R. M., 1965, *Appl. Physiol.* **20:** 621.
Portmann, G. A., 1970, in: *Current Concepts in: Pharmaceutical Sciences—Biopharmaceutics* (J. Swarbrick, ed.) Lea and Febiger, Philadelphia.
Prescott, L. F., and Nimmo, L., 1971, *J. Pharm. Exp. Therapy* **128:** 271.
Rowland, M., 1973, in: *Current Concepts in: the Pharmaceutical Sciences*, Vol. II. Chapter 6. Biopharmaceutics (Swarbrick, J., ed.), Lea and Febiger, Philadelphia.
Rowland, M., 1972, *J. Pharm. Sci.* **61:** 70.
Rowland, M., Benet, L. Z., and Graham, G., 1973, *J. Pharmacokin & Biopharm* **1:** 123, 1973.
Rowland, M., Riegelman, S., Harris, P. A., and Seholkoff, D., 1972, *J. Pharm. Sci.* **61:** 379.
Riegelman, S., Loo, J. C. K., and Rowland, M., 1968, *J. Pharm. Sci.* **57:** 117.
Sheline, R. R., 1968, *J. Pharm. Sci.* **57:** 2021.
Shand, D. G., Cavanaugh, J. H., and Oates, J. A., 1972, *Clin. Pharmacol. Therap.* **12:** 769.
Shand, D., and Rangno, R. E., 1971, *Pharmacol.* **7:** 159.
Sjoqvist, F., Alexanderson, B., Osberg, M., Bertillson, L., Borga, O., and Hamburger, B., 1971, *Acta Pharmacol. Toxicol.* **29:** 255.
Stenson, R. E., Constantino, R. T., and Harrison, P. C., 1971, *Circulation* **43:** 205.
Ther, L., and Winne, D., 1971, *Ann. Rev. Pharmacol.* **11:** 57.
Wagner, J. G., Welling, P. G., Roth, S. B., Sakmar, E., Lee, K. P., and Walker, J. E., 1971, *Intern. J. Clin. Pharmacol.* **5:** 371.
Wilkins, R. W., Culbertson, J. W., and Ingelfinger, F. J., 1951, *J. Clin. Invest.* **30:** 312.
Winne, D., and Ochsenfahrt, H., 1967, *J. Theoret.* **14:** 293.
Winne, D., and Remischorsky, J., 1970, *J. Pharm. and Pharmacol.* **22:** 640.

DISCUSSION SUMMARY

Sjoqvist opened the discussion by pointing out that the importance of the first-pass effect may vary from species to species. For example, in the rat, the extent of bioavailability for nortriptyline following intraperitoneal or oral administration is very small when a comparison is made with an *i.v.* dose. However, in man, this apparent first-pass effect is of much less importance and almost 100% of the drug appears in the general circulation as the unchanged compound. This difference may be related to the relative metabolic efficiency of the enzymatic mechanism in the liver. Sjoqvist preferred to identify the first-pass effect seen with the tricyclic antidepressants, lidocaine and propranolol, as a "first-pass disappearance" in the liver. A first-pass disappearance could be a result of binding or uptake in the liver, biliary excretion, as well as metabolism. One of Sjovist's colleagues, Dr. Von Bahr, has shown that all of the drugs listed above have a very high affinity for the T-1 binding sites on cytochrome P-450.

Riegelman responded that, because of the limited time available, he had not commented on the possible nonlinearities which might be introduced into the system by extensive protein binding. He also commented that saturation processes in the liver would be more readily seen when an oral drug is administered to a fasted patient opposed to the kinetics seen when a drug is emptied from the stomach at a slower rate. The possibility of nonlinear kinetics as well as a considerable variation in human hepatic blood flow (reported by Sjoqvist) must be seriously considered before one accepts area under the curve measurements as definitive analyses of the extent of availability.

Wagner reported the results of a bioavailability study for different oral dosage forms of para-aminosalicylic acid in a panel of human subjects where the plasma levels of the active drug and the N-acetyl metabolite were assayed. Plasma levels of the active drug following the administration of a solution of the sodium salt were about 10 times greater than those found following oral administration of a compressed tablet. Levels following the oral administration of a PAS suspension were intermediate, while no blood levels were found following dosing with an enteric coated tablet. However, the levels of metabolite found following dosing with the solution, the suspension and the compressed tablet were almost superimposable. Wagner suggested that a saturable gut wall or first-pass liver metabolic process gave rise to the equal levels of metabolites, and that this drug should only be administered in a very rapidly available form such as the sodium salt solution. He also suggested that much of the G. I. irritation seen with this drug could be eliminated by administering only $\frac{1}{10}$ of the normal daily dose, if the drug is given as the sodium salt solution.

Gillette suggested that it may be possible to identify the fraction of the first-pass disappearance in the liver due to protein binding by comparing the availability following multiple dosing with the availability from a single dose.

Williams questioned Riegelman as to the importance of drug metabolism in the gastrointestinal tract as compared to the liver. Although there have been few experiments in this area, Riegelman reported that of the 30% loss in aspirin due to first-pass effects, approximately $\frac{1}{3}$ of this could be attributed to gut metabolism. He speculated that an even greater percentage would be found following the oral administration of the organic nitrates.

Conney felt that gastrointestinal metabolism would be found to play an increasing role in drug metabolism as further studies are carried out in this area, especially for those drugs that are metabolized by an oxidative process. He reported that his laboratory was currently investigating the oxidative dealkalinization of acetophenetidin in rat intestinal mucosa and that benzpyrene hydroxylation was known to occur in the intestinal mucosa of several species.

Interspecies Scaling

R.T. Williams

Department of Biochemistry
St. Mary's Hospital Medical School
London, United Kingdom

For the testing of the safety of drugs, food additives, and other chemicals of technological importance, an animal is needed in which the absorption, distribution, excretion, and the rate and pattern of metabolism of these compounds are similar to those of man. Such an animal probably does not exist. Therefore, the question may be asked what animal or animals are likely to come close to man in these respects? To answer this question, let us look at the animals which are regarded as closest to man on an evolutionary scale and see if we can produce a hypothetical phylogenetic scale which might be used for investigating this problem. The zoologist has produced such a scale in relation to the subhuman primates. Similar scales probably exist for other groups of animals such as rodents and carnivores, some of which are our main experimental animals.

THE PRIMATE SCALE

For the primates a scale has been produced by zoologists that is based on increasing complexity of structural and behavioral organizations. On this scale the tree shrew is at the bottom and man at the top. In their book *A Handbook of Living Primates*, Napier and Napier (1967) give an illustration called "a staircase of primate evolution" and from this a primate scale can be constructed as shown in Table I.

TABLE I
A Primate Scale

1.	Man
2.	Apes (e.g., chimpanzee and gorilla)
3.	Old World monkeys (e.g., rhesus monkey and baboon)
4.	New World monkeys (e.g., capuchin, squirrel monkey and marmoset)
5.	Lemurs (e.g., lemur, loris and bushbaby)
6.	Tarsiers
7.	Tree shrew

According to Napier and Napier there are 12 families of primates, made up of six families of anthropoids and six families of prosimians. Man is included in the anthropoid group and the order, in relation to man, on the scale is shown in Table II.

The six prosimian families perhaps cannot be readily put in order on a scale except that the tree shrew would be at the bottom since it is regarded by some authors as a doubtful primate (Napier and Napier, 1967). The prosimian families are shown in Table III.

The above classifications are based on morphological and behavioral considerations which must to some extent be related to enzyme activities. It might be expected that the animals belonging to the same zoological class would have similar tissue enzymes. There is support for this view from the study of blood groups in primates for there are similarities between the serum proteins of different primate species and those of man (Goodman, 1963). If this is true they might also have similar drug metabolizing enzymes in their tissues. One could argue therefore that the animals nearest to man on the phylogenetic scale (Table I) (i.e., apes, then in turn Old World monkeys, etc.), are more likely to metabolize drugs like man than an animal far removed from man such as the rat, rabbit, or dog. However, apart from metabolism, there are other factors that do not involve the usual drug metabolizing enzymes to be considered: drug absorption, excretion, tissue distribution, and the activities of the gut flora and fauna.

TABLE II
A Scale of Anthropoids

Family	Example
1. Hominidae	Man
2. Pongidae	Chimpanzee
3. Hylobatidae	Gibbon
4. Cercopithecidae	Rhesus monkey
5. Cebidae	Capuchin monkey
6. Callitrichidae	Marmoset

TABLE III
The Prosimian Families

Family	Example
Lemuridae	Ring-tailed lemur
Indriidae	Indris
Daubentonidae	Aye-aye
Lorisidae	Slow loris
Tarsiidae	Tarsier
Tupaiidae	Tree shrew

PATHWAYS OF DRUG METABOLISM IN PRIMATES

If it is conceded that because apes and monkeys are closely related to man zoologically they are likely to possess similar drug metabolizing enzymes, then we must see what happens if such a hypothesis is put to the test. In my laboratory, attempts have been made to test this hypothesis with several compounds, including phenylacetic acid, 4-chlorophenylacetic acid, indoleacetic acid, sulfadimethoxine, phenol, benzoic acid, and quinic acid. Some of these compounds (e.g., phenylacetic acid, sulfadimethoxine, and quinic acid) were selected for study because of suggestions that they were metabolized in man differently from other species.

Phenylacetic Acid

It is well known that benzoic acid (C_6H_5COOH) is conjugated with glycine in man and many other species and excreted in the urine as hippuric acid (Bridges *et al.*, 1970). Its homolog, phenylacetic acid ($C_6H_5CH_2COOH$), however, is conjugated in man with glutamine and not with glycine. Conjugation of phenylacetic acid with glutamine also occurs in the chimpanzee (Power, 1936) and in the Old World monkeys, but not in any species lower on the scale than the marmosets (James *et al.*, 1972). The monkeys, however, differ from man in that they excrete a small amount of the glycine conjugate (Table IV) which seems to increase as we go down the primate scale. At the level of the prosimians, however, glutamine conjugation of phenylacetic acid disappears. The conjugation of phenylacetic acid in primates appears to be correlated as far as we can tell with the primate scale given in Table I.

Sulfadimethoxine

This long-acting sulfonamide drug is excreted by human beings conjugated with glucuronic acid which is attached to the sulfonamide nitrogen atom of the drug (see Formula 1). In the lower animals such as the rabbit and rat, little or none of this glucuronide is excreted. However, in all the primates examined this glucuronide is the main excretory product of the drug in the urine. The conjugation of sulfadimethoxine with glucuronic acid at the N^1-position of the drug molecule therefore occurs in the anthropoids and the prosimians including the tree shrew (Table V, Adamson et al., 1970a). It would appear that in the extent of the formation of the N^1-glucuronide of the sulfadimethoxine, all the primates examined, but not the nonprimates, are like man. Furthermore in this reaction, the doubtful primate, the tree shrew, behaves like any other primate and not like the nonprimates.

It will be noted that glutamine conjugation of phenylacetic acid occurs in the anthropoid families but not in the prosimians, whereas N^1-glucuronide formation with sulfadimethoxine occurs in both the anthropoids and prosimians.

TABLE IV
Conjugation of Phenylacetic Acid in Primates[a]

Family	Species	Percent of 24-hr excretion as conjugated with Glutamine	Glycine
Anthropoids			
1. Hominidae	Man	90	0
2. Pongidae	Chimpanzee[b]	+	?
3. Hylobatidae	—	Not tested	
4. Cercopithecidae	Rhesus monkey		
	Cynomolgus monkey		
	Green monkey		
	Red-bellied monkey		
	Mona monkey	30–90	0.1–1.0
	Mangabey		
	Drill		
	Baboon		
5. Cebidae	Capuchin monkey	64	10
	Squirrel monkey	75	2
6. Callitrichidae	Marmoset	80	1
Prosimians			
Lemuridae	Bushbaby	0	80
	Slow loris	0	87
Nonprimates			
Ten species		0	80–100

[a] Mainly the data of James et al. (1972)
[b] See Power (1936)

TABLE V
N^1-Glucuronide of Sulfadimethoxine[a]

Family	Species	N^1-Glucuronide formed as percent of 24-hr excretion
Anthropoids		
1. Hominidae	Man	65
2. Pongidae	—	Not tested
3. Hylobatidae	—	Not tested
4. Cercopithecidae	Rhesus monkey	66
	Green monkey	30
	Baboon	63
5. Cebidae	Squirrel monkey	44
	Capuchin	48
6. Callitrichidae	—	Not tested
Prosimians		
Lemuridae	Bushbaby	62
	Slow loris	49
Tupaiidae	Tree shrew	52
Nonprimates		
Nine species		0–19

[a] Data of Adamson et al. (1970a)

$$\text{Sulfadimethoxine } N^1\text{-glucuronide} \tag{1}$$

Quinic Acid

Quinic acid or 1,3,4,5-tetrahydroxycyclohexanecarboxylic acid when taken by mouth by human beings is extensively aromatized and excreted in the urine as hippuric acid. Since quinic acid is a component of tea, coffee, fruit, and vegetables, it must be an important contributor to the normal output of hippuric acid in man. The conversion of quinic acid to hippuric acid in man has been known since 1863 (Lautemann, 1863), but only in recent years has the fate of this acid has been examined in other species. Table VI shows that only in some primates, namely, the Old World

$$\underset{\text{Quinic acid}}{\text{HO}\begin{array}{c}\text{OH}\\\text{OH}\end{array}\text{COOH}\atop\text{OH}}\xrightarrow{\text{gut flora}}\underset{\text{Benzoic acid}}{\bigcirc\text{—COOH}}\xrightarrow{\text{liver}}\underset{\text{Hippuric acid}}{\bigcirc\text{—CONHCH}_2\text{COOH}}\qquad(2)$$

monkeys, does the compound behave as it does in man. In New World monkeys, prosimians, and some 12 nonprimate species, the aromatization of orally administered quinic acid occurs either to a small extent or not at all. The interesting point about the fate of the quinic acid is that aromatization occurs only when the compound is taken by mouth, for the injected compound is largely excreted unchanged and is not aromatized (Adamson et al., 1970b). Furthermore, when the intestinal flora of the rhesus monkey are suppressed by the administration by mouth of antibiotics, ingested quinic acid is not extensively aromatized. This suggests that the aromatization of quinic acid is carried out by the gut bacteria and that the

TABLE VI
The Aromatization of Quinic Acid in Primates[a]

Family	Species	Extent of aromatization percent of dose
Anthropoids		
1. Hominidae	Man	64
2. Pongidae	—	Not tested
3. Hylobatidae	—	Not tested
4. Cercopithecidae	Rhesus monkey	42
	Green monkey	45
	Baboon	40
5. Cebidae	Spider monkey	6
	Squirrel monkey	0
	Capuchin	0
6. Callitrichidae	—	Not tested
Prosimians		
Lemuridae	Bushbaby	2
	Slow loris	6
Tupaiidae	Tree shrew	0
Nonprimates		
Twelve species		0–5

[a] Data of Adamson et al. (1970b)

TABLE VII
Reactions in Man and Other Primates

	Occurrence[a] of		
Family	Quinic acid aromatization	Phenacetyl glutamine formation	Sulfadimethoxine N^1-glucuronide formation
Anthropoids			
1. Hominidae	+	+	+
2. Pongidae	n.t.	+	n.t.
3. Hylobatidae	n.t.	n.t.	n.t.
4. Cercopithecidae	+	+	+
5. Cebidae	−	+	+
6. Callitrichidae	n.t.	+	n.t.
Prosimians			
Lemuridae	−	−	+
Tupaiidae	−	n.t.	+
Nonprimates	−	−	−

[a] + means extensive; − means absent or at a relatively low level; n.t. means no member of the family has been tested.

organisms and the right conditions for their activity only occur in the gastrointestinal tracts of man and the Old World monkeys. The reaction occurs only in a limited number of primates and these are the ones nearest to man, apart from the apes and gibbons, which have not been tested.

In the above reactions, that is, glutamine conjugation, N^1-glucuronide formation, and quinic acid aromatization, the Old World monkeys are similar to man in all three reactions, the New World monkeys in two, and the prosimians in one (Table VII). The nonprimates are not like man in any of these reactions. This would suggest that as far as the pathways of metabolism of drugs are concerned, results similar to man are more likely to be found in the primates than nonprimates and the nearer the primate is to man on the evolutionary scale (see Tables I and II) the closer are the pathways of metabolism likely to be to those in man.

Other Factors

The above suggestion, however, does not take into account factors such as absorption, excretion, tissue distribution, and rate of metabolism. Although the route and extent of metabolism of a drug may be similar in man and a given nonhuman primate, other factors may be different. Thus,

TABLE VIII
Urinary Excretion of Sulfadimethoxine and Sulfadimethoxypyrimidine[a]

Drug	Species	Percent of dose excreted in 24 hr	48 hr	N^1-glucuronide excreted, percent of 24-hr excretion
Sulfadimethoxine	Man	25	—	65
	Rhesus monkey	39	55	66
	Rat	16	33	8
	Rabbit	46	73	0
Sulfadimethoxy-pyrimidine	Man	10	21	29
	Rhesus monkey	60	74	44
	Rat	6	10	7
	Rabbit	66	72	0

[a]Drugs given orally; doses, 30 mg/kg in man and 100 mg/kg in other species.

the two drugs sulfadimethoxine and sulfadimethoxypyrimidine form N^1-glucuronides as major urinary metabolites in man and the rhesus monkey (Adamson et al., 1970a; Walker and Williams, 1972), but the rates of excretion of the drugs differ completely in these two species (Table VIII). As far as the rates of excretion of these drugs are concerned, man is more comparable with the rat than with the rhesus monkey, which in turn is more comparable with the rabbit than with man. Thus, in the pattern of excretion of these drugs, man and rhesus monkey are similar but in the rate of excretion they are dissimilar. This would suggest that two species were needed to compare sulfadimethoxine in man, namely, the rhesus monkey for the pattern of biotransformation and the rat for the rate of excretion into the urine.

For scaling up to man a species is needed in which at least five parameters are similar to those in man: rate of absorption, pattern of biotransformation, rate of metabolism, tissue distribution, and rate of excretion. The higher apes and Old World monkeys may be similar to man in one of these parameters, the pattern of biotransformation, but they may differ from man in the other four. This could mean that a different species may be needed for each of the five parameters for comparison with man.

GENETIC VARIATIONS IN MAN AND SPECIES VARIATIONS

There are about three billion (3×10^9) people in the world and it would appear that there are more of the human species in the world than of any other terrestrial vertebrate species. The chances of finding genetic variations in the handling of drugs are therefore much greater in man than in any other species (insects and fish are not included).

Animal species are known that are defective in certain metabolic reactions of drugs which occur in man. For example, the cat is defective in glucuronic acid conjugation, the pig in sulfate conjugation (Capel *et al.*, 1972), and the Indian fruit bat in glycine conjugation (Bridges *et al.*, 1970; Bababunmi *et al.*, 1973). The inability of the dog to acetylate aromatic amino groups and certain hydrazines is well known (Williams, 1967). Furthermore, genetic defects in drug metabolism have been found in certain human beings (Clarke *et al.*, 1968). These include the inability to hydroxylate diphenylhydantoin, to de-ethylate phenacetin, and to conjugate bilirubin. Some groups of people have been found to be poor acetylators of isoniazid and sulfonamides and it has been reported that glycine conjugation is sometimes defective in old age and in certain mental states.

The question that these observations raise is, can those species which show defects in certain metabolic reactions of drugs be used for comparison with those groups of human beings which show similar defects in drug metabolism? This question has already been suggested by the writer (Williams, 1971) in another way in the statement: "It is possible that by studying interspecies variations in drug metabolism one could reveal the possible intraspecies variations in man."

REFERENCES

Adamson, R.H., Bridges, J.W., Kibby, M.R., Walker, S.R., and Williams, R.T., 1970a, *Biochem. J.* **118**: 41–45.

Adamson, R.H., Bridges, J.W., Evans, M.E., and Williams, R.T., 1970b, *Biochem. J.* **116**: 437–443.

Bababunmi, E.A., Smith, R.L., and Williams, R.T., 1973, *Life Sci.* **12** (II), 317–326.

Bridges, J.W., French, M.R., Smith, R.L., and Williams, R.T., 1970, *Biochem. J.* **118**: 47–51.

Capel, I.D., French, M.R., Millburn, P., Smith, R.L., and Williams, R.T., 1972, *Xenobiotica* **2**: 25–34.

Clarke, C.A., Price Evans, D.A., Harris, R., McConnell, R.B., and Woodrow, J.C., 1968, *Quart. J. Med.* **37**: 183–265.

Goodman, M., 1963, in: *Classification and Human Evolution* (S.L. Washburn, ed.), Methuen and Co. Ltd., London.

James, M.O., Smith, R.L., Williams, R.T., and Reidenberg, M., 1972, *Proc. Roy. Soc. Lond. B.* **182**: 25–35.

Lautemann, E., 1863, *Justus Liebigs Ann. Chem.* **125**: 9.

Napier, J.R., and Napier, P.H., 1967, in: *A Handbook of Living Primates*, pp. 3–5, Academic Press, London and New York.

Power, F.W., 1936, *Proc. Soc. Exp. Biol. Med.* **33**: 598–600.

Walker, S.R., and Williams, R.T., 1972, *Xenobiotica* **2**: 69–75.

Williams, R.T., 1967, *Federation Proc.* **26**: 1029–1039.

Williams, R.T., 1971, *Ann. N.Y. Acad. Sci.* **179**: 141–154.

DISCUSSION SUMMARY

Haley began the discussion by expressing his interest in William's data concerning primate metabolism, and his distress with the fact that most metabolic data today are obtained in rodents. He pointed to the danger of being misled in the extrapolation of animal data. A great deal of scrutiny should be exercised in selecting an animal to model human metabolism. For example, when many species, from the mouse to man, are given 2-fluorenylacetamide, they form the N-hydroxylated derivative and can develop various tumors. The guinea pig is an exception because the N-hydroxylation mechanism is missing and there is no tumor development. However, if the N-hydroxylated derivative is given to guinea pigs, tumors do develop. Haley suggested that human liver biopsy or autopsy material be used whenever possible to study metabolism of new or dangerous drugs.

Garrett expressed concern with the use of liver homogenates and microsomal preparations in studying drug metabolism, and stated a preference for *in vitro* studies where metabolic patterns are determined using a liver perfusion technique. He felt that most microsomal preparations do not really simulate what happens during normal liver perfusion since additional enzymes may become available during the homogenation process. Furthermore, Garrett suggested that we do not necessarily need an animal that actually simulates the metabolic distribution in man. If anatomical, distribution, and perfusion properties were appropriate in an animal model, it might be possible to account for the metabolic differences by the use of a mathematical model which considers the differences in the metabolic profiles.

Williams suggested that phenolic glucuronidation in pig liver homogenates may be amenable to such treatment. The pig conjugates phenol primarily with glucuronic acid; however, this is not meant to imply that the enzymes and cofactors necessary for sulfate conjugation are nonexistent. A means of testing whether sulfate conjugation is possible would involve an experiment with the homogenate when an inhibitor of glucuronide formation is included. Gillette responded to the points raised by Garrett and suggested that the need for concern about species differences in metabolism is dependent on the objective of the study. If the study is concerned with pharmacological response and this is only affected by unchanged drug, then metabolism differences will not be important in choosing an animal model. However, if such things as toxicity or hypersensitivity reactions are of interest, then metabolic products would be very important in choosing the appropriate animal model.

Garattini pointed out that an apparent defective metabolic pathway in a given species may sometimes be related to further metabolism of the expected metabolite. For instance, after diazepam administration there is accumulation of oxazepam in mice but not in rats, although the livers of both species contain the enzymes necessary to form oxazepam. The reason for this difference, however, is actually due to the fact that oxazepam is metabolized much faster in rats than in mice. Similarly, in the isolated perfused liver of several animal species, nitrazepam is reduced to the amino derivative and then acetylated. Once again the mouse is an exception and appreciable levels of the N-acetyl derivative cannot be found since this metabolite is rapidly hydrolyzed.

In reviewing the previous discussion, Ariens concluded that since drug metabolism causes a great deal of problems in pharmacokinetics, we may be able to resolve this complexity by designing drugs which are not metabolized. At first, this may seem an impossibility, since many drugs would essentially remain unexcreted if they were not metabolized. However, Ariens felt that this is simply a problem of drug design and something which may be solved by the medicinal chemist. Partition coefficients must be modified such that the drug has a reasonable half-life when elimination is only via urinary excretion.

LaDu pointed out that most drugs are metabolized, and this is an important facet of their safety since many drugs would not be excreted by the kidney at a fast enough rate, usually because the action of the drug is dependent on a moderately high lipid solubility so that the compound may penetrate to the site of action. LaDu posed the question as to how it would be possible to control an overdose problem with a drug which is nonmetabolized, yet is required to have a high lipid solubility in order to penetrate the brain. Ariens felt this problem could be answered simply enough, providing the drug was a weak acid or a weak base, by varying the urine pH. He suggested that some drugs could then be administered only once a month, and removed whenever desired by either acidifying or alkalinizing the urine.

Lemberger suggested that in many cases we would not want to administer drugs with long half-lives, especially if a patient could have an adverse reaction or when an analgesic was administered and the symptom of pain was necessary to judge the clinical effects. Ariens pointed out that a drug that is not metabolized does not necessarily have a long half-life. He cited curare as an example and Nodine described the pharmacokinetics of isosorbide and hydrochlorthiazide as further examples.

Wagner felt that there is insufficient basic knowledge about how and why drugs are metabolized in the body, such that we would be able to design a drug *a priori* and predict what metabolic pathway would be followed. He cited penicillin G, a drug which is excreted in the urine unchanged yet appears to have a number of available sites for metabolism when one examines the structure.

Conney suggested that the objectives which led to the rationale for proposing the design of nonmetabolized drugs could be realized for metabolized compounds also. The major difficulty in predicting efficacy and toxicity for metabolized drugs is the large variation seen in the patient population. This difficulty could be overcome if it were possible to design drugs which are metabolized by a pathway which does not vary from one person to the next.

Crout asked the group if it was generally believed that most cells across the animal kingdom have a similar sensitivity to particular drugs and that most of the variation seen in different species or within a species may be based on differences in drug metabolism. He pointed out that when one carries out dose–response relationships in isolated tissue baths, there may be a tenfold variation in the ED-50 from one specimen to another even when the experiments are carried out under carefully controlled and reproducible conditions. This large degree of variation from tissue to tissue is usually assumed to be a function of differences at the cellular level in the receptor site. However, this explanation would seem to be in opposition to the fundamental tenet of the discussion following Williams' presentation. That is, much variation from species to species may be explained on a metabolic basis instead of on the basis of variations in cellular response to drugs.

Garratini gave support to the idea that the differences in tissue response are related to differences in the response seen at the cellular or receptor site as opposed to differences in the concentration of the active drug in the bathing fluids. If one measures ED-50 levels of oxazapam as an antagonist to metrazole (pentylenetetrazole), the following brain levels are found: 600 ng/g in the rat, 200 ng/g in the guinea pig, and 100 ng/g in the mouse. In this case the levels do not correlate with the given pharmacologic effect. A more striking example is found in the C-3H strain of mice, which is insensitive to the stimulant action of amphetamine. However, both the albino and the C-3H strain give the same measured brain levels of amphetamine. Garratini did add, however, that the levels might be different if one could measure concentrations at an hypothesized critical subcellular site.

In response to the question regarding species variation, Plaa pointed out that it is not always the parent substance which is the toxic moiety. In the field of liver injury, there is considerable evidence that metabolites of certain substances are the actual inducers of toxicity. Therefore, if one attempts to correlate tissue injury with tissue drug concentrations, a lack of correlation does not necessarily indicate a species difference in cellular sensitivity. It may be that one is not measuring the correct toxic moiety. With liver injury produced by halogenated hydrocarbons, it seems that most apparent species variations observed in common laboratory animals are due to differences in "activation" or to the rate of production of toxic metabolites. Plaa speculated that if one could use only the toxic moiety in such studies, one would probably find less species variation.

Animal Scale-Up

Robert L. Dedrick

Biomedical Engineering and Instrumentation Branch
Division of Research Services, National Institutes of Health
Bethesda, Maryland

The title of this paper is freely adapted from a problem common to the art and science of chemical engineering: "plant scale-up" or "process scale-up." A chemical reaction or a set of chemical reactions is discovered which leads to a potentially useful product. The basic chemistry is worked out, often in considerable detail, at the bench in glassware. It is necessary to design a plant which will make the product economically and consistent with other constraints imposed by society.

When one addresses the scale-up problem, he finds that even detailed knowledge of the mechanism of a chemical reaction that is fully elucidated in a well-mixed flask is not sufficient. A variety of subordinate problems are introduced by the scale itself. The product may be produced under very different conditions from those in the research laboratory in order to obtain a suitable yield at an optimal rate from available raw materials. Temperatures, pressures, type of catalyst, nature of mixing, and many other factors may differ between the laboratory and the plant. Often the process is designed to run on a continuous rather than batch basis. And usually there must be a separation step to recover the product in sufficient purity.

Problems of scale are largely *physical* in character. These can be studied quite independently of any particular set of chemical reactions to which they may relate in a complete process (Himmelblau and Bischoff, 1968). Physical phenomena interact strongly with chemical reactions. For example, reactants must reach the reaction zone, and products must be removed; temperature affects both chemical kinetics and chemical thermodynamics. Interactions of mass and heat transfer can become extremely complex when heterogeneous reactions occur on porous catalysts.

In many other contexts, ranging from the mouse to the environment, chemical reactions take place which are limited or even dominated by physical processes, and the problems are often those of scale. There is little argument that a toxic material should not be disposed of by dumping it in a lake simply because, *on the average,* the concentration presents no hazard to man or wildlife. There is considerably more debate about the relevance of *in vitro* enzyme kinetics to the occurrence of the same reactions in the body.

I will discuss a formal approach to drug distribution in the body which permits consideration of scale through the individual processes that occur. Some of these are physical, such as blood flows, tissue binding, and kidney clearances. Others are chemical, such as metabolic reactions. The physical processes often vary quite predictably among mammalian species, and much is known about these, independent of any chemical reactions. Certain metabolic reactions vary greatly and unpredictably among species. The physical and chemical processes interact so that the relationship of the pharmacokinetics of any given drug between one species and another may be quite straightforward or may be rather obscure unless the correct interaction is perceived.

BASIC PRINCIPLES

Table I is a reference for physical scaling problems. It indicates that, on the basis of weight alone, only five orders of magnitude separate the elephant from the mouse while more than eight separate the mouse and a typical cell, and twelve separate the cell and a typical protein molecule. Use of a characteristic linear dimension compresses the scale but does not change the general conclusion that it is a long step from a molecule to a cell or from a cell to even a small mammal.

TABLE I
Reference Scale

Object	Weight, atomic mass units	Characteristic dimension, Å
Water molecule	18	3
Human serum albumin	6.9×10^4	36
Human red blood cell	6×10^{16}	5×10^4
Mouse	1.3×10^{25}	4×10^8
Elephant	1.8×10^{30}	2×10^{10}

Animal Scale-Up

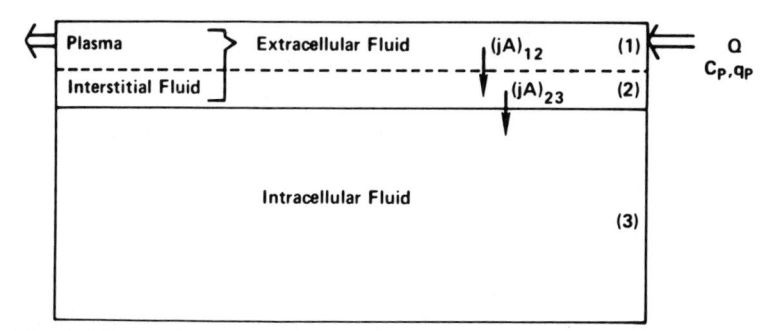

```
┌──────────────┐────────────────────────────────────────┐
│  Plasma      │   Extracellular Fluid   ↓(jA)₁₂   (1)  │⇐  Q
├──────────────┤────────────────────────────────────────│   Cp,qp
│ Interstitial │                         ↓(jA)₂₃   (2)  │
│ Fluid        │                                        │
│              │                                        │
│              │         Intracellular Fluid            │
│              │                                   (3)  │
└──────────────┴────────────────────────────────────────┘
```

Fig. 1. Schematic drawing of a compartment including subcompartments to permit analysis of intracompartment membrane transport. Q = blood or plasma flow rate; C_P = free concentration; q_P = total concentration (free plus bound); (jA) = rate of transport (Dedrick et al. 1973).

Physiologically, the mouse has a lot in common with the elephant, and we expect that a formal scheme to describe drug distribution might be suitable for either. The scheme discussed here is based on a number of physical principles including mass balances, thermodynamics, transport, and flow. Chemical reactions are included as required.

Mass Balances

Figure 1 represents an anatomic compartment in an organism. It may be a local region of tissue (Bischoff and Brown, 1966) or it may be a group of tissues which are "lumped" in the sense that they are assumed sufficiently similar for purposes of pharmacokinetic modeling (Price et al., 1960). Generally, drug enters the compartment with the flowing blood. It may also enter the compartment by direct diffusion from another compartment (Perl et al., 1965; Rackow et al., 1965). Drug moves within the compartment by diffusion, bulk flow, and membrane transport. It may undergo a variety of physical interactions, such as binding to extracellular or intracellular proteins, solubility in lipids or a variety of interactions with cell membranes. Most of the physical interactions are probably reversible; however, very high stability constants have been observed in some cases. The drug may also undergo a variety of chemical transformations catalyzed by enzymes in the compartment. The drug may leave with the blood, by diffusion to another compartment, or by a physiological process, such as urinary or biliary excretion.

A balance equation for a chemical species in any compartment is simply a statement of the conservation of mass. It is a differential equation which states mathematically that:

$$\begin{bmatrix} \text{Rate of accumulation of} \\ \text{drug in compartment} \end{bmatrix}$$

$$= \begin{bmatrix} \text{Rate of absorption} \\ \text{or injection} \end{bmatrix} + \begin{bmatrix} \text{Rate of flow in} \\ \text{with blood} \end{bmatrix}$$

$$- \begin{bmatrix} \text{Rate of flow} \\ \text{out with blood} \end{bmatrix} + \begin{bmatrix} \text{Rate of diffusion} \\ \text{in} \end{bmatrix}$$

$$- \begin{bmatrix} \text{Rate of diffusion} \\ \text{out} \end{bmatrix} + \begin{bmatrix} \text{Rate of formation} \\ \text{by chemical reaction} \end{bmatrix}$$

$$- \begin{bmatrix} \text{Rate of conversion} \\ \text{by chemical reaction} \end{bmatrix} - \begin{bmatrix} \text{Rate of excretion} \\ \text{by a physiologic process} \end{bmatrix}$$

Frequently, the balance equation simplifies considerably because many terms are not relevant. A similar balance equation is written for every compartment in the organism, and the set of differential equations is the mathematical pharmacokinetic model.

Depending on the particular drug and compartment, a variety of kinds of information is required before the equations can be solved. This information includes anatomic and physiologic data which do not depend upon the particular drug. It also includes measures of binding, excretion, transport, and metabolism for which data on the specific drug are required. Much of this may be predicted eventually or obtained from *in vitro* work;

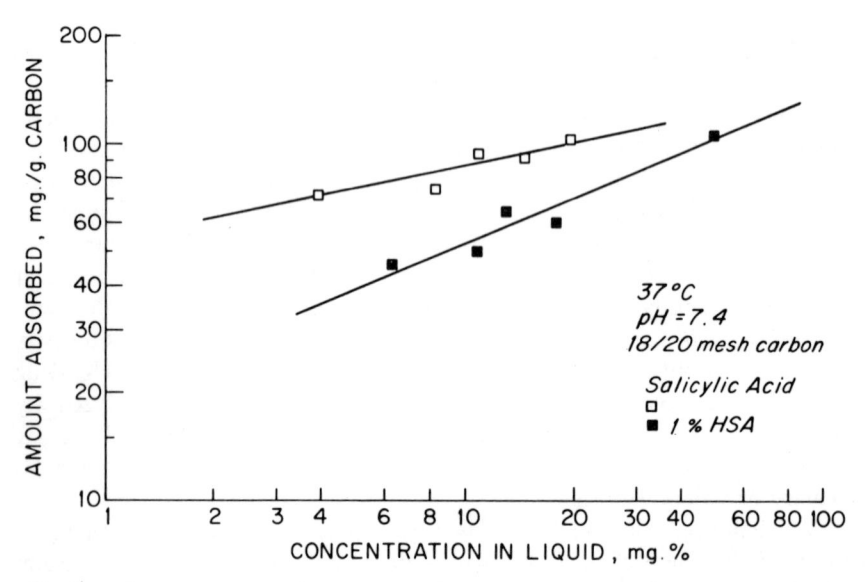

Fig. 2. Adsorption isotherms for salicylic acid on activated carbon (Dedrick *et al.*, 1967).

however, just how far general predictions or *in vitro* data can be applied is not yet clear. It is clear that the drug concentration at any actual binding or metabolic site may be very different from the measured plasma concentration. The local concentration is appropriate for correlation with binding or rate of reaction.

If sufficient information is available to permit assignment of parameters, the equations can be solved simultaneously to yield predictions of the concentration or amount of drug or metabolite in any compartment as a function of time. Urinary and biliary excretion can also be calculated.

Thermodynamics

The great importance of plasma and tissue binding in pharmacology has been discussed (Kruger-Thiemer *et al.*, 1965–1966; Gillette, 1965; Brodie *et al.*, 1950; 1952). Such binding enters the model as a thermody-

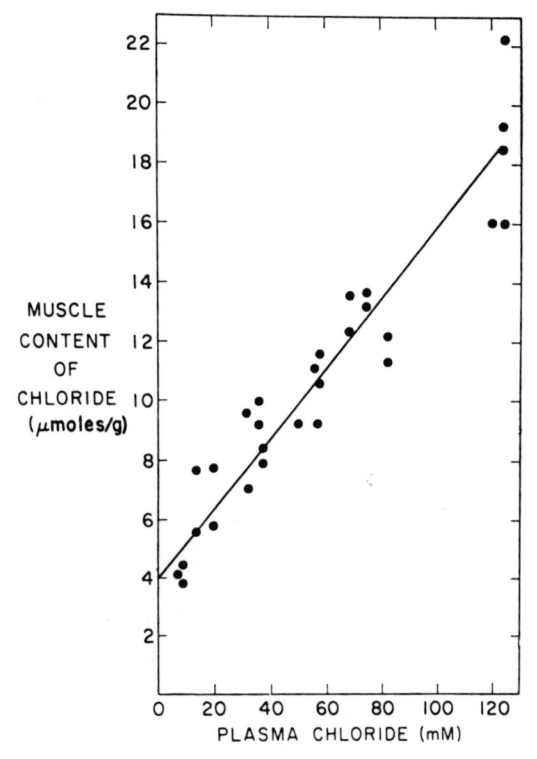

Fig. 3. Distribution of chloride between muscle and plasma of cat (Bourke *et al.*, 1970).

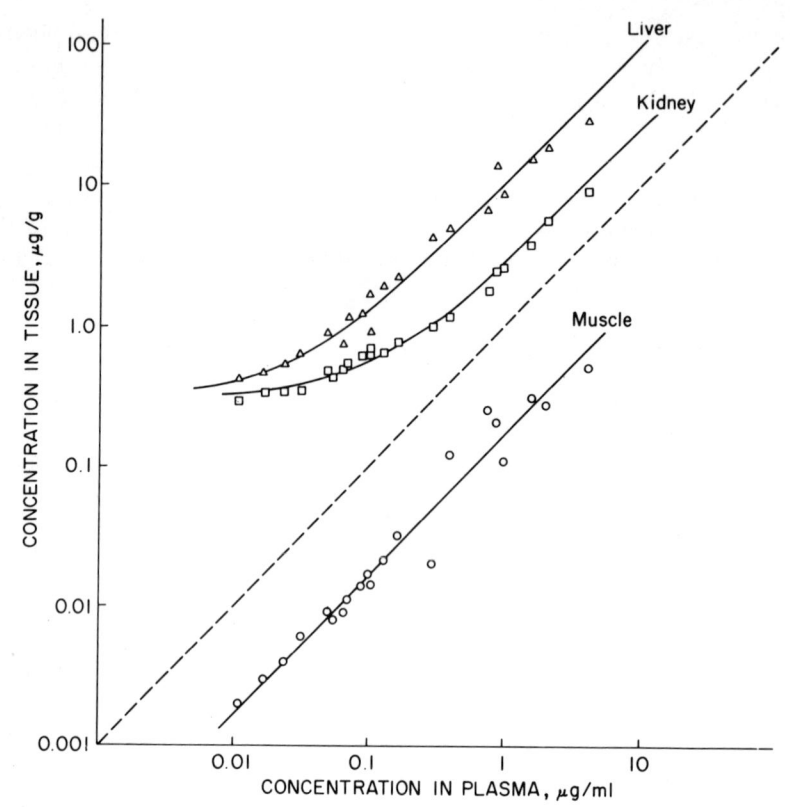

Fig. 4. Distribution of methotrexate between selected tissues and plasma of mouse (Dedrick et al.,1973).

namic relationship between the bound concentration of a drug at a particular site and the free concentration there.

The concept of binding is quite general and appears in extensive literature on adsorption in nonliving systems. For example, if activated carbon is allowed to come to equilibrium with a buffered aqueous solution of salicylate, the concentration in the solid phase is a unique function of the concentration in the liquid phase. Figure 2 presents data on such a system shown by a Freundlich plot. Addition of 1% human serum albumin (HSA) significantly shifts the isotherm to lower values of adsorbed concentration and changes the slope. The exact causes for this were not fully explored; however, binding of salicylate to the HSA is almost certainly one of these. Both isotherms have equations of the form

$$q = KC^n$$

where q is the concentration in solid; C is the concentration in liquid; n is the slope of curve; and K is the constant of proportionality.

An analogous "isotherm" may be obtained for a variety of tissues *in vivo* if they are sufficiently highly perfused so that flow does not limit the distribution of drug or metabolite between blood (or plasma) and the tissue. Figure 3 shows a plot of muscle chloride vs. plasma chloride at various times during an isosmotic dialysis of a cat against isethionate to produce hypochloremia. The slope of the curve provides a measure of chloride "space" (11.5%), while the intercept of the curve with the tissue-chloride axis is associated with intracellular chloride.

Data for the distribution of the folic acid antagonist, methotrexate (MTX), between several individual tissues and plasma of the mouse are shown in Fig. 4. This is a Freundlich-type plot (log–log) so that proportionality between tissue concentration and plasma concentration is indicated by a 45° line (slope = 1). The actual constant of proportionality is a measure

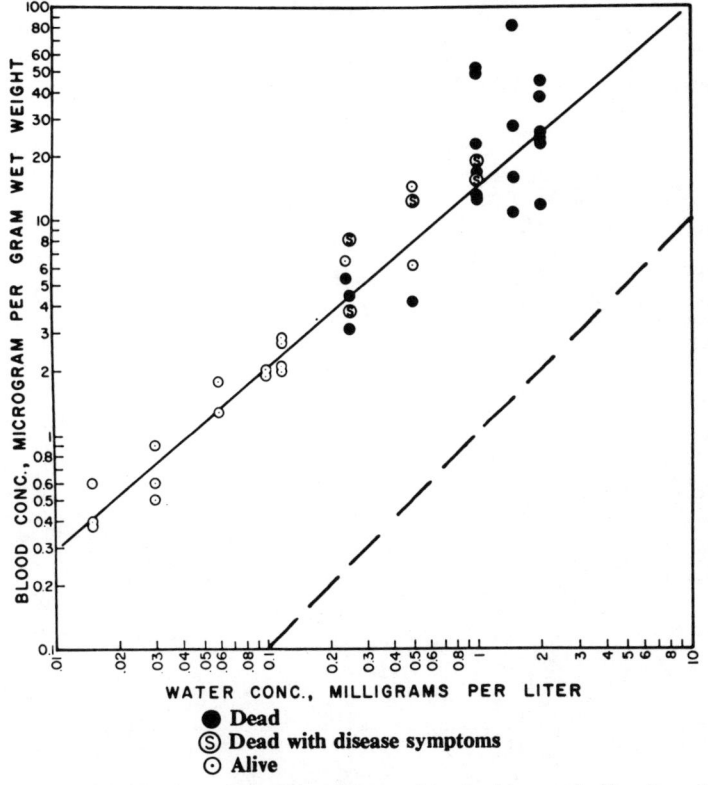

Fig. 5. Distribution of parathion between blood of brown bullheads and surrounding medium (adapted from Mount and Boyle, 1969).

of percent space. Methotrexate space in muscle is about 16% or slightly greater than the freely exchangeable chloride in cat muscle. Liver and kidney show a somewhat different behavior. The tissue to plasma concentration ratios in these are 10:1 and 3:1, respectively, at high plasma concentrations. At lower concentrations, strong binding to the tissues (presumed due to dihydrofolate reductase, DHFR) make the isotherms tend toward a constant value. The relationship between the tissue concentration, C_T, and the plasma concentration, C_P, is thus composed of a linear part plus a saturable part (Bischoff et al., 1971).

$$C_T = BC_P + \frac{aC_P}{\varepsilon + C_P}$$

where B is the tissue-to-plasma ratio at high concentration; a is the MTX equivalent of DHFR; and ε is the dissociation constant of MTX: DHFR complex.

An interesting "isotherm" has been published by Mount and Boyle (1969). They placed small brown bullheads in a large tank containing a solution of parathion. The fish were maintained until death or, at sublethal concentrations, for 30 days. Figure 5 shows the results. Blood concentration

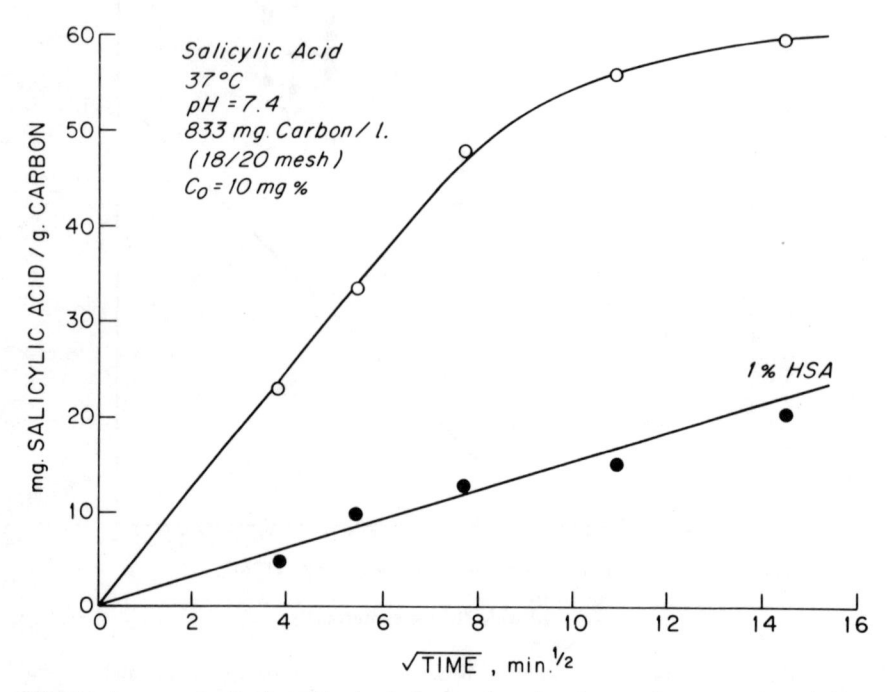

Fig. 6. Amount of salicylic acid adsorbed on activated carbon vs. the square root of time (Dedrick et al., 1967).

Kinetics

A sufficient time must elapse after the start of an experiment for equilibrium (or at least steady state) to be reached. When salicylate was adsorbed by activated carbon, under the conditions described in Fig. 6, equilibrium was not reached for well over 2 hr. The presence of 1% HSA decreased the rate of adsorption to an even more marked extent than it had decreased the adsorption capacity (Fig. 2). Adsorption data are often linearized on a plot of uptake vs. the square root of time for a significant part of the approach to equilibrium for various geometries (Crank, 1956).

The central nervous system exhibits slow uptake of a variety of substances. A general description of transport between blood and cerebrospinal fluid has been presented by Rall (1967). Various quantitative studies of transport between blood and brain or cerebrospinal fluid include those of Brodie et al. (1960), Bourke et al. (1970), and Gabelnick et al. (1970). Reed and Woodbury (1962) studied the uptake of C-14 tagged urea by the brains of functionally nephrectomized rats. Figure 7 shows the data of Reed

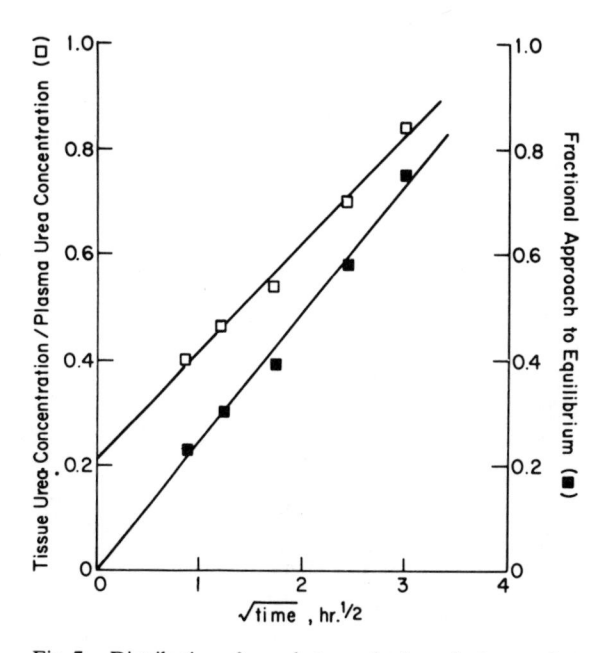

Fig. 7. Distribution of urea between brain and plasma of rat vs. the square root of time (data from Reed and Woodbury, 1962).

and Woodbury plotted in the manner of Fig. 6. Urea uptake is a very slow process with significant deviation from the equilibrium value at 9 hr. It is not certain what relationship the linear kinetic description bears to the actual detailed mechanism of urea transfer.

PHARMACOKINETIC EXAMPLES

Nonmetabolized Substances

The general balance equation is simplified if a drug is not metabolized so that all interactions are physical. The pharmacokinetics of chloride and MTX are illustrative.

Chloride Pharmacokinetics

Bourke et al. (1970) and Gabelnick et al. (1970) conducted an experiment in which they produced hypochloremic cats by isosmotic dialysis against isethionate for the purpose of studying chloride transfer in

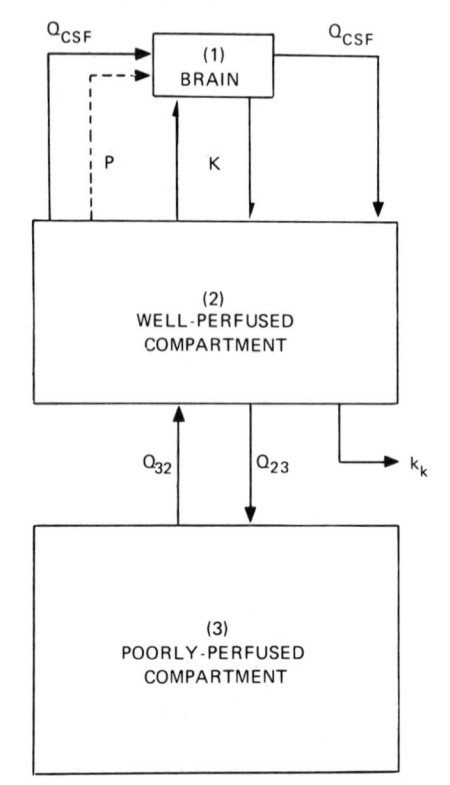

Fig. 8. Compartmental model for chloride pharmacokinetics (Gabelnick et al., 1970).

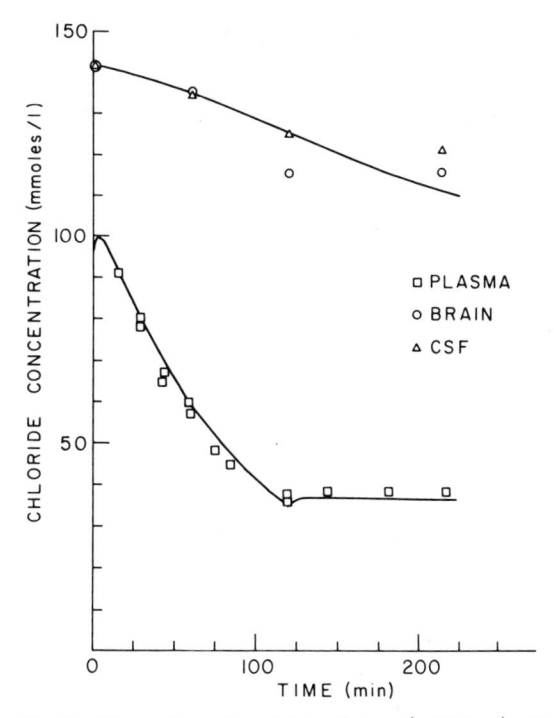

Fig. 9. Comparison of model simulations (solid lines) with experimental data from the cat during and following replacement hemodialysis (Gabelnick et al., 1970).

the brain. Figure 8 shows the three-compartment model which was used to simulate systemic chloride concentrations and to elucidate the transport mechanism between blood and brain.

The balance equation on compartment (1) is

$$V_1 \frac{dC_1}{dt} = K(C_2 - C_1) - Q_{CSF} C_1 + P$$

where V is the chloride space; C is the chloride concentration; K is the overall mass-transfer coefficient for diffusive transport between brain and well-perfused compartment; Q_{CSF} is the cerebrospinal fluid flow rate; P is the mediated transport into brain; and the subscripts refer to the compartments shown in the flow diagram.

Similar balance equations were written for the other two compartments, and these were solved simultaneously to simulate chloride concentrations in each of the three compartments as functions of time. Simulations are compared with experimental data in Fig. 9 for compartments (1) and (2). Many parameters, such as chloride spaces, flow rates, and clearance by the artificial kidney, were required for the simulation. These are all physical and determined independently of the actual concentration simulated. The transport parameters, K and P, have negligible influence on systemic chloride concentration. Thus the prediction of plasma chloride was totally *a priori*.

Methotrexate Pharmacokinetics

We have studied quantitative aspects of the distribution and disposition of MTX in several mammalian species (Bischoff *et al.*, 1970; 1971; Dedrick *et al.*, 1970) and in the sting ray (Zaharko *et al.*, 1972). It is not metabolized significantly by these species; however, metabolism by bacteria in the gastrointestinal tract has been shown in mice and rats (Zaharko and Oliverio, 1970).

Figure 10 is a flow diagram for the distribution of MTX. The drug is rapidly excreted in the bile and urine following an intravenous or intraperitoneal injection. Partial reabsorption occurs as the drug is moved by bulk flow through the gut lumen. A typical balance equation (for the kidney) is

$$V_K \frac{dC_K}{dt} = Q_K\left(C_P - \frac{C_K}{R_K}\right) - k_K \frac{C_K}{R_K}$$

where k_K has the form of a clearance and R_K is the steady-state tissue to

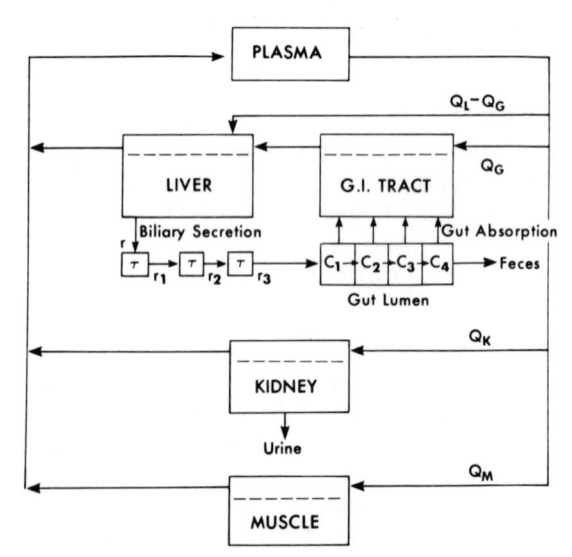

Fig. 10. Compartmental model for MTX pharmacokinetics (Bischoff *et al.*, 1971).

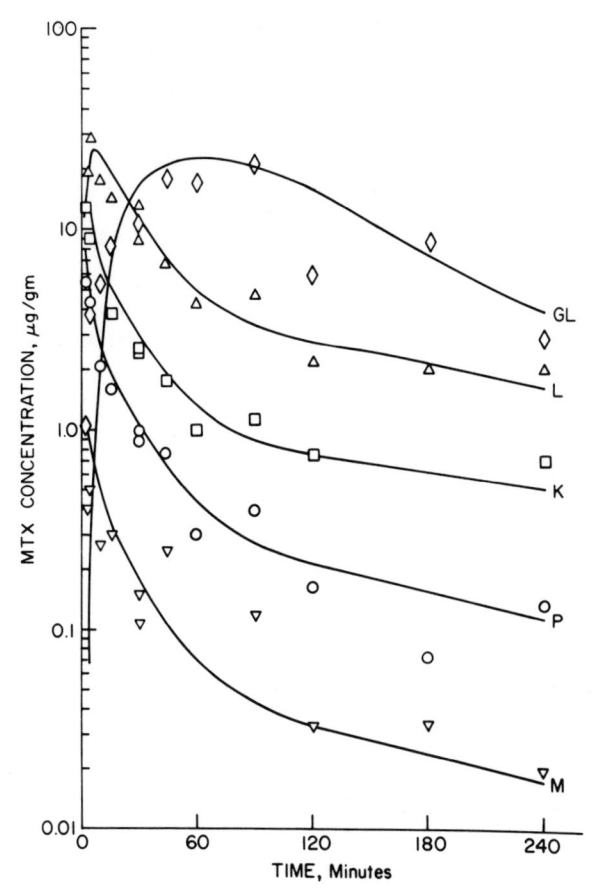

Fig. 11. Comparison of model simulations with experimental data for MTX following a dose of 3 mg/kg *in vivo* in mice (Bischoff *et al.*, 1971).

plasma ratio (e.g., from Fig. 4). Since the binding is not linear, R_K is a function of the concentration. This equation incorporates the idea of flow limitation in the sense that the drug in the plasma leaving any compartment is assumed to be in equilibrium with the tissue of that compartment.

Figure 11 illustrates a simulation of the MTX concentrations in several tissues of mice after an intravenous injection compared with experimental data. Agreement is quite good over this time scale of measurement; however, the model does not successfully extrapolate to predict plasma MTX (or DHFR equivalent) at long times, suggesting that at least one important compartment is not included in Fig. 10. Skin has some reservoir

TABLE II
Relationship Between Properties and Body Weight Among Mammals— Property ~ (Body Weight)^{Exponent}

Property	Exponent
Creatinine clearance	0.69
Inulin clearance	0.77
PAH clearance	0.80
Basal O_2 consumption	0.734
Endogenous N output	0.72
O_2 consumption by liver slices	0.77
Kidneys weight	0.85
Heart weight	0.98
Liver weight	0.87
Stomach and intestines weight	0.94
Blood weight	0.99

Abstracted from Adolph (1949).

effect in mice and rats, and reabsorption from the large intestine may be important. Further, the basic assumption of flow limitation is not valid in all tissues; significant membrane resistance to transport occurs in some (Dedrick et al., 1973).

Body Weight Relationships

Adolph (1949) observed that many anatomic and physiologic variables can be correlated among mammals as exponential functions of body weight. A few examples are shown in Table II. The anatomic variables are more nearly proportional to body weight than are the metabolic or physiologic properties. (Proportionality would be indicated by an exponent of unity.) The metabolic and physiologic properties shown exhibit exponents in the range from 0.7 to 0.8. Generally, physiologic function per unit of organ weight or per unit of animal weight thus *decreases* as size increases.

There has been considerable discussion of the use of body surface area in pharmacologic scaling. Freireich et al., (1966) observed that the maximum tolerated dose of a variety of anticancer drugs was best predicted from animal experiments if the doses were expressed on a basis of mg/m^2 of body surface area. This observation was based on data for antimetabolites, alkylating agents, and other drugs. Body surface area varies as the two-thirds power of body weight so that the use of surface area is equivalent to a body-weight correlation. Mellett (1969) called attention to the similarity of two-thirds to the range of exponents reported by Adolph. Butler (1966) has discussed some scaling concepts with particular reference to primates.

Inspection of MTX plasma concentration data from several mammalian species led us to conclude that, to a first approximation, the physical distribution effects could be separated from the kinetic and clearance effects by a simple transformation of variables. The plasma concentration data were normalized by dividing by the dose per unit body weight; the time variable was normalized by dividing by an equivalent time which is empirically proportional to body weight to the one-fourth power. Figure 12 illustrates the graphical correlation that was obtained. The figure includes data from several laboratories, by different analytical methods over a range of body sizes from 22 to 70,000 g, of dose per unit body weight of 0.1 to 450 mg/kg, and of plasma concentrations from 0.0077 to 130 µg/ml. We

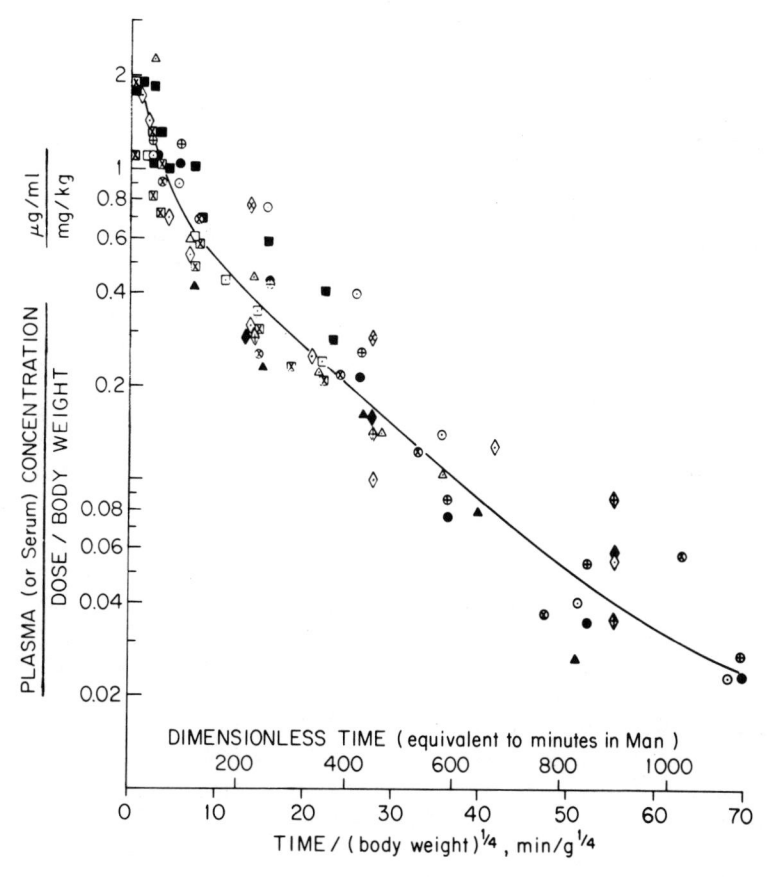

Fig. 12. Graphical correlation of plasma (or serum) concentration of MTX in mouse, rat, monkey, dog, and man (Dedrick *et al.*, 1970).

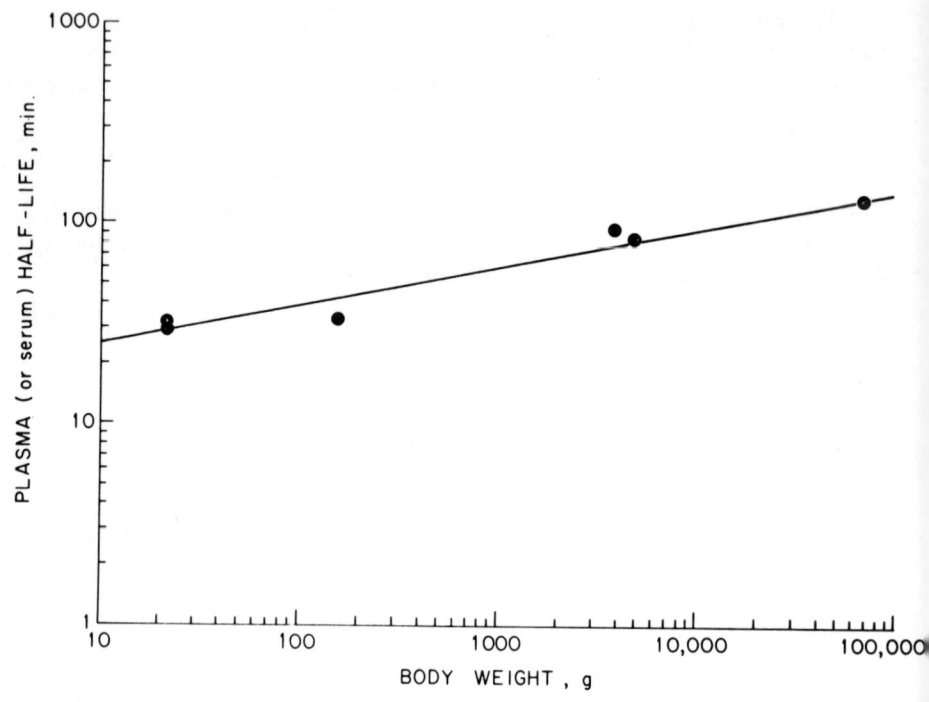

Fig. 13. Plasma (or serum) half-life of MTX *vs.* body weight for several mammals (Dedrick et al., 1970).

have found the idea of equivalent times helpful in planning kinetic experiments. For MTX distribution, one minute in the life of a mouse is equivalent to about eight minutes for man. This raises questions about the comparability of identical dose schedules in mice and men.

Whenever the type of correlation illustrated in Fig. 12 can be used, regardless of the actual function of body weight employed for normalizing the time variable, then it is possible to generalize in two ways. First, the slope of the plasma concentration curve must be a function of the body weight. Second, the area under the concentration curve must depend jointly on dose per unit body weight and the function of body weight. The former is illustrated in Fig. 13, where half-lives of MTX are plotted as functions of body weight. The slope is equal to 0.2, which is reasonably close to the expected 0.25. Disagreement may result from the fact that the concentration of MTX in plasma does not decrease as a single exponential with time so that the "half-life" depends upon the part of the curve used for calculation. The second generalization, relating to the area under the plasma concentration curve, is approximately verified by data from Mellett

(1969). The observed areas for MTX vary approximately as the 0.3 power of body weight (compare 0.25). Further, the conclusion of Wagner and Damiano (1968) concerning the proportionality of the integral with dose per unit body weight and plasma half-life for a particular drug can be obtained more generally.

Body weight is not the primary independent variable but comes into pharmacokinetics through its correlation with blood flows and clearances. We tested the ability of the model developed for mammals to simulate the distribution and disposition of MTX in the stingray. Blood flows and methotrexate clearances are very much lower in this elasmobranch than they are in a mammal of comparable size. Figure 14 shows model predictions for the plasma concentration of MTX following a dose of 3.0 mg/kg in the mouse and in the stingray. It would appear that the distribution of the drug must be very different in the two species. In fact, the physical aspects of distribution are qualitatively similar, but the time scale is changed as illustrated in Fig. 15. One minute for the mouse is comparable to about 16 min for the stingray in this context. The initial drug redistribution following an intravenous dose is over within a couple of minutes in the mouse but greatly prolonged in the ray.

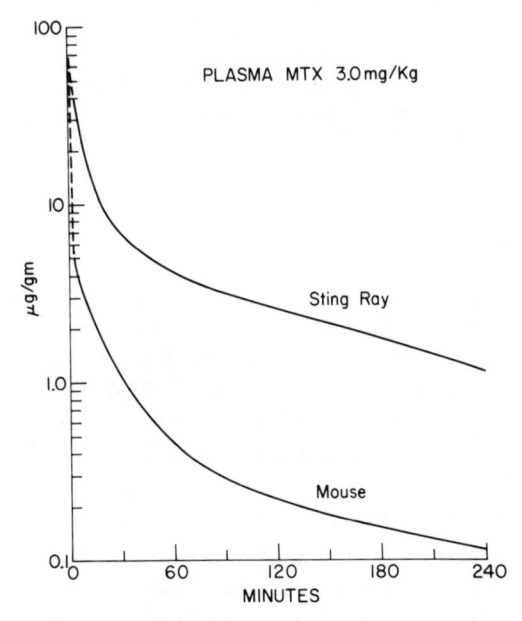

Fig. 14. Simulated plasma concentration of MTX in the mouse and the stingray (Zaharko *et al.*, 1972).

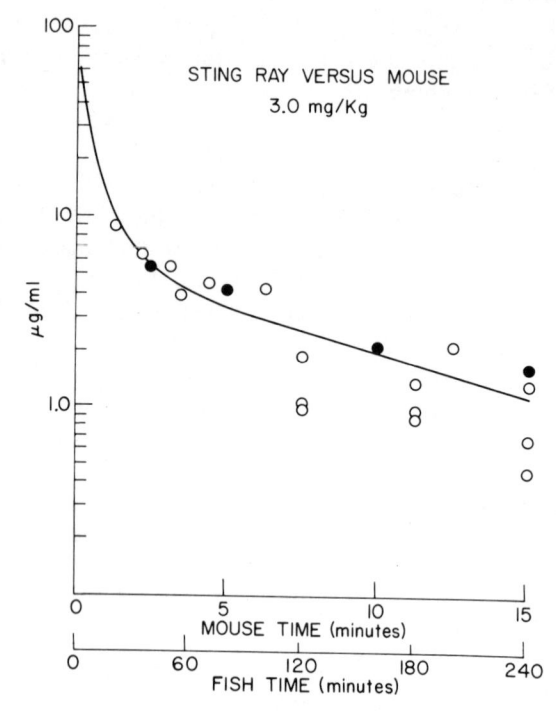

Fig. 15. Plasma MTX concentrations in the mouse (solid circles) and stingray (open circles) as functions of time. The solid line represents the model simulation for the stingray (Zaharko et al., 1972).

Metabolized Substances

If a drug is metabolized significantly, a major complication is introduced to the balance equations, because it is necessary to include suitable terms for the rate of chemical reaction. Energy metabolism bears a relationship to body size (Schmidt-Nielsen, 1970), but drug metabolism probably generally does not. Problems involving metabolism are illustrated for thiopental and cytosine arabinoside (Ara-C).

Thiopental Pharmacokinetics

The general features of thiopental distribution have been elucidated over a number of years (Brodie et al., 1950; 1952; Price et al., 1960; Mark and Brand, 1964; Saidman and Eger, 1966; Bischoff and Dedrick, 1968). It is strongly protein bound, highly lipid soluble, and rapidly metabolized in the liver. The relative roles of distribution into lean tissue, adipose tissue, and metabolism in determining pharmacologic effect have been the subject of considerable discussion.

A suitable flow diagram is illustrated in Fig. 16. It includes a well-perfused lean compartment (viscera), a poorly perfused lean compartment, and a poorly perfused adipose compartment in addition to a blood pool. This grouping is based on perfusion rates and on the different physicochemical interactions of thiopental with lean tissue and with fat. It permits the localization of the chemical reaction at least to the viscera which includes the liver. Complex balance equations are required to include both free and bound drug (Bischoff and Dedrick, 1968). Parameters relating to the physical aspects of the distribution were obtained from a variety of sources. They included consideration of nonlinear binding *in vitro* to bovine serum albumin, binding *in vitro* to rabbit tissue homogenates, the peanut oil-water distribution coefficient, and a long-time lipid-to-blood distribution coefficient *in vivo* corrected for protein binding. Compartment sizes and blood flow rates were obtained for a standard man. Only the rate of metabolism could not be determined entirely *a priori*.

Predicted thiopental concentrations in the four compartments are

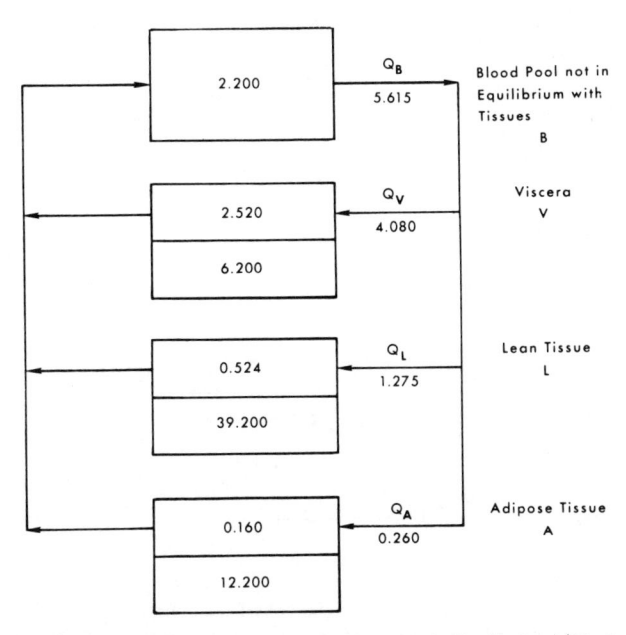

Fig. 16. Compartmental model for thiopental distribution (Bischoff and Dedrick, 1968).

compared with data from Brodie *et al.* (1950; 1952) in Fig. 17. A remarkable prediction is achieved considering that almost no dog parameters were used. The predicted concentration in the lean tissue peaks later than the observed data from the dog showing that a higher lean tissue perfusion should have been chosen. This is the expected deviation. Saturable enzyme kinetics were incorporated in the model but not fully validated.

Figure 18 shows predicted free concentrations in the four compartments. These give a better picture of the actual departure from perfusion equilibrium than the total concentrations which include effects of binding. The blood and well-perfused viscera (including brain) are quite close; perfusion equilibrium is not achieved between blood and lean tissue for

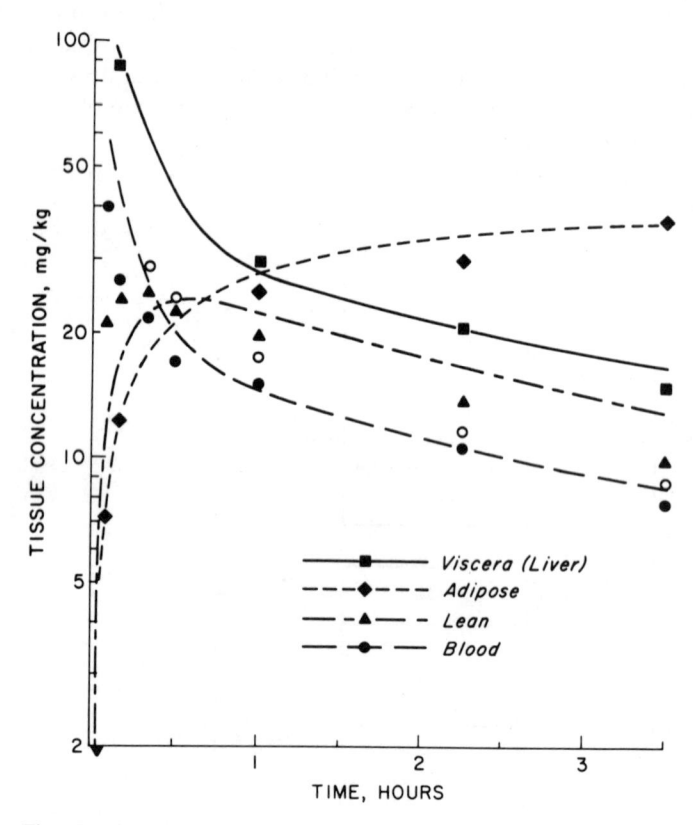

Fig. 17. Comparison of model simulations of thiopental concentrations following a dose of 25 mg/kg *i.v.* with experimental data of Brodie *et al.* (1950, 1952). The solid symbols represent the dog; the open symbols represent man (adapted from Bischoff and Dedrick, 1968).

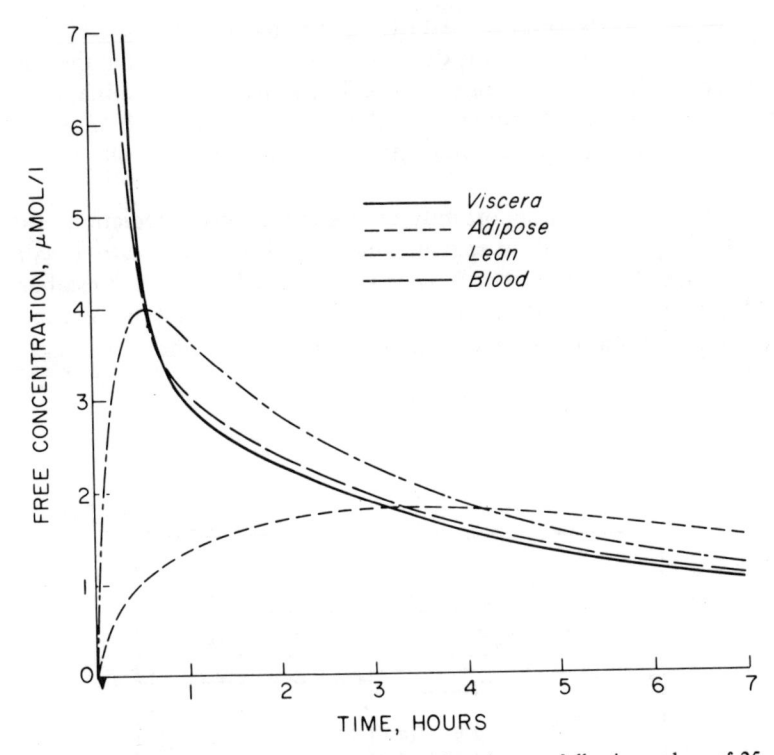

Fig. 18. Predicted free thiopental concentrations in man following a dose of 25 mg/kg *i.v.* (Bischoff and Dedrick, 1968).

about 0.5 hr; and the free concentration in the adipose tissue continues to rise for about 4 hr.

The free concentration of a drug is probably our best measure of its thermodynamic activity to correlate with binding, transport, and a variety of other biochemical interactions. If a drug is strongly and nonlinearly protein bound, the total concentration may not be a good indication of free concentration. Under conditions near saturation, a very small change in the total concentration may correspond to a large relative change in free concentration. In addition, because of the many drug–tissue interactions which do not relate to biological effect, we should question the common idea that action at a biochemical site should be associated with macroscopic drug concentration there.

Ara-C Phamacokinetics

Mellett (1969) reported plasma concentrations of Ara-C following administration of the drug to several mammalian species. He observed that there was no orderly variation with body weight and qualitatively related the interspecies variations in the disappearance of the drug from the plasma to enzyme levels that are found *in vitro*. The kinetics of deamination have been investigated extensively *in vitro* (Camiener and Smith, 1965; Camiener, 1967a; 1967b; Loo et al., 1965; Mulligan and Mellett, 1969; Tomchick et al., 1968).

Ara-C provided an opportunity to attempt a direct prediction of drug metabolism *in vivo* based on enzyme kinetics determined *in vitro* (Dedrick, Forrester, and Ho, 1972). The *in vitro* studies cited above had established that Ara-C is converted to uracil arabinoside (Ara-U) by pyrimidine nucleoside deaminase. Human liver deaminase is specific in its substrate

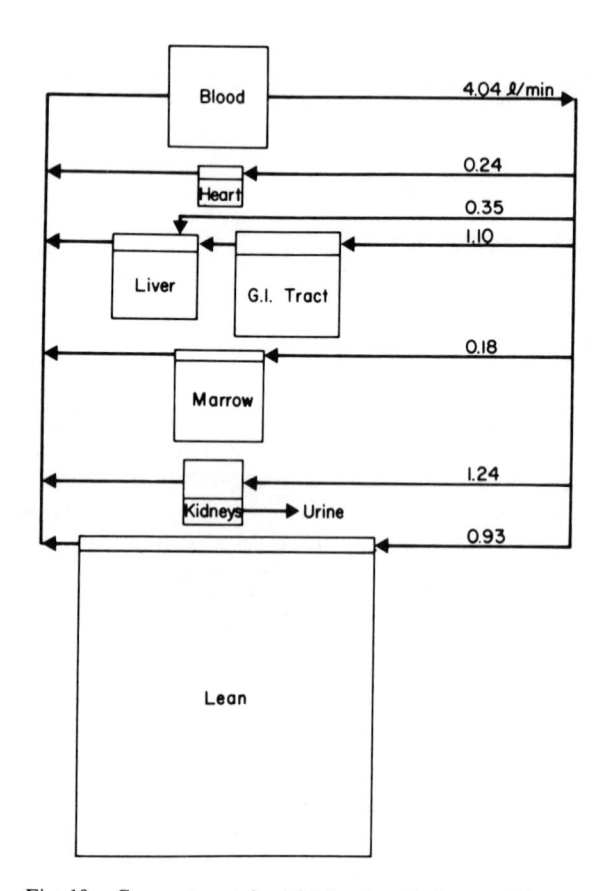

Fig. 19. Compartmental model for Ara-C pharmacokinetics (Dedrick et al., 1972).

requirement, and no direct regulatory mechanism or cofactor requirements were demonstrated. The deaminase is highly variable in location, activities, and Michaelis constants among species studied.

Figure 19 shows the flow diagram that was developed to permit prediction of concentrations in various compartments. It includes compartments which are of concern as sites of toxicity as well as those necessary to account for metabolism, excretion and distribution. A balance equation is written for each component (Ara-C and Ara-U) in each of the seven compartments. For example, the balance equation for Ara-C in the kidney

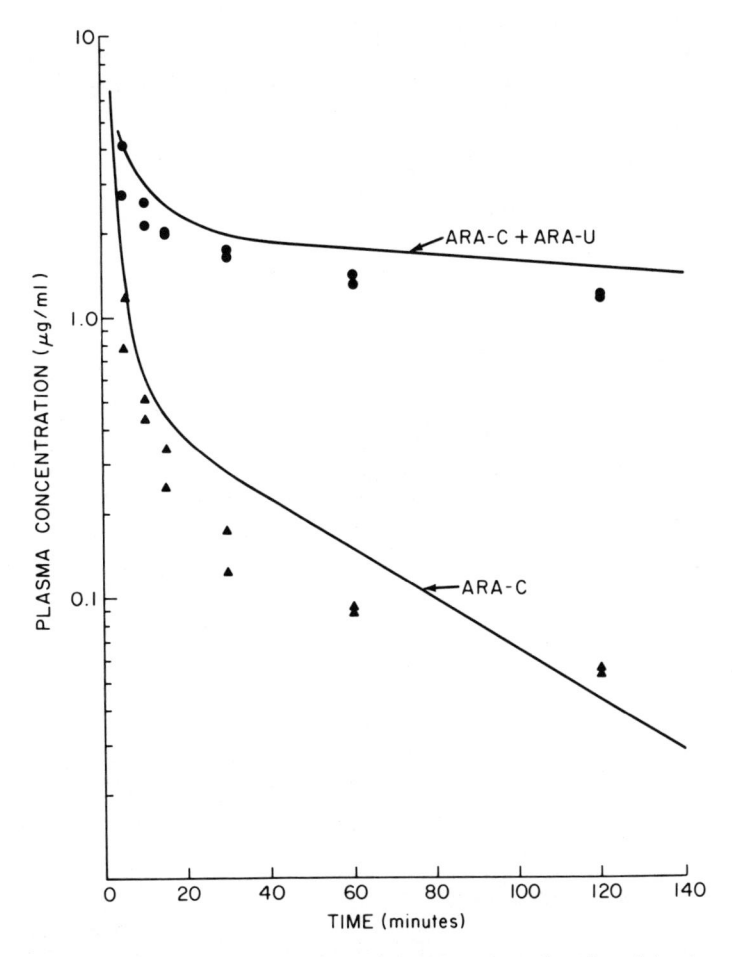

Fig. 20. Predicted concentration of Ara-C and total radioactivity in plasma of a patient compared with experimental data following a dose of 1.2 mg/kg *i.v.* (Dedrick *et al.*, 1972).

is

$$V_K \frac{dC_K}{dt} = Q_K C_B - Q_K C_K - k_K C_B - \left[\frac{v_{\max,K} C_K}{K_{m,K} + C_K}\right] V_{KT}$$

where $v_{\max}$ and K_m are the maximum reaction rate and the Michaelis constant, and the enzyme kinetics are based on kidney tissue (subscript *KT*).

Most of the variables are anatomic or physiologic and do not depend on the actual rate of metabolism. Chemical reaction rates are based upon drug concentrations at the site of metabolism which can be very different from average blood concentrations. The set of 14 differential equations was solved on a digital computer, and the solutions are the concentrations of Ara-C and Ara-U in each of the seven compartments as functions of time. Cumulative amounts in the urine are obtained by integration of $k_K C_B$ with respect to time.

Predictions of the concentrations of Ara-C and of Ara-C plus metabolite are compared with experimental data for a human in Fig. 20. All kinetic parameters were based on *in vitro* work, and all anatomic and physiologic parameters were based on data other than those predicted.

PERSPECTIVES

Detailed physiologic models of the type reviewed above have been developed for rather few drugs. Pharmacokinetic modeling of many other drugs could be attempted according to the same principles. Some of these would be quite straightforward; others would require much experimentation; and some may not be within the reach of biochemical techniques at present. The general principles force one to conduct his experiments in an operational way, i.e., one which is based on clear definitions of the terms used. This is of great help in designing experimental protocols to develop a better understanding of the physiologic, anatomic, physicochemical, and biochemical bases of drug distribution and disposition. A number of avenues of investigation are open and worthy of consideration. Some of these are direct extensions of existing theory while others are suggested by limitations on current techniques.

In Vitro–In Vivo Correlations

There is considerable discussion of the relevance of biochemical measurements conducted *in vitro* to corresponding biochemical events occurring *in vivo*. *In vitro* experimentation often has practical and scientific advantages. Physiologic modeling allows the direct incorporation of phenomena such as tissue binding and metabolism at the actual sites and in a local environment which may differ considerably from one compartment to another. The difficulties are not so much either conceptual or computational as having sufficient data obtained under appropriate experimental conditions with respect to such variables as pH and drug concentration. Complex biochemical pathways can be included in a model routinely if sufficient data exist.

Assessment of Importance of Various Effects *In Vivo*

A variety of reasons are given for limits on the effectiveness of some drugs. These include poor blood perfusion of the target tissue, low tissue permeability, strong binding, and rapid metabolism. Such concepts have no intrinsic meaning. They are useful only in some operational context. If the word "low," e.g., is used in conjunction with permeability, we must ask: "Low compared with what?" Generally we mean that the permeability poses some limitation on a particular effect *in vivo*. The same numerical value for a permeability may be low in one context and high in another depending on the time scales of related processes. Physiologic modeling enables us to examine the joint effect of a number of complex interrelated processes and assess the relative significance of each.

Individual Subject Models

No model which is based on average parameters entirely can predict pharmacokinetic events in any individual more precisely than that individual corresponds to the averages. Fortunately, large variations among individuals may significantly affect only one or a few parameters. The average model may be satisfactory for all aspects of the drug distribution except for metabolism or kidney clearance, for example, and it may be possible to obtain measures of these quite simply.

Chronopharmacology

It is generally known that many drugs can induce enzymes which catalyze chemical reactions involving them or other drugs; therefore, it is not always possible to consider enzyme kinetic parameters constant even if they are quantitated for an individual at an arbitrary time. There is a growing awareness that many biologic processes cannot be considered stationary in time and that time-dependent phenomena can have an influence on pharmacologic effect. Of particular interest are those processes which exhibit a rhythm or periodic variation with time. "Chronopharmacology" is the study of the effect of drugs on rhythm characteristics, or, conversely, the influence of biologic rhythms on drug effect (Reinberg and Halberg, 1971). These observations pose significant problems to pharmacokinetic analysis and prediction; however, they may provide additional opportunities for optimization of therapy, particularly for antineoplastic drugs. These drugs are generally toxic to sensitive normal cells, and very subtle differences in cell cycle characteristics between tumor and normal tissues may be exploitable by optimal dose scheduling. Interactions of drugs with the cell cycle may provide additional opportunities. Haus *et al.* (1972) have observed increased tolerance of leukemic mice to Ara-C when the schedule was adjusted to the circadian system.

Use of Physiologic Models with Classical Pharmacokinetics

Frequently there is no necessity to know much about the details of distribution in many tissues. It is sufficient to know and be able to control the plasma concentration. Since arterial plasma provides the input to most compartments, information on protein binding, blood flow, permeability, and specific interactions may be required at only a site of action, which can be examined in detail. There is an extensive literature on classical pharmacokinetics. Some basic sources include a review and a text by Wagner (1968; 1971).

Pharmacokinetics and Biologic Effect

One of the major goals of pharmacokinetics is to provide additional rationales for prediction of drug effect and optimization of chemotherapy. One approach is to formally relate cytokinetics to pharmacokinetics through a population balance model (Bischoff *et al.*, 1973). Another is to simulate the concentration history of a drug at a biochemical site and correlate the concentration with biochemical interactions. Brodie and Reid (1967) have emphasized the importance of plasma concentrations except for drugs such as alkylating agents. Problems related to blood flow, transport, and strong binding have been mentioned above. Frequently, the time scale is long so that poorly perfused regions and those showing some resistance to transport can be assumed to have a free drug concentration very similar to that in the plasma. Further, even though the effect of a drug such as an alkylating agent may not relate simply to its concentration at any given time, it is likely that the net effect represents some integrated result of a time-dependent local interaction.

Werkheiser (1971) has pointed out that explanation of the action of a drug *in vivo* requires consideration of many dynamic processes. He developed a mathematical model for the action of MTX *in vivo*. The model includes provision for varying plasma concentrations, passive diffusion,

DHFR synthesis and decay, oxidation and regeneration of tetrahydrofolate cofactors, and cell death in the DNA synthetic phase when cofactor concentration falls below a critical level. An important result of his simulations is that low permeability to a drug can increase toxicity because drug which enters cells at high plasma levels diffuses out slowly. Some other factors bearing on the toxicity of MTX have been discussed by Zaharko and Dedrick (1973).

ACKNOWLEDGMENTS

I thank many colleagues whose work formed a basis for this paper, particularly Kenneth B. Bischoff for his pioneering application of chemical reaction engineering to pharmacokinetics, Daniel S. Zaharko for his experimental skill and physiologic insight, and David P. Rall, who recognized the relationship of chemical engineering to problems of interspecies scaling.

REFERENCES

Adolph, E. F., 1949, *Science* **109**: 579.
Bischoff, K. B., and Brown, R. G., 1966, *Chem. Eng. Prog. Symp. Ser. No. 66*, **62**: 33.
Bischoff, K. B., and Dedrick, R. L., 1968, *J. Pharm. Sci.* **57**: 1346.
Bischoff, K. B., Dedrick, R. L., and Zaharko, D. S., 1970, *J. Pharm. Sci.* **59**: 149.
Bischoff, K. B., Dedrick, R. L., Zaharko, D. S., and Longstreth, J. A., 1971, *J. Pharm. Sci.* **60**: 1129.
Bischoff, K. B., Himmelstein, K. J., Dedrick, R. L., and Zaharko, D.S., 1973, *Advances in Chemistry Series 118*, American Chemical Society, Washington, D. C., p. 47.
Bourke, R. S., Gabelnick, H. L., and Young, O., 1970, *Exp. Brain Res.* **10**: 17.
Brodie, B. B., Bernstein, E., Mark, L. C., 1952, *J. Pharmacol. Exp. Therap.* **105**: 421.
Brodie, B. B., Kurz, H., and Shanker, L. S., 1960, *J. Pharmacol. Exp. Therap.* **130**: 20.
Brodie, B. B., Mark, L. C., Papper, E. M., Lief, P. A., Bernstein, E., and Rovenstine, E.A., 1950, *J. Pharmacol. Exp. Therap.* **98**: 85.
Brodie, B. B., and Reid, W. D., 1967, *Federation Proc.* **26**: 1062.
Butler, T. C., 1966, in: *Conference on Nonhuman Primate Toxicology*, p. 68 (C.O. Miller, ed.), Department of Health, Education, and Welfare, FDA, Washington, D.C.
Camiener, G. W., 1967a, *Biochem. Pharmacol.* **16**: 1681.
Camiener, G. W., 1967b, *Biochem. Pharmacol.* **16**: 1691.
Camiener, G. W., and Smith, C. G., 1965, *Biochem. Pharmacol.* **14**: 1405.
Crank, J., 1965, *The Mathematics of Diffusion*, Oxford, London.
Dedrick, R. L., Bischoff, K. B., and Zaharko, D. S., 1970, *Cancer Chemotherapy Rep. Part I*, **54**: 95.
Dedrick, R. L., Forrester, D. D., and Ho, D. H. W., 1972, *Biochem. Pharmacol.* **21**: 1.
Dedrick, R. L., Vantoch, P., Gombos, E. A., and Moore, R., 1967, *Trans. Am. Soc. Artificial Internal Organs* **13**: 236.
Dedrick, R. L., Zaharko, D. S., and Lutz, R. J., 1973, *J. Pharm. Sci.* **60**: 882.
Freireich, E. J., Gehan, E. A., Rall, D. P., Schmidt, L. H., and Skipper, H. E., 1966, *Cancer Chemotherapy Rep.* **50**: 219.

Gabelnick, H. L., Dedrick, R. L., and Bourke, R. S., 1970, *J. Appl. Physiol.* **28:** 639.
Gillette, J. R., 1965, in: *Drugs and Enzymes*, p. 9, *Proc. 2nd Int. Pharmacol. Mtg.*
Haus, E., Halberg, F., Scheving, L. E., Pauly, J. E., Cardosa, S., Kuhl, J. F. W., Sothern, R. B., Shiotsuka, R. N., and Hwang, D. S., 1972, *Science* **177:** 80.
Himmelblau, D. M., and Bischoff, K. B., 1968, *Process Analysis and Simulation*, John Wiley, New York.
Krüger-Thiemer, E., Bunger P., Dettli, L., Spring, P., and Wempe, E., 1965-1966, *Chemotherapia.* **10:** 61, 129, 325.
Krüger-Thiemer, E., Diller, W., and Bunger, P., 1966, in: *Antimicrobial Agents and Chemotherapy—1965* (G.L. Hobby, ed.), American Society of Microbiologists, Ann Arbor, Mich.
Loo, R. V., Brennan, M. J., and Talley, R. W., 1965, *Proc. Am. Assoc. Cancer Res.* **6:** 41.
Mark, L. C., and Brand, L., 1964, *Bull. N.Y. Acad. Med.* **40:** 476.
Mellett, L. B., 1969, *Prog. Drug Res.* **13:** 136.
Mount, D. I., and Boyle, H. W., 1969, *Environ. Sci. Tech.* **3:** 1183.
Mulligan, L. T., and Mellett, L. B., 1969, *J. Chromatog.* **43:** 376.
Perl, W., Rackow, H., Salanitre, E., Wolf, G. L., and Epstein, R. M., 1965, *J. Appl. Physiol.* **20:** 621.
Price, H. L., Kovnat, P. J., Safer, J. N., Conner, E. H., and Price, M. L., 1960, *Clin. Pharmacol. Therap.* **1:** 16.
Rackow, H., Salanitre, E., Epstein, R. M., Wolf, G. L., and Perl, W., 1965, *J. Appl. Physiol.* **20:** 611.
Rall, D. P., 1967, *Federation Proc.* **26:** 1020.
Reed, D. J., and Woodbury, D. M., 1962, *J. Physiol.* **164:** 252.
Reinberg, A., and Halberg, F., 1971, *Ann. Rev. Pharmacol.* **11:** 455.
Saidman, L. J., and Eger, E. I., 1966, *Anesthesiology* **27:** 118.
Schmidt-Nielsen, K., 1970, *Federation Proc.* **29:** 1524.
Tomchick, R., Saslaw, L. D., and Waravdekar, V. S., 1968, *J. Biol. Chem.* **243:** 2534.
Wagner, J. G., 1968, *Ann. Rev. Pharmacol.* **8:** 67.
Wagner, J. G., 1971, *Biopharmaceutics and Relevant Pharmacokinetics*, Drug Intelligence Publications, Hamilton, Illinois.
Wagner, J. G., and Damiano, R. E., 1968, *J. Clin. Pharmacol.* **8:** 102.
Werkheiser, W. C., 1971, *Ann. N.Y. Acad. Sci.* **186:** 343.
Zaharko, D. S., and Dedrick, R. L., 1973, *Proc. 5th Int. Congr. Pharmacol.* S. Karger, Basel, Vol. 3, p. 316.
Zaharko, D. S., Dedrick, R. L., and Oliverio, V. T., 1972, *Comp. Biochem. Physiol.* **42A:** 183.
Zaharko, D. S., and Oliverio, V. T., 1970, *Biochem. Pharmacol.* **19:** 2923.

DISCUSSION SUMMARY

Gillette questioned the relative importance of diffusion rates vs. perfusion rates with specific reference to fatty tissues. The model as used by Dedrick assumes that equilibrium is obtained between the perfused tissue and the emergent venous supply. Thus, it is only necessary to know the partition coefficient between the tissues and blood and the blood flow rate to each tissue. Rowland commented that the error propagated as a consequence of assuming this equilibrium is relatively small for the drugs with which he is familiar. Dedrick explained that although most of the models have been derived on the basis of flow limitation, in the sense that one assumes there is equilibrium in the free concentration between the venous blood and the tissue, it is fairly straightforward from a modeling point of view to put in finite membrane permeabilities. This was done in several important tissues for methotrexate, but none of these values play a really important role in changing the systemic pharmacokinetics.

Melmon commented on the usefulness and desirability of the perfusion models described by Dedrick and Rowland, since these models maintain their tenability in a disease state in which the kinetics of the drug may be greatly altered. Melmon felt this type of model would be extremely valuable if a feedback mechanism were incorporated to account for physiological changes induced by a drug, which might result in a change in kinetics. Such models would allow the clinician to adjust subsequent doses with respect to the pharmacokinetic changes observed.

Wagner asked to what degree blood flow rates vary from individual to individual. He felt that predictions may be insensitive to variations in individual parameters since blood level predictions are made on the basis of a large number of different parameters. Nodine responded by citing some of the experimental blood flow measurements found in his laboratory. Blood flow in muscle tissue of a normal resting man is 1 to 2 ml/min/100g; however, after moderate exercise, these values increase to 50 to 60 ml/min/100g. He also cited values for the increase in blood flow in the thyroid from 3 ml/min/100g in the normal state up to 10 to 20 ml/min/100g in hyperthyroidism.

Bischoff suggested that the reliability of the predictions in the animal scale-up models may not be as sensitive as one would expect to variations in blood flow, since the actual equations contain the blood flow to a particular tissue divided by the mass of that tissue. As may be expected, the larger the size of the tissue, the greater the flow to the tissue,, and therefore the ratio may remain fairly constant irrespective of the individual variation seen in flow parameters.

Crout asked whether changes in blood flow in a physiological range, such as following the eating of a meal, were sufficient to alter the pharmacokinetics of a drug. Rowland noted that blood flow to the liver is almost doubled in going from a prone to an upright position. The importance of this increase depends on the individual drug and the degree to which liver blood flow contributes to the drug's total clearance. Wagner pointed out that experimental conditions, such as position, could be very important when comparing different dosage forms of a drug such as seen in oral vs. *i.v.* administration. He noted that in his laboratory the subject is always maintained in the same position, whether that be prone or upright, from one experiment to the next. Riegelman reminded the group that position can also have an effect on stomach emptying, which may influence drug absorption, since the small intestine appears to be the predominant site for absorption of most drugs. For example, the absorption of tetracyclines is profoundly influenced by stomach emptying and this is probably the rate-limiting step, rather than blood flow.

Drug Metabolism in Normal and Disease States

A. H. Conney, B. Craver, and R. Kuntzman

Research Division
Hoffman-La Roche, Inc.
Nutley, New Jersey

and

E. J. Pantuck

Department of Anesthesiology
Columbia University College of Physicians and Surgeons and Presbyterian Hosptial
New York, New York

The concept that most patients have the same response to the usual therapeutic dose of a given drug is a plausible but dangerous myth. People differ in their responsiveness to drugs because of differences in receptor sensitivities, because of differences in the absorption and transport of drugs to their receptors, and because of individual differences in rates and pathways of drug metabolism. Table I shows that marked interindividual variations in steady-state blood levels and half-lives occur in different individuals receiving the same dose of a drug. In a recent study, bishydroxycoumarin, antipyrine, and phenylbutazone were administered successively to seven sets of identical twins and seven sets of fraternal twins (Vesell and Passananti, 1971; Vesell et al., 1971); the range of plasma half-lives was tenfold for bishydroxycoumarin, threefold for antipyrine, and sixfold for phenylbutazone. These marked variations were attributed to genetic factors, since they were greater in the fraternal twins than in the identical

TABLE I
Variability in Plasma Half-Lives and Steady-State Plasma Concentrations of Drugs in Different Individuals

Drug	Plasma half-life, hr	Steady-state plasma level, ng/ml
Ethylbiscoumacetate (Brodie et al., 1952)	0.7–14	
Bishydroxycoumarin (Vesell and Page, 1968a; Weiner et al., 1950)	7–74	
Antipyrine (Kolmodin et al., 1969; Vesell and Page, 1968b)	5–35	
Diphenylhydantoin (Arnold and Gerber, 1970)	7–73	
Phenylbutazone (Vesell and Page, 1968a; Burns et al., 1953)	29–175	
Desmethylimipramine (Hammer et al., 1967; Hammer and Sjöqvist, 1967)		8–290
Nortriptyline (Hammer and Sjöqvist, 1967)		10–275
Chlorpromazine (Curry and Marshall, 1968)		<10–107

twins. Similar results have been obtained in twins during studies with nortriptyline (Alexanderson et al., 1969).

It is well known that a portion of the human population is made up of slow acetylators of drugs, whereas another portion comprises fast acetylators (Evans, 1971; Kalow, 1962). The slow acetylators are more apt to develop peripheral neuropathy after taking the "usual" dose of isoniazid, since these individuals develop higher blood levels that persist longer. In some individuals, a prolonged period of apnea results from administration of succinylcholine because their plasma contains an abnormal variant of pseudocholinesterase instead of the usual form of this enzyme (Kalow, 1962). The genetic differences in esterases and in the acetylation of drugs have been studied extensively and will be discussed by Dr. La Du later at this conference.

Although the plasma concentration of diphenylhydantoin, procainamide, lidocaine, quinidine, or nortriptyline required for pharmacological activity does not vary over a large range, the dose required to achieve the desired plasma level may vary as much as tenfold or more (Koch-Weser, 1972; Vesell and Passananti, 1971). These observations suggest that determination of the concentration of drug in the blood can help the physician avoid a toxic dose on the one hand or a therapeutically ineffective dose on the other.

Thus far, we have considered the marked variations in rates of metabolism and plasma concentrations of drugs that occur in normal people given the same dose of a drug. Since most drugs are given to patients with a disease, and more often than not the patient receives several drugs at the same time, it is important to know how various disease states and concomitant drug therapy influence drug metabolism.

EFFECT OF KIDNEY DISEASE ON DRUG METABOLISM

Kidney disease slows the urinary excretion of many drugs. Examples include digoxin, bretylium, tetracycline, kanamycin, penicillin G, gentamycin, streptomycin, and other drugs that are eliminated from the body primarily by excretion in urine (Dollery, 1960; Reidenberg, 1971). The effect of kidney disease on the half-lives of various antibiotics is shown in Table II. Because of impaired elimination of these drugs in patients with kidney disease, the dose must be lowered or toxicity will occur. For instance, failure to make adjustments in the dose of streptomycin in patients with kidney disease has produced deafness. The importance of kidney function for the elimination of tetracycline from the body is shown in Table III. Individuals with a creatinine clearance of 100 ml/min had a tetracycline half-life of six hours, whereas patients with a creatinine clearance of 2 ml/min had a tetracycline half-life of 42 hours. Indeed, there was an excellent correlation between the decrease in creatinine clearance

TABLE II
Effect of Kidney Disease on the Half-Lives of Antibiotics Excreted in the Urine[a]

| | Half-lives, hr | |
Drug	Normal	Severe kidney disease
Penicillin G	0.5	10
Streptomycin	2–3	28–111
Kanamycin	2–3	20–43
Gentamycin	2–3	24
Vancomycin	6–10	144
Tetracycline	6	42

[a]Data taken from Reidenberg (1971) and from Orme and Cutler (1969).

TABLE III
Tetracycline Half-Lives in Patients with Kidney Disease[a]

Creatinine clearance, ml/min	Tetracycline half-life, hr
100	6
50	9
40	11
30	13
20	14
10	16
5	22
2	42
anuric	4 days

[a] Taken from Kunin and Finland, 1959.

and the prolongation of tetracycline half-life. The impact of renal disease on the cumulative excretion of digoxin, another drug excreted primarily unmetabolized in the urine, is shown in Fig. 1. The excretion of digoxin was markedly slowed in patients with kidney disease (Bloom and Nelp, 1966). In the patients with the worst renal damage, the fecal excretion (usually an unimportant route of elimination of digoxin) exceeded the renal, and the sum of the two was less than half of the total excretion by normal subjects.

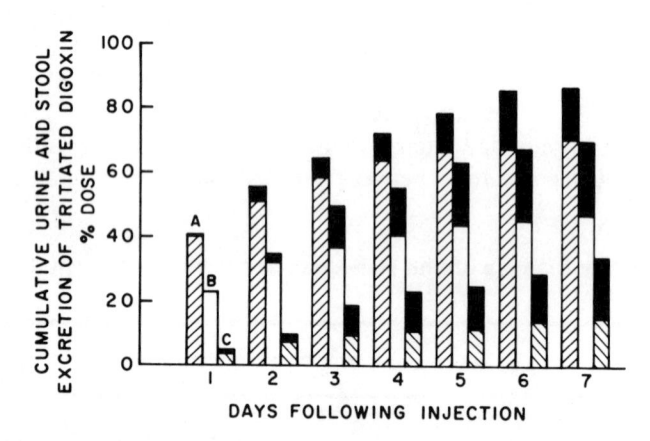

Fig. 1. The cumulative urine and stool excretions of tritium for seven days after the administration of tritiated digoxin. Mean values have been plotted for the following subjects: (A) four normal subjects; (B) three patients with a creatinine clearance of 50 to 60 ml/min; and (C) three patients with a creatinine clearance of less than 8 ml/min. The solid areas on top of each bar represent the recoveries of tritium in stool. The clear or cross-hatched portions of the bars represent urinary excretions. Taken from the data of Bloom and Nelp, 1966.

The observations described above indicate the importance, when treating patients with renal disease, of decreasing the dose of drugs eliminated by urinary excretion. The measurement of the plasma level of these drugs in patients with renal disease would help the physician in his determination of the proper dose.

Metabolism of drugs by certain pathways is slowed in uremia, and drugs metabolized by these pathways should be given in reduced dosage to uremic patients. These pathways include acetylation of sulfisoxazole (Reidenberg et al., 1969), the reduction of cortisol (Englert et al., 1958), and the hydrolysis of esters such as procaine, metabolized by plasma pseudocholinesterase (Reidenberg et al., 1972). The available evidence suggests that the concentration of plasma pseudocholinesterase is low in uremia, and not that the enzyme is inhibited by some unexcreted waste product (Reidenberg et al., 1972). In contrast, the oxidations of tolbutamide, phenobarbital and phenacetin, and the glucuronide conjugation of chloramphenicol, occur at normal rates in uremic patients (Reidenberg, 1971). The half-life of diphenylhydantoin is decreased in uremic patients (Letteri et al., 1971)—possibly because this drug binds poorly to the plasma proteins from uremic patients (Reidenberg et al., 1971). In one epileptic with severe kidney disease, the percent of unbound diphenylhydantoin was fourfold higher than normal (Odar-Cederlöf et al., 1970). Similarly, sulfonamides, barbituates, fluorescein, and tryptophan—all weak acids—also bind poorly to the plasma proteins in uremic subjects. Desmethylimipramine and quinidine—both weak bases—bind normally to plasma proteins from uremic subjects (Reidenberg et al., 1971). The possibility of a change in the protein binding of a drug in uremic plasma should be considered during drug therapy in patients with renal disease.

EFFECT OF LIVER DISEASE ON DRUG METABOLISM

Reports on the effect of liver disease on drug metabolism have not been in agreement, and Levi et al. (1968) were able to show that this was due to a disregard of the effects of concomitantly taken drugs on the metabolism of the drug under study. They determined the plasma half-lives of phenylbutazone, a drug hydroxylated by hepatic microsomal enzymes, and of isoniazid, a drug metabolized by a nonmicrosomal acetylase. A comparison of the phenylbutazone half-lives in 55 normal subjects and in 95 patients with liver disease revealed no differences between the two groups, except for a greater variability in half-lives among different patients in the liver disease group (Fig. 2). However, after Levi had subdivided the subjects according to drug intake and considered only those individuals

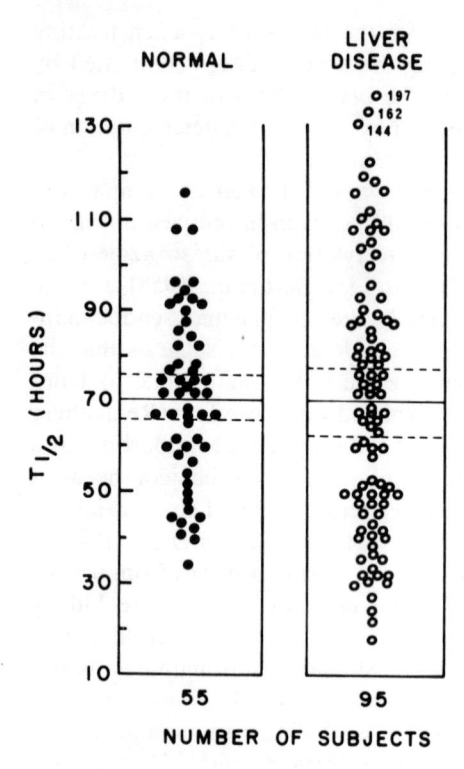

Fig. 2. Phenylbutazone half-lives in normal subjects and in patients with liver disease. [Mean (±2 S.E.M.) is shown.] Taken from Levi et al., 1968.

who had not taken drugs, those patients with liver disease metabolized phenylbutazone more slowly than did normal subjects (Fig. 3). Treatment with several drugs known to induce microsomal enzymes that hydroxylate phenylbutazone shortened its half-life but had no effect on the half-life of isoniazid. Levi concluded that genetic differences were more important than liver disease in explaining the variability in isoniazid metabolism that occurred among different patients. Although liver disease impaired the acetylation of isoniazid, no effect of liver disease on the acetylation of p-aminobenzoic acid or of sulfadiazine was observed (Gershberg and Kuhl, 1950).

Cookesley and Powell (1971) concluded that the effects of hepatic disease on drug metabolism varied with the nature and severity of the disease. They recommended treating hepatitis with prednisolone and not with prednisone, which requires biotransformation by the liver to the active metabolite prednisolone. This metabolic pathway is impaired in people with liver disease.

Niridazole (nitrothiamidazol), a schistosomicide, is usually well tolerated, but Faigle (1972) found that the higher concentrations of drug in the blood of patients with severe bilharziasis resulted in a higher incidence of

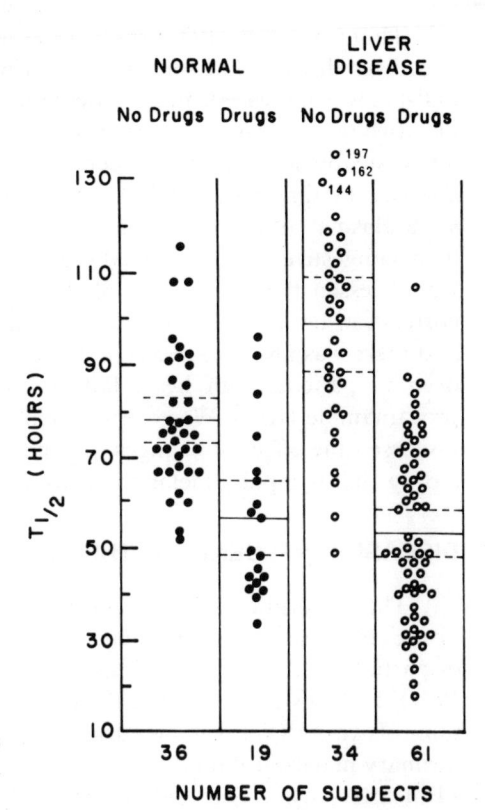

Fig. 3. Effect of drug treatment on phenylbutazone half-lives in normal subjects and in patients with liver disease. Taken from Levi et al., 1968.

adverse effects. This was due to the formation of portal-systemic shunts as the result of parasitic damage to the liver. Since the drug bypassed the liver, metabolism of the drug was delayed and higher blood levels resulted. Ueda et al. (1963) reported that the plasma half-life for tolbutamide was prolonged in patients with hepatic disease, but Nelson (1964) was unable to confirm this observation because of the high individual variations in plasma half-lives.

In mice, a high dose of paracetamol (N-acetyl-p-aminophenol) produces hepatotoxicity. The occurrence of this toxicity requires biotransformation of paracetamol to a reactive metabolite (perhaps a hydroxylamine) which reacts with macromolecules in the liver (Mitchell et al., 1972). Prescott et al. (1971) reported that an overdose of paracetamol caused hepatic necrosis in man, with a resultant lengthening of the plasma half-life of the drug. Normal subjects metabolized paracetamol with a plasma half-life of 2.0–2.9 hr, whereas in patients with liver disease the average half-life was 7.6 hr. Prescott used the rate of metabolism of paracetamol as an index of liver toxicity in patients who had taken an overdose of this drug.

Thomson et al. (1971) studied the metabolism of lidocaine in patients with liver disease. The volume of distribution was normal, but the plasma half-life was increased, and the clearance was reduced. A change in the rate of infusing the drug into normal individuals required 6 to 10 hours before a new steady-state plasma concentration was reached; in subjects with liver disease, the time required was much longer. The time to achieve a steady-state plasma concentration of lidocaine would be even longer in patients with congestive heart failure, because poor circulation through the liver would lessen the metabolism of this and other drugs. There was a good correlation between the hepatic blood flow and the clearance of lidocaine, and there was also a decrease in the apparent volume of distribution of the drug in patients with heart failure. Similar results were obtained with procainamide (Koch-Weser and Klein, 1971). Gillette (1971) has recently discussed the effect of changes in hepatic blood flow on the elimination of a drug that is rapidly metabolized by the liver.

DISEASES INFLUENCING THE ABSORPTION OF DRUGS

The absorption of vitamin E is impaired in patients with biliary obstruction, pancreatic insufficiency, steatorrhea, cystic fibrosis, or a history of partial gastrectomy (MacMahon and Neale, 1970; Harries and Muller, 1971). It seems probable that these conditions adversely affect the absorption of various fat-soluble drugs. Patients with idiopathic steatorrhea (primary malabsorption disease) excreted much less ^{35}S-thiamine in the first 24 hr after dosing than did normals (Thomson, 1966). In 1964, Brain and Booth showed that the absorption of pyridoxine was impaired by the same disease. Patients with regional ileitis (Crohn's disease) had impaired absorption of vitamin B_{12} but normal absorption of thiamine.

EFFECT OF AGE ON DRUG METABOLISM

A tendency for older patients to have a reduced intestinal blood flow may delay absorption. The elderly are apt to be more sensitive to depressants, cardiac glycosides, and to a number of other drugs (Macgregor, 1965; Aagaard, 1972). In the older patient, the metabolism and excretion of drugs in general may be slowed; consequently, the dose of some drugs should be decreased in elderly patients to avoid toxic effects. An example of a decreased rate of drug metabolism in the elderly has been described for antipyrine (Stevenson et al., 1972; O'Malley et al., 1971). These observations in man are in agreement with animal studies by Kato and Takanaka (1968), who found impaired hepatic metabolism of drugs in old rats. In a sense, the increased response of the aged to drugs (a subject heretofore little studied) reflects the impact of disease, since multiple degenerative changes occur with the passing decades. In the aged, the glomerular filtration rate may be low, and as a result the plasma half-lives of some drugs, e.g., digoxin and kanamycin, may be more than doubled.

Newborn animals possess very low drug-metabolizing enzyme activity, and they metabolize drugs very slowly *in vivo* (Fouts and Adamson, 1959; Jondorf et al., 1958). The very young are susceptible to the toxic effects of some drugs due to the inadequate development of drug-metabolizing enzymes. Many years ago, serious toxicity to chloramphenicol occurred in newborn infants given the fraction of the adult dose dictated by the body weight of the child. This toxicity occurred because chloramphenicol is metabolized more slowly in the newborn than in the adult (Weiss et al., 1960). In addition to impaired drug metabolism in the newborn, renal tubular function in the infant is poorly developed, suggesting that drugs excreted in the urine will have prolonged half-lives.

ENVIRONMENTAL CHEMICALS AND DRUG METABOLISM

Metabolic interactions between drugs are well recognized and should be considered when patients are receiving more than one drug. Examples include the stimulatory effect of phenobarbital on bishydroxycoumarin metabolism (Cucinell et al., 1965), and the inhibitory effect of chloramphenicol on tolbutamide metabolism (Christensen and Skövsted, 1969). The pharmacokinetics of drug interactions will be discussed at this conference by Dr. Malcolm Rowland.

In recent years, man has been exposed to increasingly large amounts of environmental chemicals, and many of these substances stimulate or inhibit drug metabolism (Conney and Burns, 1972). Examples of stimulators of drug metabolism in animals include halogenated hydrocarbon pesticides, polycyclic aromatic hydrocarbons, herbicides, industrial chemicals, food additives, tobacco smoke, and normal constituents of food. Environmental chemicals that inhibit drug metabolism include organophosphorus insecticides, pesticide synergists of the methylenedioxyphenyl type, carbon tetrachloride, ozone, and carbon monoxide. Most studies on the interactions between environmental chemicals and drugs have been done in animals, but there have been some studies in man.

Insecticides

Halogenated hydrocarbon insecticides in our environment are potent stimulators of drug metabolism. Figure 4 shows the range in half-lives of antipyrine after it had been administered to control subjects and to individuals working in a factory manufacturing DDT and lindane (Kolmodin et al., 1969). It is apparent that there was wide variability in plasma

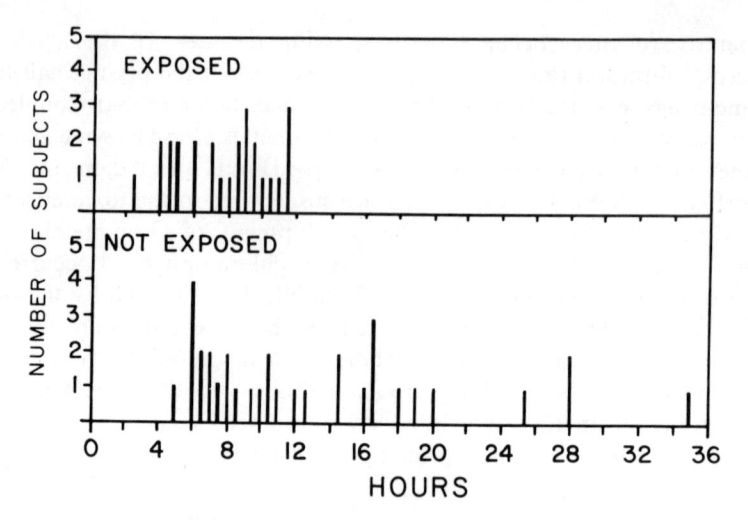

Fig. 4. Plasma half-lives of antipyrine in subjects exposed to insecticides and in nonexposed control subjects. Taken from Kolmodin et al., 1969.

half-lives of antipyrine in different individuals. In the control population, the half-lives of antipyrine varied from about 5 hr to 35 hr. In the individuals that had been exposed to insecticide, the average half-life was about half of that in the control population, and the half-lives were grouped in a narrower range. Another group of individuals working in a factory that manufactured only DDT had an enhanced rate of phenylbutazone metabolism (Poland et al., 1970). In this study, the half-life of phenylbutazone was decreased 19% and the urinary excretion of 6β-hydroxycortisol was increased 57%.

Cigarette Smoking

Recently, we studied the effects of cigarette smoking on the metabolism of phenacetin. Nine nonsmokers and nine individuals who smoked more than 15 cigarettes per day were given 900 mg of phenacetin, and the concentration of phenacetin in the blood was measured at various intervals (Pantuck et al., 1972). The plasma levels of phenacetin in the smokers were markedly lower than those in the nonsmokers (Table IV), but the average half-life of phenacetin was not changed. We showed that the lower plasma levels were not due to an altered absorption of the phenacetin, since the urinary excretion of its major metabolite, N-acetyl-p-aminophenol (paracetamol), was unaltered (Pantuck et al., 1972). We attributed the effect of cigarette smoking to an enhanced metabolism of phenacetin, either when it

TABLE IV
Plasma Levels of Phenacetin in Cigarette Smokers and Nonsmokers at Various Intervals After the Oral Administration of 900 mg of Phenacetin[a]

Hours after phenacetin administration	1	2	3½	5
Subjects	\multicolumn{4}{c}{Phenacetin in plasma, µg/ml}			
Nonsmokers	0.81 ± 0.20	2.24 ± 0.73	0.39 ± 0.13	0.12 ± 0.04
Smokers	0.33 ± 0.23	0.48 ± 0.28	0.09 ± 0.04	0.02 ± 0.01

[a]Each value represents the mean ± S.E. for nine subjects. Taken from Pantuck et al., 1972.

passed through the gastrointestinal tract or during its first few passes through the liver. This interpretation was strengthened by data obtained from measuring the levels of N-acetyl-p-aminophenol in the plasmas of the smokers and nonsmokers. The plasma levels of unconjugated or total N-acetyl-p-aminophenol in the plasmas of the smokers were only slightly lower than those in the nonsmokers (Table V), and the ratios of the plasma concentration of total N-acetyl-p-aminophenol to phenacetin were increased severalfold in the smokers (Table VI). These results indicated that cigarette smoking stimulated the metabolism of phenacetin to N-acetyl-p-aminophenol, but the results did not demonstrate where the enhanced metabolism occurred.

In order to learn whether polycyclic hydrocarbons in cigarette smoke could influence the gastrointestinal metabolism of phenacetin, we studied the effects of 3,4-benzpyrene administration on the metabolism of C^{14}-

TABLE V
Concentration of Unconjugated and Total N-Acetyl-p-Aminophenol (APAP) in Plasmas from Cigarette Smokers and Nonsmokers at Various Intervals After the Oral Administration of 900 mg of Phenacetin[a]

Hours after phenacetin administration	1	2	3½	5
Subjects	\multicolumn{4}{c}{Free APAP in plasma, µg/ml}			
Nonsmokers	4.08 ± 0.54	7.82 ± 0.85	5.84 ± 0.79	3.80 ± 0.58
Smokers	3.67 ± 0.87	5.62 ± 0.84	3.76 ± 0.54	2.29 ± 0.32
	\multicolumn{4}{c}{Total APAP in plasma, µg/ml}			
Nonsmokers	6.26 ± 0.84	13.52 ± 1.51	13.76 ± 1.00	10.25 ± 0.76
Smokers	5.66 ± 1.38	11.37 ± 1.60	11.44 ± 1.39	7.49 ± 0.95

[a]Total APAP was measured after hydrolysis of APAP conjugates by treatment of the plasma with Glusulase. Each value represents the mean ± S.E. for nine subjects. Taken from Pantuck et al., unpublished observations.

TABLE VI
Ratios of Concentration of Total N-Acetyl-p-Aminophenol (APAP) to Concentration of Phenacetin in Plasmas of Cigarette Smokers and Nonsmokers at Various Intervals After the Oral Administration of 900 mg of Phenacetin[a]

Hours after phenacetin administration:	1	2	3½	5
Subjects	Ratio of total APAP/phenacetin in plasma			
Nonsmokers	7.7	6.0	35.3	85.4
Smokers	17.2	23.7	127.1	374.5

[a] Each value represents the mean for nine subjects. Taken from Pantuck et al., unpublished observations.

phenacetin by enzymes in the intestinal mucosa of the rat. The data indicate that O-dealkylation of phenacetin did occur, to a small extent, by an enzyme system in the small intestine, and that the activity of this enzyme was stimulated by treatment of rats with 3,4-benzpyrene (Table VII).

Cigarette smoking enhances the *in vivo* metabolism of nicotine in man (Beckett and Triggs, 1967), which may explain the tolerance to nicotine that occurs in smokers. Long-term marihuana smokers metabolize Δ^9-tetrahydrocannabinol more rapidly than nonsmokers (Lemberger et al., 1971), and cigarette smokers require a larger dose of pentazocine for analgesia than do nonsmokers (Keeri-Szanto and Pomeroy, 1971). The results that we have presented concerning phenacetin's metabolism, and the other studies cited above, indicate that it is important to find out if cigarette smoking stimulates the metabolism of other commonly used drugs and whether this effect adversely influences the actions of these drugs.

TABLE VII
Effect of Pretreatment of Rats with 3,4-Benzpyrene on the *In Vitro* Metabolism of Phenacetin by Intestinal Mucosa[a]

	N-Acetyl-p-aminophenol formed (ng/500 mg intestinal mucosa/30 min)			
Treatment	Experiment 1	Experiment 2	Experiment 3	Average
Control	12	45	50	36
3,4-Benzpyrene	100	134	139	124

[a] Male Long Evans rats weighing 190–210 g were treated with corn oil or 3,4-benzpyrene (40 mg/kg in corn oil, p.o.) once daily for two days. The rats were killed 24 hr after the last dose. The intestinal mucosas were homogenized and incubated with 10 μg of C^{14}-phenacetin and an NADPH-generating system. N-Acetyl-p-aminophenol was isolated by chromatography on glass aluminum oxide thin-layer plates, and the C^{14}-N-acetyl-p-aminophenol was quantified in a liquid scintillation spectrometer. Each value was obtained with pooled intestinal mucosas from 4 to 6 rats. Taken from Pantuck et al., unpublished observations.

TABLE VIII
Effect of Vegetables on Benzpyrene Hydroxylase Activity in Small Intestine[a]

Addition to purified diet	Benzpyrene hydroxylase activity, units/mg wet weight
None	0.1
Cauliflower	1.0
Broccoli	3.5
Turnips (greens)	5.4
Cabbage	11.6
Brussels sprouts	23.8

[a] Diets containing 25% dried vegetable powder were fed to rats for 7 days. Taken from Wattenberg, 1971.

DIETARY FACTORS

Starvation inhibits hepatic drug metabolism in rodents (Dixon et al., 1960), and vitamin C deficiency inhibits hepatic drug metabolism in guinea pigs (Conney et al., 1961; Degkwitz and Staudinger, 1965; Degkwitz et al., 1968; Kato et al., 1968; Zannoni, 1972; Avenia, 1972). Although dietary factors are important in studies of drug metabolism, very little systematic research has been done in this area. Some years ago, Dr. R. Brown and Drs. J.A. and E.C. Miller at the University of Wisconsin found that certain peroxides in stored food stimulated the hepatic metabolism of an aminoazo dye (Brown et al., 1954). More recently, Wattenberg et al. (1968) found that some flavones present in food stimulated the metabolism of 3,4-benzpyrene in the liver and in nonhepatic tissues. Wattenberg (1971) also reported that feeding certain vegetables to rats markedly enhanced benzpyrene hydroxylase activity in the small intestine. The results of these studies have been summarized in Table VIII. A very large increase in hydroxylating activity was observed after substances such as Brussels sprouts and cabbage had been fed to rats; the largest increase was more than two-hundredfold. The observations made in rats may have important implications for the metabolism of drugs in animals and in man. There is a great need to determine whether Brussels sprouts, cabbage, or other foods can stimulate the metabolism of drugs in man.

CONCLUDING REMARKS

Many factors influence the metabolism of drugs in man, and these should be considered during drug therapy. We have discussed a few of these factors, and many others exist. Because marked genetic differences in drug metabolism occur among normal individuals, one person may metabolize a drug much more rapidly than another. These observations indicate that it is important to tailor the dose to the individual patient. The measurement of blood levels of drugs can be of considerable help in selecting the dose that will be safe and effective for each patient. In addition to large, genetically determined differences in drug metabolism in normal individuals, the effects of disease states, of concomitant drug therapy, and of environmental chemicals can markedly influence drug metabolism. The many factors that influence drug metabolism indicate the importance of developing rapid and simple methods for measuring the concentrations of drugs in blood and for the wide-scale monitoring of blood levels in individuals that undergo drug therapy.

ACKNOWLEDGMENT

We thank Mrs. MaryAnn Augustin for her excellent assistance in the preparation of this manuscript.

REFERENCES

Aagaard, G. N., 1972, *Postgrad. Med.* **52**: 115.
Alexanderson, B., Evans, D. A. P., and Sjöqvist, F., 1969, *Brit. Med. J.* **4**: 764.
Arnold, K., and Gerber, N., 1970, *Clin. Pharmacol. Therap.* **11**: 121.
Avenia, R. W., 1972, *Federation Proc.* **31**: 547.
Beckett, A. H., and Triggs, E. J., 1967, *Nature* **216**: 587.
Bloom, P. M., and Nelp, W. B., 1966, *Am. J. Med. Sci.* **251**: 133.
Brain, M. C., and Booth, C. C., 1964, *Gut* **5**: 241.
Brodie, B. B., Weiner, M., Burns, J. J., Simson, G., and Yale, E. K., 1952, *J. Pharmacol. Exp. Therap.* **106**: 453.
Brown, R. R., Miller, J. A., and Miller, E. C., 1954, *J. Biol. Chem.* **209**: 211.
Christensen, L. K., and Skövsted, L., 1969, *Lancet* **2**: 1397.
Conney, A. H., and Burns, J. J., 1972, *Science* **178**: 576.
Conney, A. H., Bray, G. A., Evans, C., and Burns, J. J., 1961, *Ann. N.Y. Acad. Sci.* **92**: 115.
Cookesley, W. G. E., and Powell, L. W., 1971, *Drugs* **2**: 177.
Cucinell, S. A., Conney, A. H., Sansur, M., and Burns, J. J., 1965, *Clin. Pharmacol. Therap.* **6**: 420.
Curry, S. H., and Marshall, J. H. L., 1968, *Life Sci.* **7**: 9.
Degkwitz, E., and Staudinger, Hj., 1965, *Hoppe-Selyer's Z. Physiol. Chem.* **342**: 63.
Degkwitz, E., Luft, D., Pfeiffer, U., and Staudinger, Hj., 1968, *Hoppe-Selyer's Z. Physiol. Chem.* **349**: 465.
Dixon, R. L., Shultice, R. W., and Fouts, J. R., 1960, *Proc. Soc. Exp. Therap.* **103**: 333.
Dollery, C. T., Emslie-Smith, D., and McMichael, J., 1960, *Lancet* **1**: 296.
Englert, E., Jr., Brown, H., Willardson, D. G., Wallach, S., and Simons, E.L., 1958, *J. Clin. Endocrinol.* **18**: 36.
Evans, D. A. P., 1971, *Acta Pharmacol. Toxicol.* **29**: (Suppl. 3), 156.
Faigle, J. W., 1972, *Acta Pharmacol. Toxicol.* **29**: (Suppl. 3), 233.
Fouts, J. R., and Adamson, R. H., 1959, *Science* **129**: 897.

Gershberg, H., and Kuhl, W. J., Jr., 1950, *J. Clin. Invest.* **29**: 1625.
Gillette, J. R., 1971, *Ann. N.Y. Acad. Sci.* **179**: 43.
Hammer, W., and Sjöqvist, F., 1967, *Life Sci.* **6**: 1895.
Hammer, W., Idestrom, C. W., and Sjöqvist, F., 1967, *Excerpta Medica*, p. 301. *Proc. First International Symposium on Antidepressant Drugs*, Milan, 1966.
Harries, J. T., and Muller, D. P. R., 1971, *Arch. Diseases Childhood* **46**: 341.
Jondorf, W. R., Maickel, R. P., and Brodie, B. B., 1958, *Biochem. Pharmacol.* **1**: 352.
Kalow, W., 1962, *Pharmacogenetics: Heredity and the Response to Drugs*, W.B. Saunders Company, Philadelphia.
Kato, R., and Takanaka, A., 1968, *Japan J. Pharmacol.* **18**: 389.
Kato, R., Takanaka, A., and Oshima, T., 1969, *Japan J. Pharmacol.* **19**: 25.
Keeri-Szanto, M., and Pomeroy, J. R., 1971, *Lancet* **1**: 947.
Koch-Weser, J., and Klein, S. W., 1971, *J. Am. Med. Assoc.* **215**: 1454.
Koch-Weser, J., 1972, *N. Engl. J. Med.* **287**: 227.
Kolmodin, B., Azarnoff, D. L., and Sjöqvist, F., 1969, *Clin. Pharmacol. Therap.* **10**: 638.
Kunin, C. M., and Finland, M., 1959, *Am. Med. Assoc. Arch. Intern. Med.* **104**: 1030.
Lemberger, L., Tamarkin, N. R., Axelrod, J., and Kopin, I. J., 1971, *Science* **173**: 72.
Letteri, J. M., Mellk, H., Louis, S., Kutt, H., Durant, P., and Glazko, A., 1971, *New Engl. J. Med.* **285**: 648.
Levi, A. J., Sherlock, S., and Walker, D., 1968, *Lancet* **1**: 1275.
Macgregor, A. G., 1965, *Proc. Roy. Soc. Med.* **58**: 943.
MacMahon, M. T., and Neale, G., 1970, *Clin. Sci.* **38**: 197.
Mitchell, J. R., Potter, W. Z., Jollon, D., Davis, D. C., Gillette, J. R., and Brodie, B. B., 1972, *Federation Proc.* **31**: 539.
Nelson, E., 1964, *Am. J. Med. Sci.* **248**: 657.
Odar-Cederlöf, I., Lunde, P., and Sjöqvist, F., 1970, *Lancet* **2**: 831.
O'Malley, K., Crooks, J., Duke, E., and Stevenson, I. H., 1971, *Brit. Med. J.* **3**: 607.
Orme, B. M., and Cutler, R. E., 1969, *Clin. Pharm. Therap.* **10**: 543.
Pantuck, E. J., Kuntzman, R., and Conney, A. H., 1972, *Science* **175**: 1248.
Pantuck, E. J., Hsaio, K.-C., Kuntzman, R., and Conney, A.H., 1972, unpublished observations.
Poland, A., Smith, D., Kuntzman, R., Jacobson, M., and Conney, A. H., 1970, *Clin. Pharmacol. Therap.* **11**: 724.
Prescott, L. F., Roscoe, P., Wright, N., and Brown, S. S., 1971, *Lancet* **1**: 519.
Reidenberg, M. M., 1971, *Renal Function and Drug Action*, W. B. Saunders Company, Philadelphia.
Reidenberg, M. M., Kostenbauder, H., and Adams, W., 1969, *Metabolism* **18**: 209.
Reidenberg, M. M., Odar-Cederlöf, I., vonBahr, C., Borgå, O., and Sjöqvist, F., 1971, *New Engl. J. Med.* **285**: 264.
Reidenberg, M. M., James, M., and Dring, L. G., 1972, *Clin. Pharmacol. Therap.* **13**: 279.
Stevenson, I. H., O'Malley, K., Turnbull, M. J., Ballinger, B. R., 1972, *J. Pharm. Pharmacol.* **24**: 577.
Thomson, A. D., 1966, *Clin. Sci.* **31**: 167.
Thomson, P. D., Rowland, M., and Melmon, K. L., 1971, *Am. Heart J.* **82**: 417.
Ueda, H., Sakaurai, T., Ota, M., Nakajima, A., Kamii, K., and Naezawa, H., 1963, *Diabetes* **12**: 414.
Vesell, E. S. and Page, J. G., 1968a, *J. Clin. Invest.* **47**: 2657.
Vesell, E., and Page, J. G., 1968b, *Science* **161**: 72.
Vesell, E., and Passananti, G. I., 1971, *Clin. Chem.* **17**: 851.
Vesell, E., Passananti, G. T., Greene, F. E., and Page, J. G., 1971, *Ann. N.Y. Acad. Sci.* **179**: 752.

Wattenberg, L. W., 1971, *Cancer* **28**: 99.
Wattenberg, L. W., Page, M. A., and Leong, J. L., 1968, *Cancer Res.* **28**: 934.
Weiner, M., Shapiro, S., Axelrod, J., Cooper, J. R., and Brodie, B. B., 1950, *J. Pharmacol. Exp. Therap.* **99**: 409.
Weiss, C. F., Glazko, A. J., and Weston, J. K., 1960, *New Engl. J. Med.* **262**: 787.
Zannoni, V. G., Flynn, E. J., and Lynch, M., 1972, *Biochem. Pharm.* **21**: 1377.

DISCUSSION SUMMARY

In response to the question of whether men living in urban and rural environments differed in drug-metabolizing capacity, Conney said such studies had been done with pentazocine and that to produce the same effect individuals in an urban environment required larger doses of pentazocine than those living in a rural environment.

Vesell stated that in addition to the diseases mentioned by Conney, thyroid disorders also cause alterations in rates of drug metabolism. In hyperthyroid patients, antipyrine metabolism is accelerated, whereas in hypothyroid patients, antipyrine metabolism is retarded compared to rates in euthyroid volunteers.

Axelrod inquired whether thyroid hormone affects drug metabolism in animals. Conney replied that the situation in the rat was complicated, depending on sex and the particular drug being investigated. Thyroxin enhances zoxazolamine metabolism in male rats, but for hexobarbital the effect is opposite. Conney stated that this observation provides additional evidence that different drugs are metabolized by different hepatic microsomal enzymes and that they are under separate regulatory control.

Drug Action: Target Tissue, Dose–Response Relationships, and Receptors

E.J. Ariëns and A.M. Simonis

Pharmacological Institute
University of Nijmegen
Nijmegen, The Netherlands

In the complex processes of drug action three main phases can be distinguished (Fig. 1): the pharmaceutical phase, the pharmacokinetic phase and the pharmacodynamic phase. They form a suitable frame for the discussion of the chemical basis of drug action.

THE PHARMACEUTICAL PHASE

This phase includes the disintegration of the drug application form, the dissolution of the drug, and the decay due to instability of the drug at the site of application and absorption (e.g., in the tractus intestinalis). The efficacy of a drug application form is dependent on the fraction of the dose which becomes available for absorption (the *pharmaceutical availability*) and the availability profile which takes the time factor into account. In the design of drug application forms the objective is a pharmaceutical availability which is as high as possible and an availability profile adapted to the therapeutic requirements. Drug–drug interactions which result in a decrease of the pharmaceutical availability, i.e., in a pharmaceutical incompatibility, must therefore be avoided. The pharmaceutical availability of a drug is dependent on a variety of factors, such as the crystal type and size of the drug, the additives used, and the technical procedure followed in the production of the application form. Chemical equivalence of drug preparations therefore is no guarantee of biological equivalence.

Scheme 1

| I Pharmaceutical phase | II Pharmacokinetic phase | III Pharmacodynamic phase |

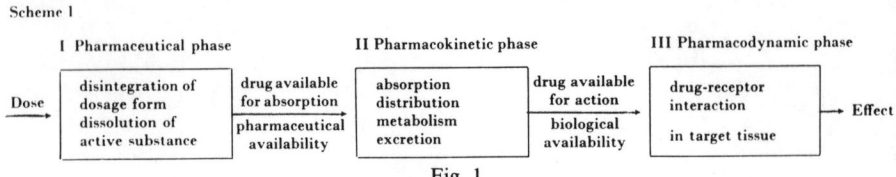

Dose → | disintegration of dosage form / dissolution of active substance | drug available for absorption / pharmaceutical availability | absorption / distribution / metabolism / excretion | drug available for action / biological availability | drug-receptor interaction in target tissue | → Effect

Fig. 1

THE PHARMACOKINETIC PHASE

This phase comprises the processes of absorption, metabolism, binding to plasma and tissue proteins, distribution, and elimination. These are determinant for the concentration of the drug in its active form reached in the various compartments. A parameter often used in this respect is the *biological availability* (bioavailability). This can be defined as that part of the dosage of the drug that reaches general circulation in its active form and thus is available for systemic action (Ritschel, 1972). In this definition the elimination of the drug due to metabolism at first passage through the liver after oral administration is taken into account. Also, the surface under the time–plasma concentration curve is used as a parameter to indicate the bioavailability or systemic availability of the drug. Two drug preparations with an equal biological availability may differ greatly in their therapeutic efficacy since they may differ essentially in their *bioavailability profile*, the form of the time–plasma concentration curve. In the design of drugs and drug application forms, specifications for the bioavailability profile required for optimal therapeutic efficacy should be taken into account. This implies that, besides a study of the pharmacokinetics and therewith the bioavailability profiles of existing drugs and drug preparations to which much effort is devoted, clinicians together with pharmacokineticists should try to formulate general specifications for the bioavailability profile of various types of therapeutics. This, then, might contribute to the development of drugs with built-in optimalized availability profiles.

For a variety of drugs it is known that not the compound applied, but some metabolite is partly or mainly responsible for therapeutic and/or side effects. In these cases the compound applied is a pro-drug, a pharmacogen, which is converted in the body to the active product. The availability profile of this active product is determinant. This holds true, for instance, for the various transport forms of drugs, such as drugs with disposable facilitating moieties, disposable restricting moieties, disposable desolubilizing moieties, disposable masking moieties, etc. (Ariëns, 1971b).

One particular type of side effect is to be mentioned explicitly: the *chemical lesions* caused by reactive short-living intermediate products in drug metabolism. Such reactive intermediate products (e.g., epoxides, free radicals, and peroxides) act as biologically alkylating or acylating agents, binding covalently to cell constituents, or as oxidants, and thus cause irreversible changes: chemical lesions (Brodie, 1972; Symposium, 1973). Such lesions may be involved in carcinogenic and mutagenic actions, tissue necrosis, allergic sensitization, and photosensitization. A certain degree of protection against the reactive intermediate products of drug metabolism is possible by means of glutathion and probably by radio-protective agents. These then will appear in the urine coupled to the biologically alkylating intermediate metabolites, bound at the reactive site in these metabolites. If this type of bioactivation is involved, the tissue in which the reactive intermediate product is generated as a rule will also be the tissue where the lesion is induced, the response tissue. The rate of product formation, then, is a relevant parameter. Species differences in the response and tissue differences in the localization of the response will be often based on species and tissue differences in drug-metabolizing capacity.

The concentration of the active product in the general circulation in certain cases is suitable, but in many cases is only a poor measure for the concentration of the active product in the target organs.

THE PHARMACODYNAMIC PHASE

This phase covers the interaction of the drug molecules with the molecular sites of action, the specific receptors for the drug in the target tissue (the target compartment or biophase), resulting in the induction of a stimulus which finally leads to the response in the effector organ (Fig. 2). Target tissue and effector organ are not necessarily identical. Most convulsants, for instance, have their sites of action in the central nervous system while the effect is observed in the voluntary muscular system. One drug may induce a whole spectrum of actions. The various components in this spectrum are not necessarily induced on one type of specific receptors. In those cases that components in the spectrum of action of a drug are induced on different types of receptors, separation and thus elimination of particular components will be possible by suitable molecular manipulation.

Pharmacodynamic Phase

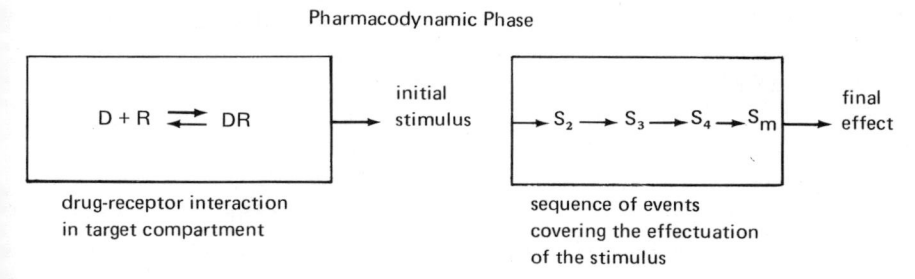

D + R ⇌ DR → initial stimulus → $S_2 \rightarrow S_3 \rightarrow S_4 \rightarrow S_m$ → final effect

drug-receptor interaction
in target compartment

sequence of events
covering the effectuation
of the stimulus

Fig. 2

The Drug Concentration in the Target Compartment

From the fact that the bioavailability profile in certain cases supplies useful information with regard to the efficacy of a drug product, it may be concluded that in these cases there is a relatively simple relationship between the concentrations of the drug in the extracellular field, the plasma, and the various target compartments. There have been effective efforts to eliminate particular components from the spectrum of actions of drugs by restricting their distribution with regard to particular target compartments. Introduction of a highly ionized onium group in anticholinergic, cholinergic, or antihistaminic agents, for instance, results in an elimination of the effects on the central nervous system (Fig. 3) (Hansson et al., 1961). The highly ionized groups serve as restricting moieties. Efforts to promote particular actions by selective bioactivation in the target compartment have been less successful up to now. The use of phosphates of estrogenic compounds, to be activated by acidic phosphatase in the target compartment, the prostate tissue in the case of cancer of that organ, has not been fully successful, since bioactivation also takes place in the liver and kidney which are also rich in the enzyme concerned. More effective were the efforts to obtain selectivity in action by designing compounds preferentially and rapidly bioinactivated outside the target compartments, namely, by introduction of suitable vulnerable moieties. As such serve the carboxy-ester groups in local anesthetics, rapidly hydrolyzed and thus bioinactivated once they reach the general circulation, and in selective organic phosphates—insecticides—rapidly hydrolyzed in the economic species (mammalian tissues are rich in carboxy-esterases) and only slowly hydrolyzed by insects. Both the bioavailability profile in the extracellular fluid or general circulation and the partition over the various compartments can be modulated by suitable chemical modification (Ariëns, 1971b).

The occurrence of particularly high concentrations of a drug in a particular tissue does not mean that this tissue can be regarded as target tissue. A number of bisonium compounds (curariform drugs), for instance, accumulate selectively in cartilage (acidic mucopolysaccharides) (Fig. 4) (Wieriks, 1972). Neither do low concentrations of a drug in a particular compartment as compared to the concentrations in plasma necessarily imply that selective transport or barrier mechanisms are involved. As indicated, the blood–brain barrier is involved in the restriction in the distribution of the quaternary onium compounds. In many cases, however, differences in the concentrations of a drug in plasma and cerebrospinal fluid have little to do with the blood–brain barrier but are mainly due to the plasma protein binding. Then the total plasma concentration of the drug

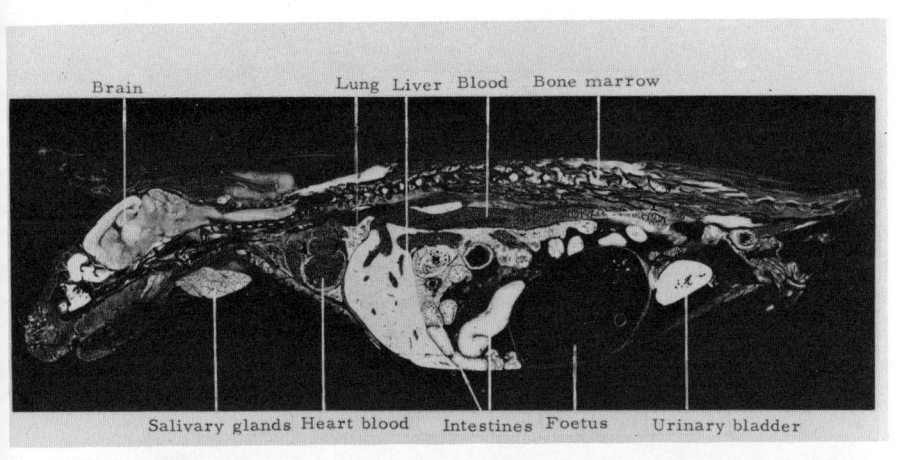

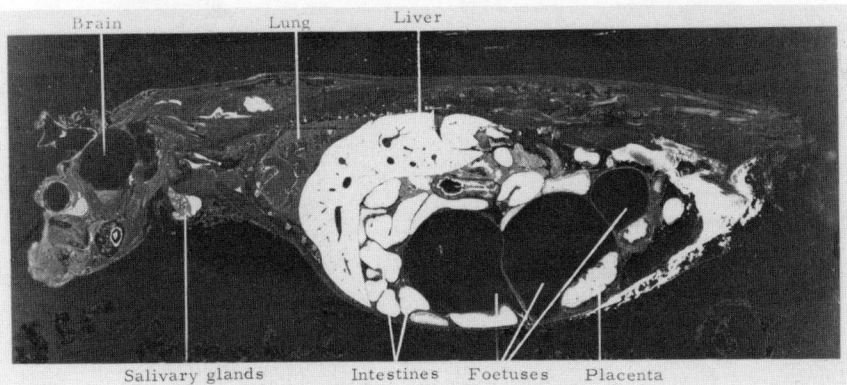

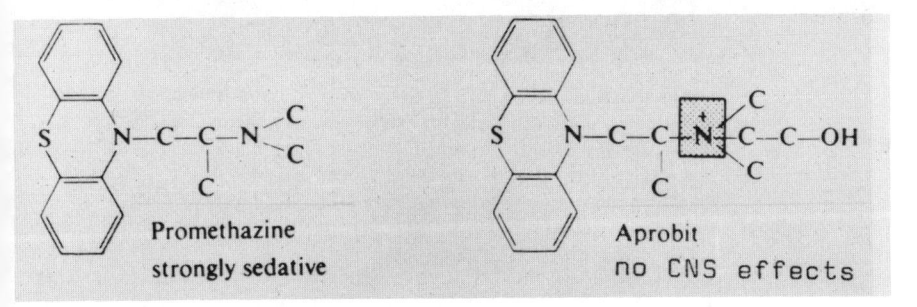

Fig. 3. A comparison of the distribution and excretion of two antihistaminics, the tertiary promethazine (a) and the quaternary Aprobit (b), both phenothiazine compounds labeled with ^{35}S. Note the high concentration of the tertiary amine in brain tissue and the restriction in the distribution of the quaternary compound mainly to the liver and the intestines (Hansson and Schmiterlöw, 1961).

(a)

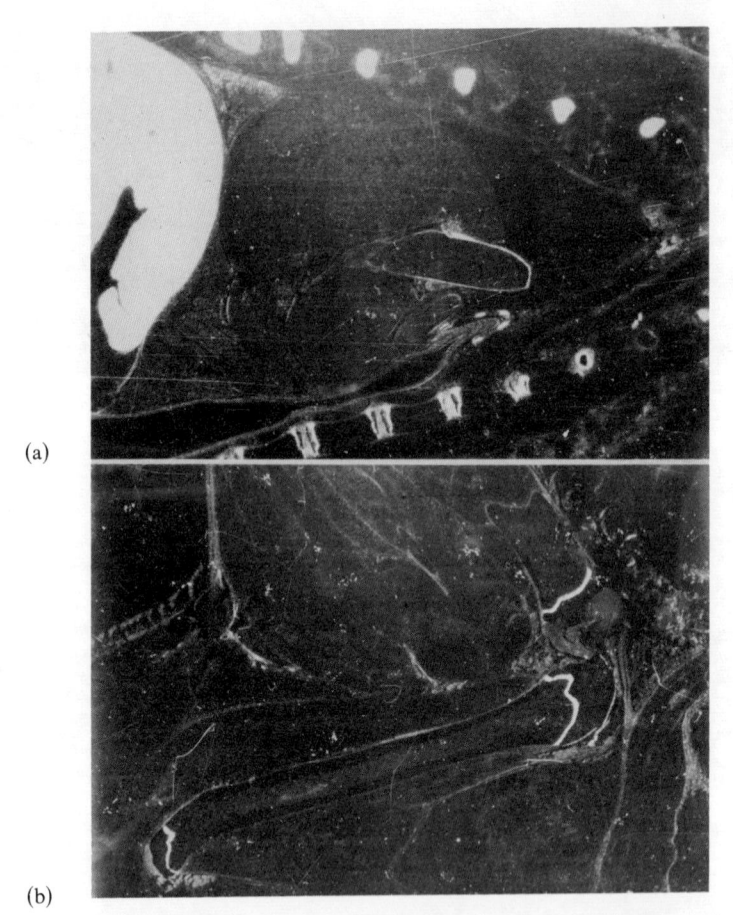

(b)

Fig. 4. Autoradiogram obtained after intravenous administration of a radioactive labeled curariform bisonium base (*N*-ethyl-4,7-dehydroconessine; Myc 1080) to a rat. Note: the radioactive base accumulates especially in cartilage tissue rich in acidic mucopolysaccharides: (a) costal and intervertebral cartilage; (b) epiphyseal cartilage of hindleg bones (Wieriks, 1972).

(plasma protein-bound and free) is higher than the concentration in the cerebrospinal fluid which is poor in protein. The free concentration in the plasma, however, is practically equal to the free concentration in the cerebrospinal fluid so that the differences in total concentrations are mainly due to differences in drug-binding protein contents in these compartments.

If drugs are eliminated from the plasma compartment by biochemical processes, such as active excretion in the kidney or enzymatic degradation

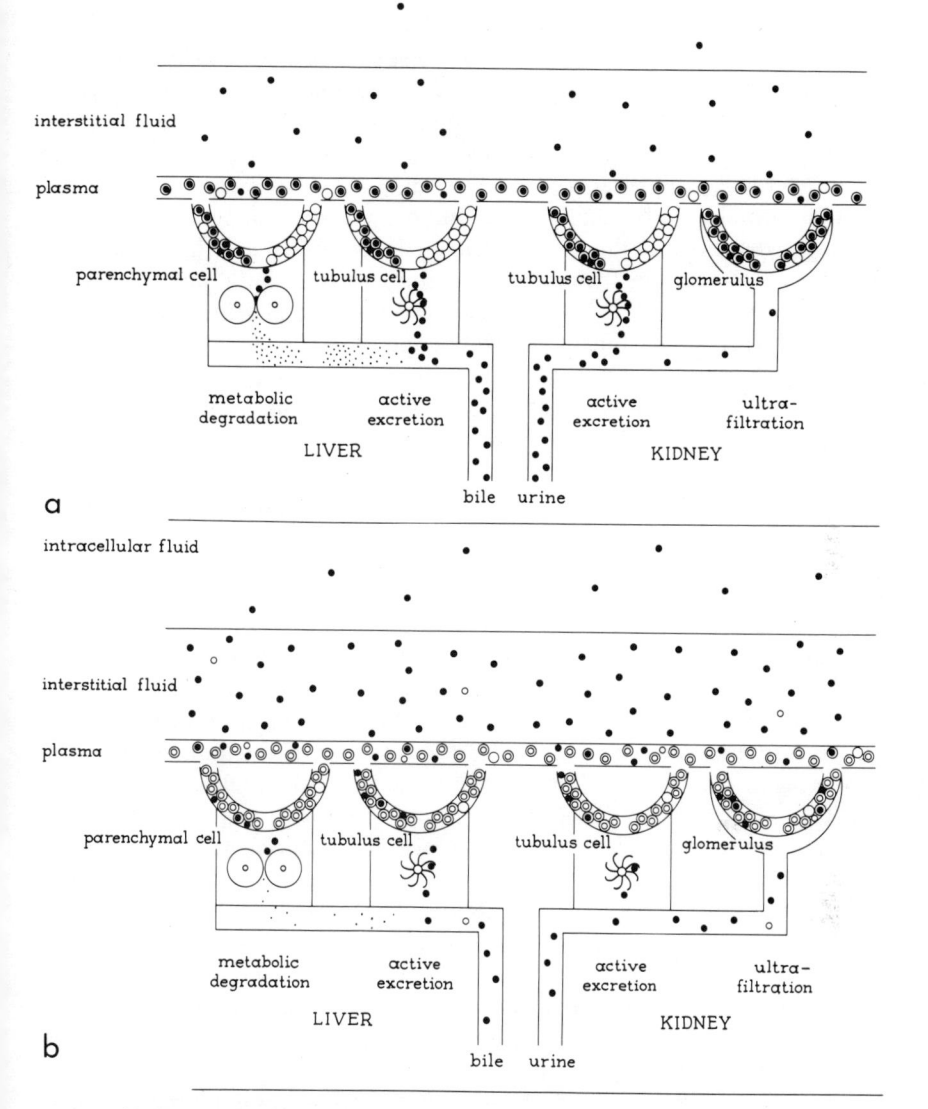

Fig. 5. (a) Schematic representation of the excretion in liver and kidney of a drug with strong protein-binding but a high rate of dissociation of the drug-protein complex. The glomerular filtration is restricted to the unbound drug. Active excretion and metabolic degradation extend themselves to the total plasma concentration of the drug. The concentration in the interstitial fluid and the unbound concentration in plasma are both low. (b) As (a), but now in the presence of a second drug displacing the original one from the plasma proteins. The excretion by glomerular filtration is increased because of the increase in the concentration of unbound drug. The active excretion and metabolic degradation are decreased owing to the decrease in plasma concentration of the drug, which is the result of the redistribution, leading to increased interstitial and possibly intracellular concentrations after displacement (Ariëns, 1971a).

in the liver, protein binding has as a consequence an increase in the load offered to these eliminating systems. This is especially the case if the rate of dissociation of the drug from the plasma protein is sufficiently high, which indeed it often appears to be. The renal excretion of a drug by ultrafiltration is hampered by its plasma-protein binding. Displacement of a strongly protein-bound drug by another one causes a redistribution which results in a strong decrease in the total plasma concentration and a smaller, but significant, increase in the concentration of the drug in its unbound form, both in plasma and other extracellular fluid compartments including possible target compartments. Another consequence of such a displacement will be an increase in the rate of drug elimination by ultrafiltration and a decrease in the rate of elimination by active excretion and biodegradation (Fig. 5) (Ariëns, 1971*a*).

The Drug Concentration in the Target Compartment and the Response

Information on the bioavailability profile of the active compound in general circulation or even in the target compartment does not always allow straight conclusions with regard to the response. This holds true for drugs which act by irreversible, covalent binding to their specific receptors, and, in general, for drugs which cause chemical lesions. Then an accumulation in the response and a persistence of the response after elimination of the drug may occur. In other cases complicated and time-related factors are involved in the sequence of events leading from the drug–receptor interaction to the response. There is, for instance, the phenomenon of tachyphylaxis for drugs that act as releasers of particular mediators, which is due to exhaustion of the stores of the mediators. This is the case for histamine-releasing agents and indirectly acting adrenergic and cholinergic agents; renin application leads to exhaustion of the angiotensinogen from which it generates angiotensin I. The opposite situation is a delay in the response of a drug due to the availability of a stock of mediators (e.g., the indirectly acting anticoagulants which inhibit the synthesis of certain coagulation factors). The effect, e.g., the prolongation of the prothrombin time, becomes manifest only after consumption of a certain fraction of the coagulation factors in circulation. Measurement of the inhibition of the formation of mediator compounds—the rate of synthesis of the factors—may result in a clearer relationship of the concentration of the drug and the response. In the case of drug interactions the relationship between the concentration of the interfering drug and its effect (the change it brings about in the effect of the other drug) can be particularly complex. An example is the enhancement of the warfarin-induced hypoprothrombinemia by trichloroethanol (hypnotic). The hypnotic is metabolized to trichloroacetic acid, which strongly binds to plasma albumin and thus gradually accumulates. The anticoagulant, also strongly protein-bound, is displaced by this acid from its binding sites, thus is redistributed such that its inhibiting effect on the synthesis of coagulation factors is enhanced. This in its turn, with a certain delay, becomes manifest finally as the effect, an enhanced prolongation of the prothrombin time (Sellers *et al.*, 1972).

The Stimulus–Effect Relationship

The relationship between the concentration of a drug in the target compartment and the response will be at least partially describable on basis of the mass–action law. There are, however, complicating factors, for instance in the case of a so-called receptor reserve. This implies that in the earlier steps in the sequence of biochemical events between drug–receptor interaction (the induction of the stimulus) and final response there is a reserve capacity such that a maximal response is obtained after only a partial occupation or activation of the receptor system concerned (Ariëns, 1964). Dependent on the size of the receptor reserve, a smaller or larger fraction of the receptors can be blocked irreversibly without a reduction in the maximal response obtainable with the drug concerned. After such a partial irreversible blockade, however, the concentration at which the maximal response is obtained, is increased. The fraction of the receptors that can be blocked irreversibly before a reduction in the maximal response obtainable takes place is a measure for the receptor reserve. An analysis of the intermediate steps in the sequence of events between drug–receptor interaction (stimulus induction) and final effect may throw light on the biochemical basis of this phenomenon. With ACTH, for instance, there is a spare capacity with regard to the formation of cyclic AMP; a maximal response (i.e., maximal cortisol synthesis) is obtained at concentrations of ACTH which only partially activate the adenyl cyclase system, while ACTH derivatives with a relatively low capacity to activate this system equal ACTH with regard to the maximal cortisol synthesis obtained (Seelig *et al.*, 1972*a,b*). As a matter of fact the point of measurement along the sequence of events initiated by the drug–receptor interaction, and therewith the "response," may be chosen arbitrarily according to the objectives of the investigator. The closer the parameter chosen as response is biochemically tied up with the drug–receptor interaction, the simpler the concentration–response relationship will be. The indirectly acting anticoagulants already mentioned may exemplify this. The intermediate steps in the sequence of events between the initial stimulus and the final response can be indicated as intermediate stimuli or as response.

Although species differences and individual differences in sensitivity to drugs in many cases have to be related to differences in pharmacokinetics, especially in drug metabolism, differences in sensitivity, e.g., under normal and pathological conditions, may well be due to differences in the response systems. Examples are the differences in sensitivity for sedatives and hypnotics among healthy, hyperthyroid, and hypothyroid individuals, and the differences in the diuretic effect dependent on the plasma pH and electrolyte composition of the extracellular fluid. The same holds true for differences between infantile and adult individuals with regard to their response to sex hormones, differences between slowly growing and quickly growing tissues in their responses to cytostatic agents, etc.

After this general discussion of various kinetic aspects of the pharmacodynamic phase of drug action it may be worthwhile to pay more attention to drug–receptor interaction as such.

DRUG–RECEPTOR INTERACTION

Here one of the most fundamental questions in pharmacology is touched on: "How do drugs act?" The pharmacodynamic effect of a drug originates from an interaction of the drug molecules with specific molecules, molecular complexes or parts of them in the biological object. On the molecules of the drug as a rule, plenty of information is available on the structure as well as the inherent chemical properties. These are determinant for the specific pharmacological characteristics of the drug. On the molecules in the biological object with which the drug molecules *must* interact in order to induce their effect (the specific receptors), little or no information is available. The use of the term receptor to indicate them underlines our lack of knowledge in this respect. The receptor concept, however, is essential in a discussion of drug action on a molecular level. It was Langley who in 1905 introduced the notion of a specific receptive substance: that part of the myoneural junction that serves as site of action for drugs such as curare.

The use of the term receptor makes sense only in relation to particular bioactive compounds and their particular effects. In a number of cases the specific receptors for a drug may be found to be located on enzyme molecules. These are changed by the drug molecules in their characteristics (e.g., by blockade of the active site or by an allosteric interaction). In other cases the receptors may be found to be functional proteins, lipoproteins, or protein-lipid complexes in membranes. There is a whole gamut of possibilities with, at one side, the interaction of drug molecules with preformed, stereospecific receptors. requiring a highly specific charge distribution and sterical configuration in the drug molecule, and at the other side, the diffuse interaction with water molecules in particular compartments as in the case of plasma extenders and osmotic diuretics where the receptor concept loses its strict sense. In between there are the interposition of drug molecules between the molecules composing the semifluid lipid membrane structures, which is probable for the local anesthetics, and the dissolution of drug molecules into particular lipid fractions of cell membranes, which is probable in the case of various general anesthetics. In these cases the structural requirements for action are low and extremely low, respectively.

The receptor concept has been most useful in the efforts to study structure–action relationship, in the classification of different types of drugs and drug actions, the analysis of drug interactions on the pharmacodynamic level, and drug design, while it also has challenged scientists to locate, isolate, and identify specific receptors. The study of dose–response relationships for single and combined drugs is an integral part of this approach (Ariëns and Simonis, 1964). In various papers dealing with isolation of specific receptors, the term receptor is used for the receptor molecule or even molecular complexes on which the site of action for the drug is located. In the studies of structure–action relationship, the term receptor is used in the sense of the site of action or, better, of interaction, the area on the receptor molecule on which the drug molecule initiates the conformational changes in the receptor molecule leading to the response. This site is to a certain degree chemically complementary to the drug molecule. It is suggested that the term *specific receptor* be used for the receptor molecule or molecular complexes as a whole and the term *specific receptor site* for the areas on the receptor primarily involved in the drug–receptor interaction.

The Induction of Stimulus and Effect

Drug–receptor interaction must be seen as a mutual molding of drug and receptor, similar to the enzyme–substrate interaction. While in the latter case, however, the conformational changes in the substrate molecule—resulting in a chemical activation and thus chemical reaction—are essential, in the case of the drug–receptor interaction conformational changes in the receptor molecules, resulting in an activation thereof, are of primary importance. As a rule the drug molecule will dissociate from the receptor site without being changed. Exceptions are the drugs acting by covalent bond formation. In certain cases the drug–receptor interaction will have as a consequence only a blockade of the receptor site without induction of essential conformational changes in, or activation of, the receptor. This is similar to the interaction of an enzyme and a reversibly acting antimetabolite, a competitive antagonist for the substrate. Examples are the reversible competitive antagonists blocking the specific receptor sites for agonists such as neurotransmitter substances, hormones, etc.

The changes induced by the agonistic compound in the conformation of the receptor molecules in membranes, for instance, are assumed to result in propagated changes in the surrounding molecules leading to changes in the membrane properties and thus to the final effect: the muscle contraction or muscle relaxation. As mentioned, the choice of the parameter considered as effect is subjective; for cholinergic agents, for instance, the change in the membrane potential, in the ionflux, or in the contraction state of the muscle fibers, may be regarded as effect.

A great advantage of the receptor concept is that it implies by its own nature the application of the principles of the mass–action law to drug action. One of the main parameters in the analysis of drug action therefore is the affinity constant: the concentration of the drug required to obtain a certain fraction (e.g., 50%) of the maximal response obtainable with that drug. This constant is determined by the rate of association (mainly dependent on the rate of diffusion of the drug molecules to the receptor) and the rate of dissociation (mainly dependent on the binding forces at action in the drug–receptor complex). Since the drug–receptor interaction may or may not result in the conformational changes and therewith the activation of the receptor required for action, a second parameter evolves, "the intrinsic activity" (Ariëns, 1964): a measure for the efficacy of the drug–receptor interaction. There can be distinguished between full agonists, those members of a family of drugs (drugs interacting with common receptors) which fully activate the receptors and thus have a maximal intrinsic activity, competitive antagonists, those members which only have an affinity to the receptors, and thus lack an intrinsic activity, and partial agonists, the members which activate the receptors they occupied only fractionally. This may be due to the requirement of an activation energy for the receptor activation such that of the receptors occupied by a partial agonist only a fraction is activated. An only partial activation of each of the receptors occupied is much less feasible. Interesting is the dualism, synergism and antagonism, observed if a partial agonist is combined with a full agonist from the same family of drugs (Fig. 6a–d) (Ariëns, 1964).

A variety of models can underlie the mechanisms involved in receptor activation. The conformational change essential for the receptor activation and the induction of the initial stimulus may last only as long as the drug molecule is bound to the receptor, or it may be triggered by a hit-and-run mechanism and last for a certain time, namely, until the receptor is regenerated. It may be that the rate at which the receptors are activated is determinant for the stimulus induced (Paton, 1961), for instance, for drugs which take part in turnover processes. In the latter case a rate of dissociation appreciably smaller than the rate of regeneration of the receptors implies a low intrinsic activity for the compound concerned. The

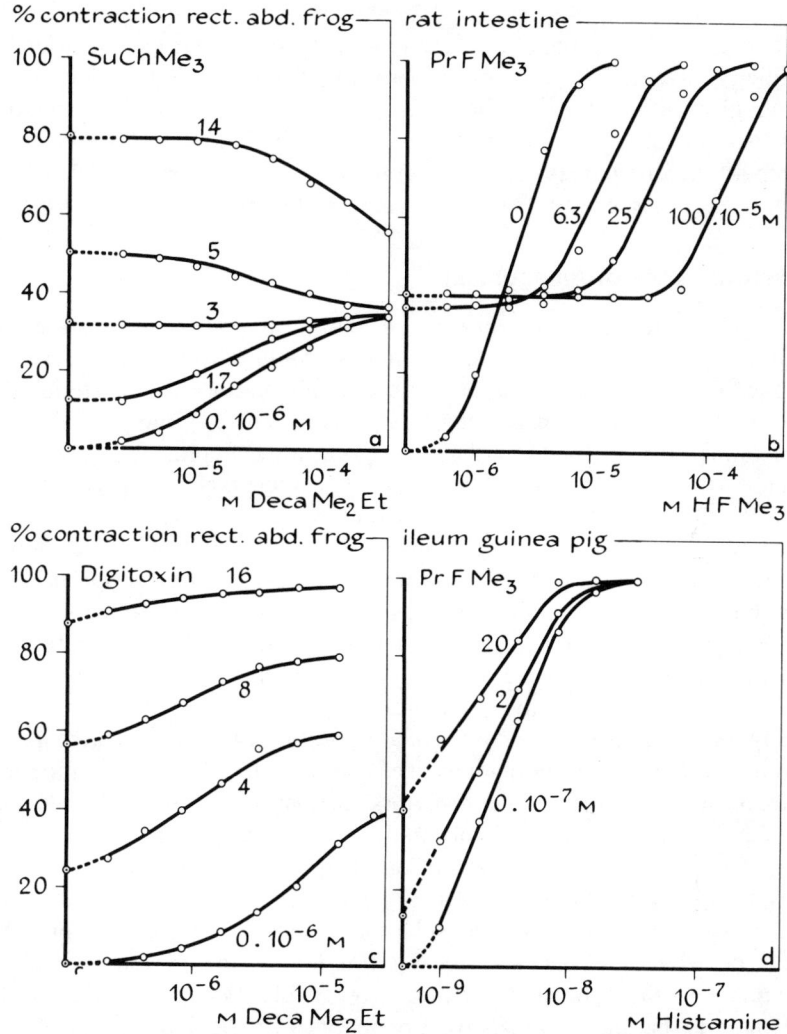

Fig. 6. Cumulative log concentration–response curves for: (a) a partial agonist (the bis-N-ethyl derivative of decamethonium, DecaMe$_2$Et) in the presence of various concentrations of the full agonist suxamethonium (SuChMe$_3$); (b) the full agonist oxapropanium (HFMe$_3$) in the presence of various concentrations of the partial agonist PrFMe$_3$ (a propyl derivative of oxapropanium); (c) the partial agonist DecaMe$_2$Et in the presence of various concentrations of the full agonist digitoxin; (d) the full agonist histamine in the presence of various concentrations of the partial agonist PrFMe$_3$. ⊙ indicates the responses obtained with the various concentrations of SuChMe$_3$ (a), PrFMe$_3$ (b), digitoxin (c) and histamine (d). Note the remarkable differences in the sets of concentration–response curves for the cases that the drugs combined belong to one family of drugs (a) and (b) and to different families of drugs (c) and (d), as expected from the concepts of competitive and functional interaction (Ariëns, 1964).

fact that certain competitive antagonists, due to strong hydrophobic binding, have a low rate of dissociation does not imply that a rate mechanism is involved in the receptor activation by the corresponding agonists. Definitely not if, as for the cholinergic receptors, for instance, competitive antagonists (anticholinergic agents) are known which show a high rate of dissociation from the receptors (Ariëns and Simonis, 1967).

Different Types of Antagonism

The existence of a sequence of bio- and physicochemical events leading from the induction of the initial stimulus to the final response implies that drugs may interfere with the effectuation of that stimulus at different points along this sequence of events. There is the principle of a noncompetitive interaction, e.g., antagonism. Different noncompetitive antagonists, i.e., acting on different specific receptor sites, may interfere with the induction of the response by one agonist. On the other hand, one noncompetitive antagonist, for instance, a musculotropic spasmolytic agent, may interfere with the response to different types of spasmogens, members of different families of drugs like cholinergic, histaminergic, and α-adrenergic agents inducing their effect on different specific receptors but having part of the sequence of events in common.

Besides the competitive antagonists blocking the specific receptors for the agonist in a reversible way, there also exist blocking agents blocking the specific receptors for the agonist irreversibly. The reversible competitive antagonists can protect the receptors against the irreversibly blocking agents. These are used as tools in the detection of a receptor reserve, mentioned earlier in the section on drug concentration in the target compartment. In that case there is an overcapacity with regard to the induction of the initial stimulus such that a maximal response is obtained with the effector organ with only a fraction of the receptors available occupied by the agonist. Only after irreversible blockade of the surplus receptors is the maximal response obtainable with the agonist reduced.

A particular type of antagonism is that between two agonists acting on different, specific receptor systems. The parameter representing one of the intermediate stimuli or the response of the one type of agonist may be changed in an opposite direction by the other one, the antagonizing agonist. For didactic reasons one differentiates between a physiological antagonism (the agonists induce effects which contribute in an opposite way to a resultant effect, for instance, an increase in cardiac output and a decrease in peripheral resistance with respect to the blood pressure), and a functional antagonism, where the antagonists contribute in an opposite way to a common intermediate stimulus and thus contribute in an opposite way to the final response (Ariëns, 1971a). An example of a functional antagonism is the antagonism between cholinergic and β-adrenergic agents with regard to the state of contraction of tracheal smooth muscle tissue. The final response in the presence of high doses of both agonists greatly depends on the intrinsic activities of both (Van den Brink, 1973).

A type of antagonism between drugs without direct receptor involvement is the antagonism by neutralization or chemical antagonism. In this case the antagonistic drug reacts with the agonistic drug and thus eliminates it. While in competitive antagonism, noncompetitive antagonism, and functional antagonism, the potency of the antagonist is dependent on its affinity to the respective receptors and independent of the agonist, in chemical antagonism the potency of the antagonist is dependent on its affinity for the particular agonistic compound involved. The differentiation between competitive antagonism and functional or physiological antagonism has as a parallel the differentiation between competitive synergism, analogous to the substrate competition in enzymology, and functional or physiological synergism where the agonists combined act on different receptors but contribute in the same sense to a common stimulus or induce effects contributing in the same sense to a resultant effect. This differentiation becomes especially evident with combinations of a full agonist and a partial agonist belonging to different drug families (Fig. 6c and d) (Ariëns, 1964).

It is not unusual that one drug interacts with different types of receptors, and at different concentrations (different affinities). A compound with such a multiple action may be, for instance, a competitive antagonist of two or more types of agonists. Examples are the compounds which have an anticholinergic, an antihistaminic as well as an α-adrenergic blocking action found among the group of the phenothiazines. It may be emphasized that there are no multipotent agonists, i.e., compounds with a cholinergic, a histaminergic as well as an α-adrenergic action. This is peculiar. The receptors for the different types of competitive antagonistic actions, although supposed to be identical to the receptors for the corresponding types of agonistic actions, apparently are much less selective than the receptors for the agonists. In fact the various competitive antagonists show little or no structural relationship with their corresponding agonists (Fig. 7), while the various types of antagonists undoubtedly show a certain structural relationship. This dilemma will be analyzed later in this paper.

The Receptors and Receptor Sites

Up to now receptor sites are not chemically identifiable nor can the affinity or the intrinsic activity be interpreted in detail in terms of chemical interactions. Some progress has been made on the level of receptor

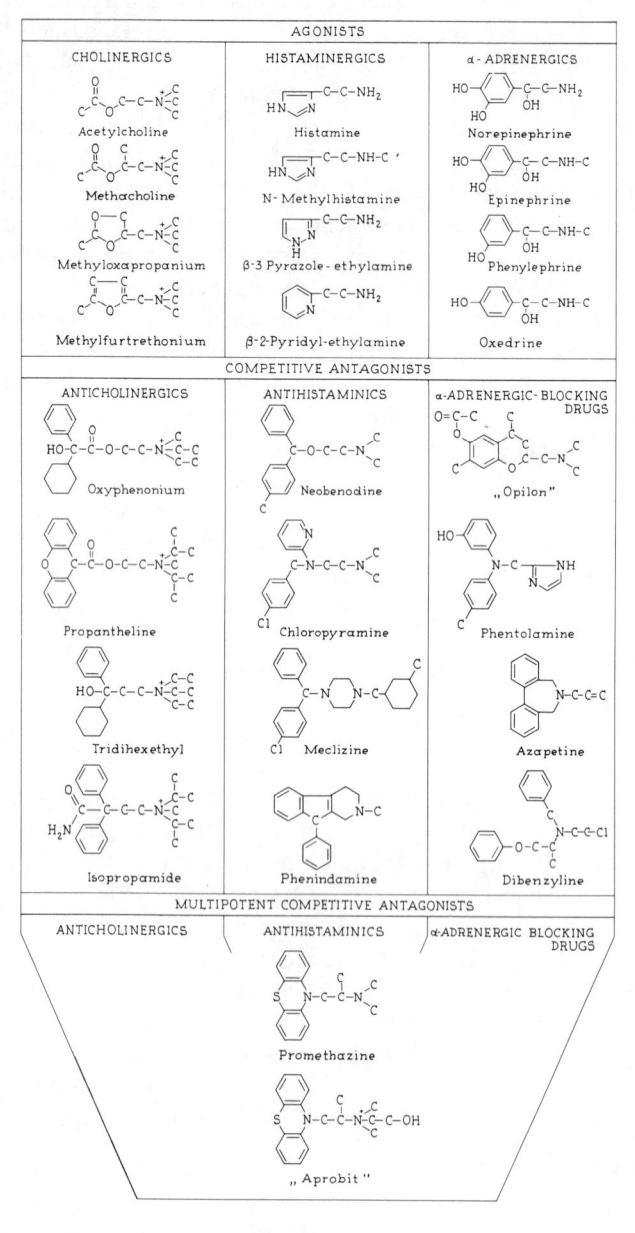

Fig. 7. Structure–action relationships of agonists and their competitive antagonists (Ariëns and Simonis, 1967).

localization, isolation, and identification. The same holds true for the analysis of the receptor-site characteristics. Some aspects of this work will be discussed in more detail. Information on receptors and receptor sites can be obtained through a number of approaches. The most direct are receptor isolation, with selective labeling of the receptors with covalently bound radioactive markers (indicated as affinity labeling), and affinity chromatography. The question is whether after isolation the receptors are functionally comparable to the receptors *in situ*, a problem which is similar to that encountered in the solubilization of enzymes which normally are part of membrane structures. While in the isolated enzyme, the affinity constant and the turnover constant for the substrates and thus the functional state of the enzyme can be evaluated, it is hard to say which parameter has to be used to evaluate the functional condition of isolated receptors. One of the characteristics which at least should be taken into account in receptor isolation is the stereoselectivity of the receptors. How far isolated receptors may serve as tools in the analysis of drug action is an open question.

It is certain that the analysis of the parameters for drug action obtained in systematic structure–action relationship studies has given interesting information on receptor sites. The cholinergic receptor may serve as an example here.

If the molecule of acetylcholine is reduced to only the tetramethylammonium moiety, the remaining compound still can bring about a 100% contraction in various smooth-muscle preparations. The dosages required, however, are about one hundred times that of the cholinergic agent. If, on the other hand, the quaternary ammonium group is omitted from acetylcholine, cholinergic activity is lost. This indicates that the onium group is essentially involved in the activation of the cholinergic receptor. Substitution of the methyl groups on the onium group in cholinergic agents by heavier substituents such as ethyl and isopropyl groups results in a conversion of these agents via partial agonists into competitive blockers of the cholinergic receptors. As compared to acetylcholine these anticholinergic agents have a relatively low affinity for the cholinergic receptors and a high rate of dissociation from these receptors.

The Receptor Sites for Cholinergic and Anticholinergic Agents

If the highly polar character of the various groups in the agonistic agents is taken into account, the receptor sites for the agonists may be assumed to be composed of clusters of complementary polar groups. In the surrounding thereof hydrophobic moieties are to be expected. The formation of polar bonds in a medium of water rich in ions, as a rule implies substitution of existing bonds by new ones such that only a small

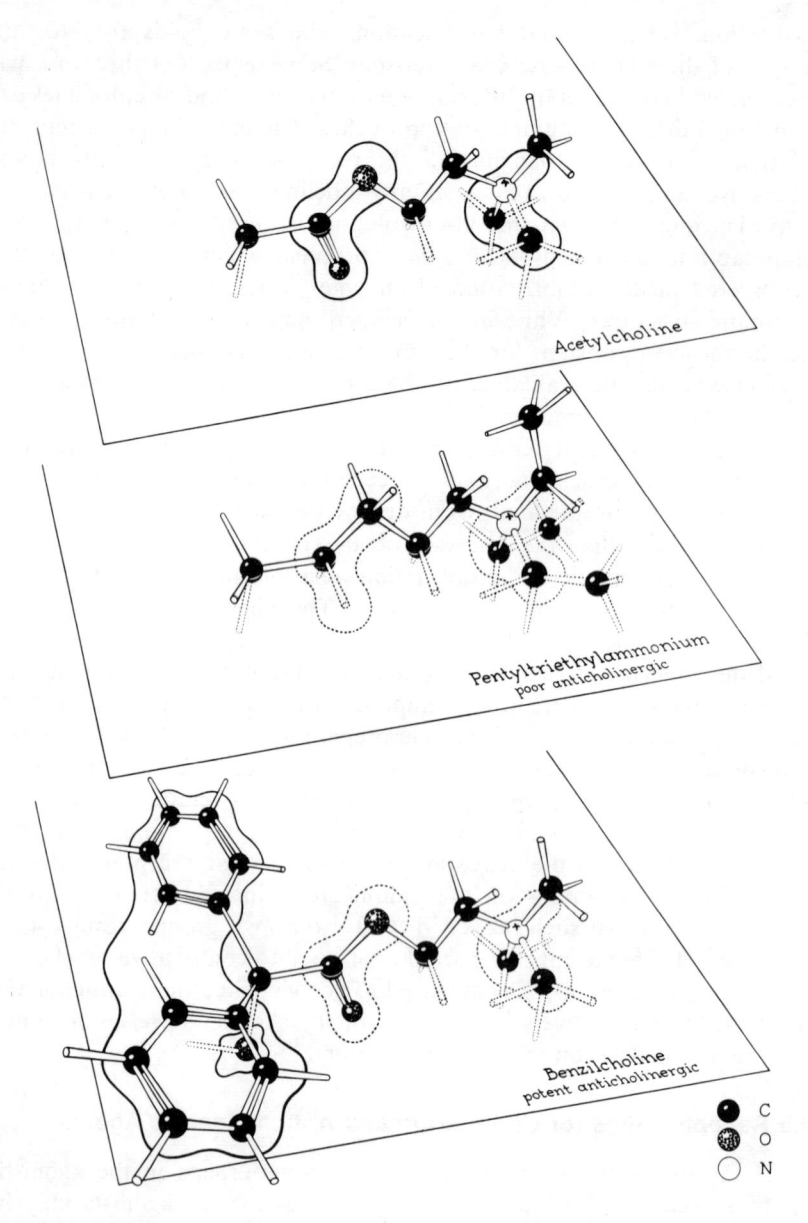

Fig. 8. Relation between the chemical structure of the cholinergic compound acetylcholine, the weak anticholinergic pentyltriethyl ammonium and the potent anticholinergic benzilylcholine respectively, projected on an imaginary complementary receptor surface. Note the extension of the receptor for the potent anticholinergic compound with an accessory receptor area lodging the hydrophobic ring system (Ariëns and Simonis, 1967).

contribution to the binding energy may be expected from these groups. From the hydrophobic groups, as present in the anticholinergic agents, however, large contributions may be expected. The high affinity of the blocking agents (which often is a thousand times higher than that of the agonistic agents) and their relatively low rate of dissociation (Paton, 1961), therefore, are understandable.

A comparison of the chemical structures of acetylcholine and the potent anticholinergic agents projected on imaginary complementary receptor surfaces makes a topographical identity of the receptor sites for both types of agents highly doubtful (Fig. 8). The same holds true if in a similar way histaminergic agents and various antihistaminics, and α-adrenergic agents and various α-adrenergic blocking agents are compared (Fig. 7). It may be postulated that the hydrophobic ring systems of the blocking agents interact with hydrophobic receptor areas located close to the receptor sites for the agonistic agents. The postulate of the hydrophobic accessory binding areas in the vicinity of the receptor sites of the various agonists (cholinergic, histaminergic, α-adrenergic agents) also makes understandable the existence of multipotent blocking agents (as a rule molecules containing hydrophobic phenyl rings) which block various types of receptors by binding to the hydrophobic accessory receptor areas of the respective receptor sites (Fig. 7).

In acetyl-β-methylcholine a high ratio (about a factor 300) is found for the cholinergic activity of both stereoisomers. In the corresponding benzilyl esters, which are highly potent anticholinergics, the ratio for the isomers is close to one (Table I). Apparently for the cholinergic action a close fit of the amino alcohol moiety of the drug and the receptor site is required, while for the anticholinergic action this appears not to be the case at all. The large degree of freedom with regard to N-substitution in the anticholinergic agents, e.g., atropine, propantheline, isopropamide, etc., in contrast to the loss of cholinergic action already with small N-substituents in the cholinergic agents also indicates an only loose interaction of the amino alcohol moiety in the anticholinergic agents and the cholinergic receptor site. This makes probable the theory that the blocking agents are strongly bound to the hydrophobic accessory receptor areas, and interfere with the action of the agonistic agents mainly through sterical hindrance by the moiety which bears the onium group in the anticholinergic agent. If indeed the moiety with the phenyl rings in these agents plays such a predominant role, introduction of a center of asymmetry in that part should result in optical isomers with a high ratio for their activities. This is indeed what is found (Table I) (Ellenbroek *et al.*, 1965). Anticholinergics with two centers of asymmetry, one in the amino alcohol moiety and one in the phenyl-bearing

TABLE I[a]
Structure and Activity of Choline Esters and Carbo Choline Esters

est/org.	$pA_2 \pm P_{95}$		config.	activity ratio	config.		$pA_2 \pm P_{95}$	est/org.
19/18	9.6 ± 0.26	(structure)	R_A	25	S_A	(structure)	8.2 ± 0.14	24/23
22/21	7.3 ± 0.17	(structure)	R_A	100	S_A	(structure)	5.3 ± 0.20	14/12
27/23	6.8 ± 0.15	(structure)	R_A	60	S_A	(structure)	5.0 ± 0.18	10/8

[a] The ± figures give the P_{95} for the mean value, est./org. = number of estimations/number of organs used. The data were obtained by testing the compounds on the isolated jejunum of the rat. Note the dependence of the activity ratios on the location of the centers of asymmetry in cholinergics and anticholinergics (Ellenbroek et al., 1965; Ariëns and Simonis, 1967).

Drug Action

ACTIVITY RATIOS

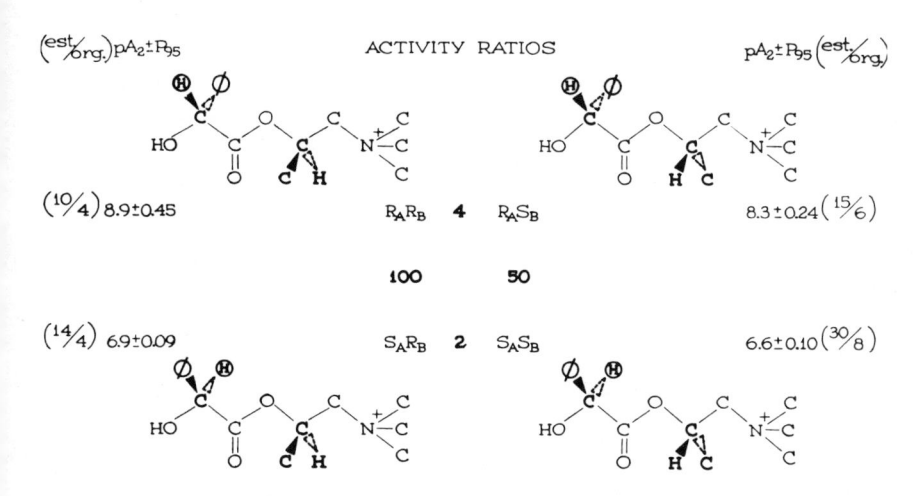

$(^{10}/_4)\ 8.9\pm0.45 \qquad R_AR_B \quad 4 \quad R_AS_B \qquad 8.3\pm0.24\ (^{15}/_6)$

100   50

$(^{14}/_4)\ 6.9\pm0.09 \qquad S_AR_B \quad 2 \quad S_AS_B \qquad 6.6\pm0.10\ (^{30}/_8)$

Fig. 9. The test organ is the rat jejunum. The ± figures give the P_{95} level for the mean value; est./org. = number of estimations/number of organs used. Note that the activity ratios are high if the center of asymmetry in the acid moiety differs in its configuration, and are low if the center of asymmetry in the choline moiety differs in its configuration. This indicates a close fit to the receptors for the acid moiety and the absence of such a fit for the choline moiety (Ellenbroek *et al.*, 1965; Ariëns and Simonis, 1967).

moiety, give further evidence (Fig. 9) (Ellenbroek, 1965) for the concept outlined before and summarized in Fig. 10 (Ariëns and Simonis, 1967).

It is even questionable whether the onium function in the anticholinergic agents plays any essential role in the anticholinergic action. Substitution of the onium group by nononium moieties results in still potent anticholinergic agents with the same stereospecificity with regard to the center of asymmetry in the phenyl ring-bearing moiety as observed for the mother compounds (Table II) (Ariëns and Simonis, 1967; Funcke *et al.*, 1959). These data indicate that anticholinergic agents cannot just be considered as cholinergic agents with a low rate of dissociation as postulated by the rate theory. As mentioned, for the *N*-alkyl substitution in the anticholinergics there is a relatively large degree of structural freedom allowed, indicating an absence of a close fit to the receptors. One may expect that if these substituents are gradually increased in size, they will get in close contact with the receptors again. At a certain critical size the contact will be reestablished. Since spatial arrangements are involved, a stereoselectivity for the substituted onium moiety may well be the result then. This is indeed what happens. If anticholinergic compounds with a tropanol moiety instead of a choline moiety are studied, introduction of substituents increasing in size on the onium group results in a stereospeci-

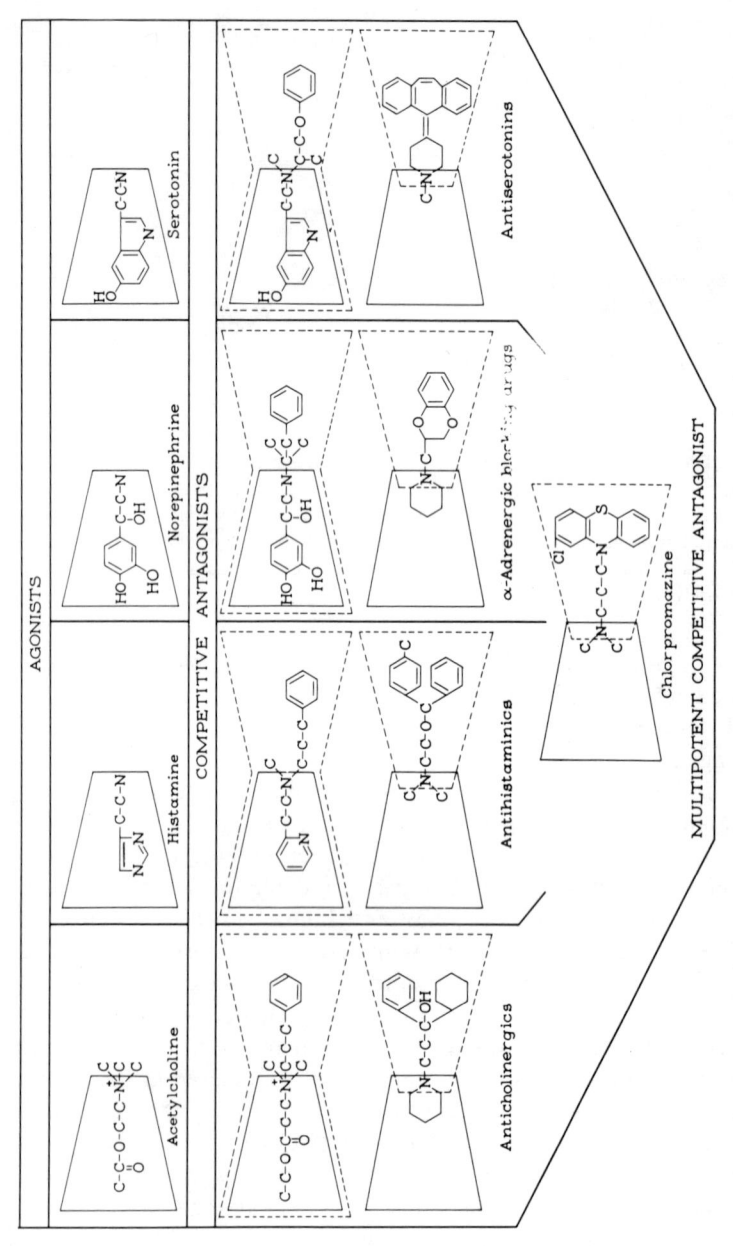

Fig. 10. Structure–action relationship for agonists, their competitive antagonists, and their receptors (Ariëns and Simonis, 1967).

TABLE II[a]
Stereoisomers and Biological Activity of Choline Esters

est./org.	$pD_2 \pm P_{95}$		config.	activity ratio	config.		$pD_2 \pm P_{95}$	est./org.
	7.0						7.0	
11/7	6.8 ± 0.14		S_B	320	R_B		4.1 ± 0.23	7/4
	$pA_2 \pm P_{95}$						$pA_2 \pm P_{95}$	
28/9	8.0 ± 0.14		S_B	5/6	R_B		8.1 ± 0.10	31/10
26/5	8.6 ± 0.18						8.6 ± 0.18	26/5
19/18	9.6 ± 0.26		R_A	25	S_A		8.2 ± 0.14	24/23

[a] The ± figures give the P_{95} for the mean value. est./org. = number of estimations/number of organs used. The data were obtained by testing the compounds on the isolated jejunum of the rat. Note: the onium group is not essential for anticholinergic action (Ellenbroek et al., 1965; Ariëns and Simonis, 1967).

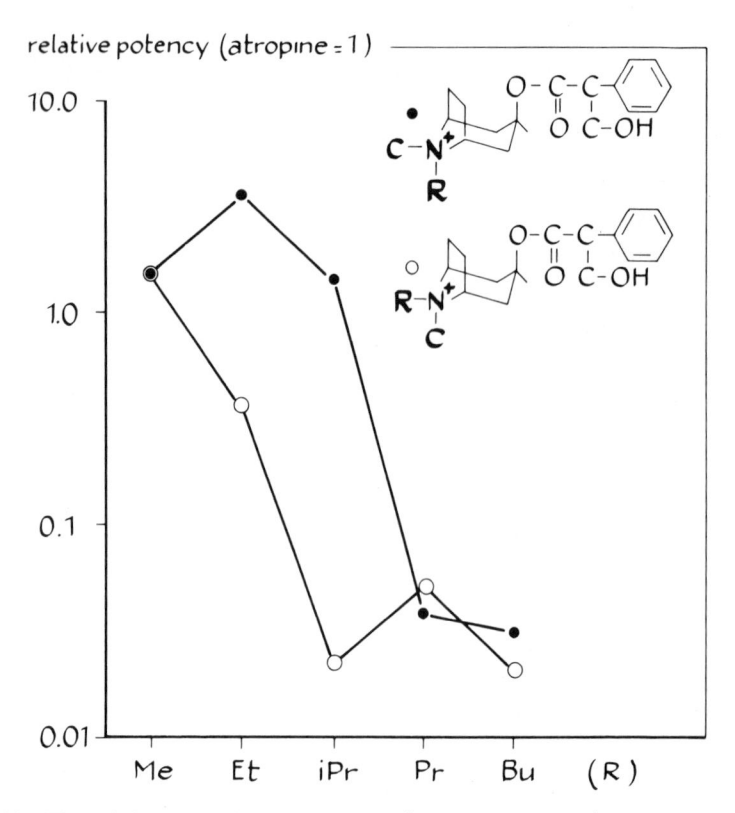

Fig. 11. The relative potencies of two series (geometrical isomers) of *N*-alkyl atropine derivatives tested against acetylcholine on the isolated gut of the guinea pig. Note the large ratio for the potencies of the isopropyl-substituted isomers due to the loss in potency of one of these isomers. For the propyl and butyl derivatives both isomers show a loss in potency, and thus a ratio of about 1. Apparently with an increase in the size of the alkyl substituent stereoselectivity with regard to drug–receptor interactions becomes manifest. (Wick, 1972).

ficity based on the differences in sterical structures of the geometrical isomers thus obtained (Fig. 11) (Wick, 1972). A next step may be the synthesis of anticholinergic β-alkyl choline derivatives with alkyl groups of increasing size. Analysis of the anticholinergic activity of such compounds probably will show a reappearance of the stereospecificity present in the original agonist (acetyl-β-methylcholine), namely, when the alkyl groups come into contact with the receptor site again.

The hydrophobic accessory receptor areas of the different types of receptor sites may be expected to differ in their sterical properties. A highly flexible molecule such as diphenhydramine appears to fit the accessory

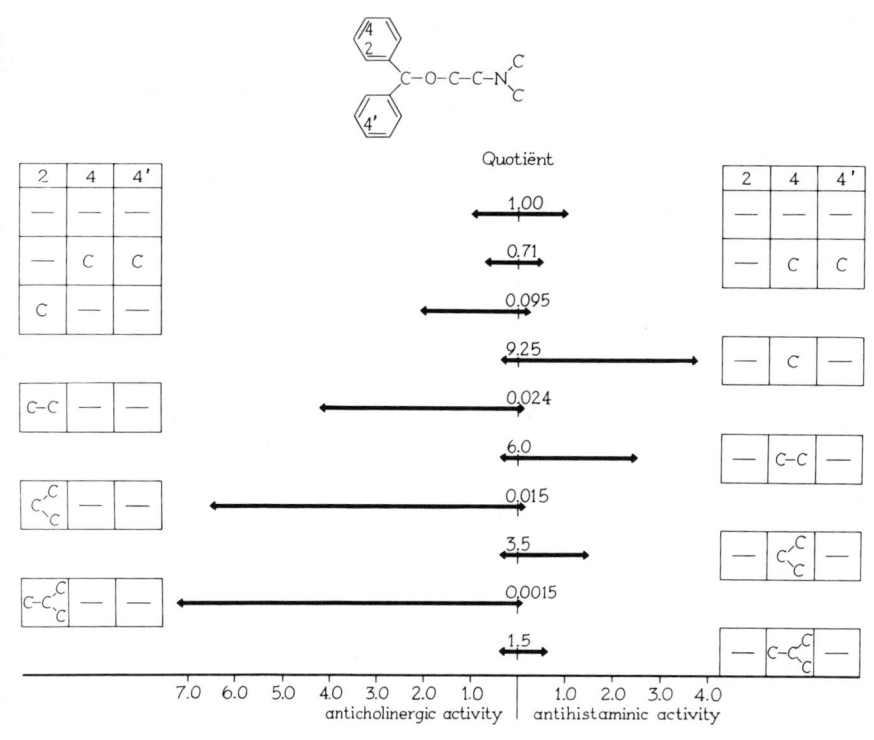

Fig. 12. Increase of specificity in action of diphenhydramine derivatives as a result of a decrease in the degree of conformational freedom (Harms and Nauta, 1960).

receptor areas of both the cholinergic and the histaminergic receptors. The compound has both anticholinergic and antihistaminic activity. Introduction of substituents in the 2-position in one of the rings—which results, especially if the size of the substituent is increased, in a rigidity of the double ring system—has as a consequence an increase in the anticholinergic and a decrease in the antihistaminic activity. Introduction of such alkyl substituents in the 4-position results in a decrease of the anticholinergic activity and an increase in the antihistaminic activity (Fig. 12). This indicates that indeed the accessory receptor areas of the cholinergic and histaminergic receptor sites, although having a hydrophobic character in common, differ in their sterical configuration (Harms and Nauta, 1960; Ariëns and Simonis, 1967).

The relationship between the dose of the drug, its systemic bioavailability profile, the availability profile in the target compartment (biophase), the drug-receptor interaction, the induction of the stimulus, and finally the response is very complex and dependent on a variety of interlinked part-processes often complicated by feedback mechanisms. In order to relate in a quantitative way the various factors involved in drug application to the effect obtained, a number of simplifying preassumptions must be made. Using a computer-simulated program Smolen *et al.* (1972) have worked out a theoretical basis for the computation of dose forms and regimens optimalized with regard to the requirements for a high therapeutic efficacy. The integrated use of the information gained from an empirical approach, the insights gained on pharmacokinetics and pharmacodynamics, and suitable theoretical models will point the way in the development of more effective therapeutics.

ACKNOWLEDGMENT

The valuable assistance of Miss A.R.H. Wigmans in the preparation of the manuscript is acknowledged.

REFERENCES

Ariëns, E. J., 1964, *Molecular Pharmacology*. Academic Press, New York.
Ariëns, E. J., 1971a, *Drug Design, Vol. I.*, Academic Press, New York.
Ariëns, E. J., 1971b *Drug Design, Vol. II*, Academic Press, New York.
Ariëns, E. J., and Simonis, A. M., 1964, *J. Pharm. Pharmacol.* **16:** 137, 289.
Ariëns, E. J., and Simonis, A. M., 1967, *Ann. N.Y. Acad. Sci.* **144:** 842.
van den Brink, F. G., 1973, Part I and II. *European J. Pharmacol.*, **22:** 270 and 279.
Brodie, B. B., 1972, Abstracts of Invited Presentations, p.5. 5th International Congress on Pharmacology, San Francisco, California.
Ellenbroek, B. W. J., Nivard, R. J. F., van Rossum, J. M., and Ariëns, E. J., 1965, *J. Pharm. Pharmacol.* **17:** 393.
Funcke, A. B. H., Rekker, R. F., Ernsting, M. J. E., Tersteege, H. M., and Nauta, W. Th., 1959, *Arzneim. Forsch.* **9:** 573.
Hansson, E., and Schmiterlöw, C. G., 1961, *Arch. Int. Pharmacodyn.* **131:** 309.
Harms, A. F., and Nauta, W. Th., 1960, *J. Med. Pharm. Chem.* **2:** 37.
Paton, W. D. M., 1961, *Proc. Roy. Soc. (Biol.)* **154:** 21.
Ritschel, W. A., 1972, *Drug Intell. Clin. Pharm.* **6:** 246.
Seelig, S., Sayers, G., Beall, R., and Schwyzer, R., 1972a, *Abstracts of Volunteer Papers*, p. 207, 5th International Congress on Pharmacology, San Francisco, California.
Seelig, S, and Sayers, G., 1972b, personal communications.
Sellers, E. M., Lang, M., Koch-Weser, J., and Colman, R. W., 1972, *Clin. Pharmacol. Therap.* **13:** 911.
Smolen, V. F., Turrie, B. D., and Weigand, W. A., 1972, *J. Pharm. Sci.* **61:** 1941.
Symposium on Mechanisms of Toxicity by Therapeutic and Environmental Agents, 1973, Vol. 2, Proceedings, 5th International Congress on Pharmacology, San Francisco, California, Karger, Basel.
Wick, H., 1972, unpublished data. Research Institute, C.H. Boehringer Sohn, Ingelheim am Rhein, Germany.
Wieriks, J., 1972, Thesis, Medical School of Rotterdam, The Netherlands.

DISCUSSION SUMMARY

Axelrod commented on recent progress in the purification and isolation of drug receptor sites which previously had to be considered in a purely theoretical manner. He referred to isolation and purification of the cholinergic receptor and also of the beta adrenergic receptor. The insulin receptor has been well characterized and work has progressed on isolation of opiate receptors. Such achievements should permit pharmacokinetic experiments on the interaction between drugs and their receptor sites. Ariëns replied that some caution in interpretation of such experiments was required because the function of the receptor *in vitro* might differ from its function *in vivo*.

Segre noted that it is possible to combine, in the same compartmental model, the kinetics of a drug and the kinetics of its effect by deriving the drug concentration at the receptor biophase from the dose–effect relationship.

Berman raised another point related to quantitative evaluation of drug effects. He and his associates recently studied the action of lithium on thyroid hormone metabolism in hyperthyroids and showed through careful modeling of the kinetics that there are at least two sites of action of lithium: (1) a slowdown of the rate of secretion of hormone from the thyroid, and (2) a slowdown of the rate of disappearance of thyroxine (and T_3?) from the circulation. The net effect of the two modes of action can be an increase, a decrease, or no change in the level of hormone in blood, depending on which site is more responsive, and large variations in hormone levels can result from relatively small changes at each of the sites of action. Several pathways can be recognized for the disappearance of the T_4-deiodination, fecal excretion, metabolism, and conversion to T_3. It is not yet known which of the paths are affected by lithium. It is obvious, however, that the biological effectiveness of the drug will greatly depend on which of these pathways are affected. This raises still another point, namely, that a single drug may act as if it were two drugs given simultaneously.

Pharmacokinetics and Pharmacodynamics of Acetazolamide in Relation to Its Use in the Treatment of Glaucoma*

Per J. Wistrand

University of Uppsala
Department of Medical Pharmacology
Uppsala, Sweden

Many speakers have alluded to the problem of describing the kinetics of the events at the drug receptor in relation to the time course of the physiological response. I would like to give an example of a drug action where it might be possible to unify the pharmacokinetic and the pharmacodynamic events.

Figure 1 describes a scheme of events that occurs from the moment a patient with glaucoma takes his tablet of acetazolamide up to the moment when the eye pressure has reached its new reduced level. Acetazolamide is an ideal substance from a pharmacokinetic point of view. Thus, all of an oral dose is absorbed and excreted unchanged in the urine and a great deal is known about its distribution kinetics in man (Lehman et al., 1969). We also know the characteristics of its plasma protein binding and the approximate rate by which it equilibrates between plasma and ciliary epithelium. This rate is rapid and probably similar to that measured for the erythrocytes. The inhibitory activities toward human carbonic anhydrases have been determined, including the association and the dissociation rate constants for the formation of the inhibitor-enzyme complex. It would, therefore, seem possible to construct a rather detailed pharmacokinetic model in which could also be included the kinetics of the enzyme inhibition. This model would give, at any moment, the concentration of free inhibitor, I_{free}, inside the secretory cells, which together with the knowledge of the

---

*This work was supported by grant 02X-2874 from the Swedish Medical Research Council.

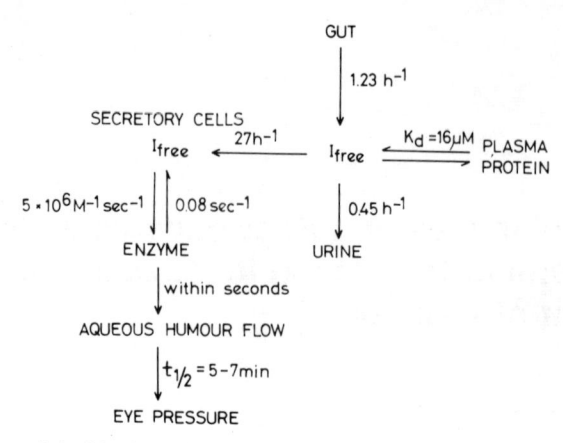

Fig. 1. Scheme of the kinetics of body distribution, enzyme and eye pressure effects in man of the carbonic anhydrase inhibitor, acetazolamide. For explanation of symbols see text.

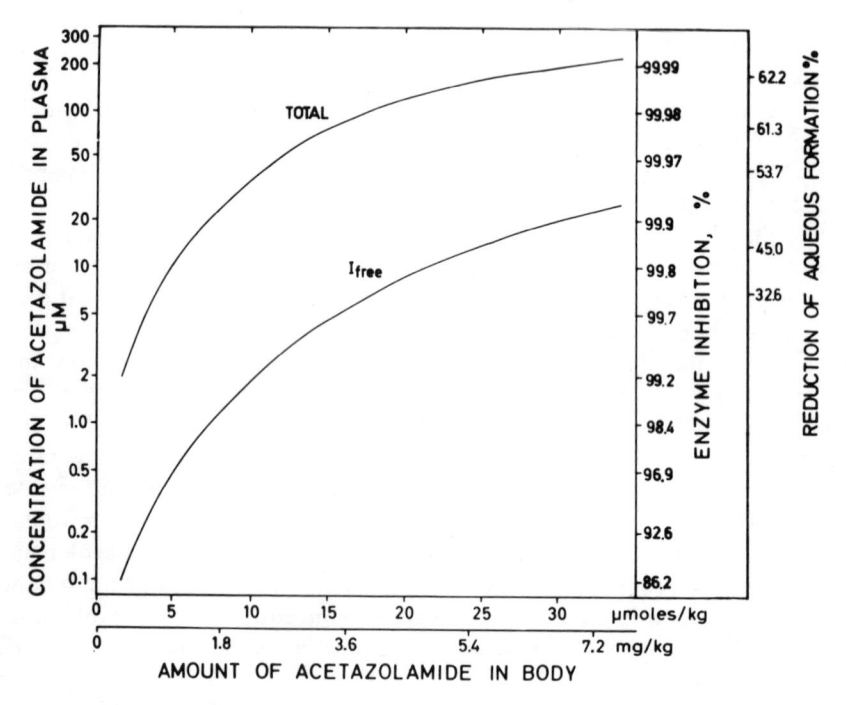

Fig. 2. The relation between the total amount of acetazolamide in the human body, the total and free, I_{free}, plasma concentration, the degree of enzyme inhibition in the ciliary epithelium and the effect of aqueous humour formation at steady state.

inhibitor constant K_i [taken to be $1.6 \times 10^{-8} M$ and similar to that of the erythrocyte isoenzyme HCA C at 37°C (Wistrand and Lindahl, unpublished observation)] permits the calculation of the fractional enzyme inhibition. Such a model, which relates the amount of drug given with the degree of enzyme inhibition, is seen in Fig. 2.

In order to include the pharmacodynamic events in our model we first need to know the relation between the amount of drug given, the plasma concentration, and the eye pressure response. This is best studied under steady state conditions (Lehman et al., 1969).

The eye pressures of patients with glaucoma were measured at different plasma concentrations of acetazolamide. The levels of acetazolamide were kept constant for 1 hr to ensure diffusion equilibrium between the inhibitor in plasma and the secretory cells and to allow the eye pressure to reach its new steady state in response to the changes in the plasma inhibitor level and aqueous humour flow. It was then possible to relate the eye pressure response to the plasma concentration and, therefore, also with the degree of enzyme inhibition. Moreover, since we know the relation between eye pressure and aqueous humour flow at steady state, the enzyme inhibition can also be related to the reduction of aqueous flow. The relation between aqueous humour flow and the eye pressure at steady state can be written as $P_0 - P_v = F \times R$, where P_0 is the measured eye pressure, P_v is the episcleral venous pressure, R is the resistance to aqueous outflow, and F is the aqueous humour flow; P_v and R are assumed to be constants. It can be seen from the model of Fig. 2 that the aqueous formation becomes reduced only when the enzyme has been inhibited by more than 99%. In order to reach the maximal effect, about 60–70% flow reduction, the enzyme must be inhibited by more than 99.9%. This is analogous to the situation in the kidney and the erythrocytes (Maren, 1967).

To complete the combined model we must also be able to formulate the course of the eye pressure drop in response to changes in the aqueous humour formation. This seems to be possible since we know that the eye pressure falls along an approximately exponential curve with a half time for the establishment of the new steady-state level of between 5–7 minutes after the parenteral administration of acetazolamide. Since this time constant is similar to that seen after rapidly induced disturbances of the eye pressure equilibrium (Bárány, 1947), this implies that the rate of aqueous flow rapidly responds to changes in enzyme activity. It has also been shown that the eye pressure starts to drop within seconds after an intravenous or intracarotid infusion of acetazolamide. The kinetics of the eye pressure response could therefore be included in a unified model together with the kinetics of the drug distribution and the kinetics of the enzyme effects.

Using a computer we should find it possible to solve, simultaneously, all parts in this model.

REFERENCES

Lehman, B., Linnér, E., and Wistrand, P. J., 1969, The pharmacokinetics of acetazolamide in relation to its use in the treatment of glaucoma and to its effects as an inhibitor of carbonic anhydrases, in: *Advances in the Biosciences* Vol. 5, pp. 197-217 (G. Raspé, ed.), Pergamon Press, Oxford.

Maren, T. H., 1967, Carbonic anhydrase: chemistry, physiology and inhibition, *Physiol. Rev.* **47**: 595-781.

Bárány, E., 1947, The rate of equilibration of intraocular pressure: On the boundary between transient and stationary intraocular pressure changes, *Acta Ophthal.* **25**: 175-193.

The Role of the Lungs in the Metabolism of Vasoactive Substances*

John R. Vane[†]

Department of Pharmacology, Institute of Basic Medical Sciences
Royal College of Surgeons
London, England

The lungs are in an excellent and strategic position for cleansing the blood, for it all passes through them several times a minute. Apart from their respiratory function (removing carbon dioxide from the pulmonary circulation), the lungs also have other important cleansing mechanisms, including phagocytosis by alveolar macrophages, the filtering of emboli and circulating leucocytes, and excretion of other volatile substances (Said, 1968; Heinemann and Fishman, 1969). Work from my laboratory in recent years has highlighted the less widely appreciated but probably equally important function of the lungs: the removal of some vasoactive hormones from blood and the synthesizing of others. This paper will bring earlier reviews up-to-date (Vane, 1968; 1969).

INACTIVATION OF AMINES

5-Hydroxytryptamine

Almost fifty years ago Starling and Verney (1925) found that they could not maintain adequate circulation through an isolated perfused kidney with a simple perfusion circuit. A substance was present in

*This review was completed in 1972.
[†]Present address: Wellcome Research Laboratories, Langley Court, Beckenham, Kent, England.

defibrinated blood which caused intense vasoconstriction in the kidneys. They removed this substance by perfusing the kidney from a heart–lung preparation and concluded that the blood was "detoxicated" in the lungs. The isolation of the serum vasoconstrictor substance and its identification as 5-hydroxytryptamine (5-HT or serotonin) by Rapport et al. (1948a,b) started a whole field of new research; it was some years later that Gaddum et al. (1953) showed that the perfused lung of the cat removed the pharmacological activity of 5-HT from the blood. Isolated perfused lungs of the dog also metabolize 5-HT (Eiseman et al., 1964) and Davis and Wang (1965) showed that both liver and lung remove 5-HT *in situ* but that inhibition of monoamine-oxidase did not alter the rate of removal. Thomas and Vane (1967) investigated removal of 5-HT in the circulation of dogs by using infusions rather than injections, in order to study the steady-state effects. They estimated the removal of 5-HT by the blood-bathed organ technique (Vane, 1964; 1969) which is a dynamic bioassay method in which heparinized blood is removed continuously from the anesthetized animal, assayed for its hormone content without processing and then returned intravenously. The hormones are assayed by superfusing (Gaddum, 1953) the blood continuously over smooth muscle preparations chosen for their sensitivity and specificity to the substance being assayed. Over the years, we have developed a whole range of bioassay tissues with which we can estimate many different vasoactive substances, using up to six tissues at a time, bathed either in blood or in the saline effluent from a perfused isolated organ. The specificity and sensitivity of this parallel pharmacological assay technique is reviewed by Vane (1969 and 1973). Its main advantage is that it allows continuous "on-line" estimation of changes in concentration of a hormone in amounts that are likely to occur physiologically.

Thomas and Vane (1967) found that up to 98% of an intravenous infusion of 5-HT into the anesthetized dog disappeared in a single passage through the pulmonary circulation and that this disappearance was unaffected by monoamine-oxidase inhibition. Alabaster and Bakhle (1970a) found that isolated lungs from the rat perfused with Krebs' solution removed 92% of 5-HT perfused through them. This degree of removal was independent of concentration in the range from 5–100 ng/ml. When labeled 5-HT was infused for four minutes, 10% of the radioactivity appeared in the lung effluent as 5-HT within the first five minutes, and the rest of the radioactivity could be recovered as a metabolite, probably 5-hydroxyindoleacetic acid, over the next 50 minutes. Monoamine-oxidase inhibitors inhibited the initial removal only slightly but their main effect was to preserve the 5-HT taken up and this slowly reappeared into the effluent from the lungs. Inhibitors of 5-HT uptake by platelets such as amitriptyline and desmethylimipramine substantially prevented the removal of 5-HT by the lungs. Alabaster and Bakhle concluded that the removal process involves uptake followed by metabolism rather than uptake followed by storage. Junod (1971) showed that the removal process for 5-HT in rat lungs was saturable, with transport of 5-HT into the cell as the rate-limiting step. Cold, anoxia, but not lack of glucose inhibited uptake, as did cocaine, imipramine, and chlorpromazine. A lowered sodium concentration also reduced the uptake, and he suggested that the transport of 5-HT is carrier-mediated. Gillis (1971) homogenized rat lungs immediately after infusions of 5-HT. In agreement with Alabaster and Bakhle (1970a), he found that the lungs retained radioactivity after infusion of 5-HT but that as time passed, there was a preferential release of metabolized 5-HT.

Gruby et al. (1971), using isolated lungs from guinea pigs, found that 50% of infused 5-HT disappeared in one passage. This disappearance could be abolished by cooling the lungs to 5°C but was unaffected by mono-amine-oxidase inhibitors. They also concluded that the primary inactivation process was uptake, followed by slow metabolism within the cell. Gillis and Iwasawa (1972) studied uptake of 5-HT in rabbit perfused lungs. The removal was inhibited by cocaine, 17-β-estradiol, hydrocortisone, and other steroids. Gillis et al. (1972) studied removal of 5-HT by the lungs of man, before and after cardiopulmonary bypass. The mean percentage extraction in 9 patients was 65% before bypass and this increased somewhat immediately after the bypass was over.

Thus in all species studied, including man, 5-HT is substantially removed by the lungs, whether they are perfused with saline solution *in vitro* or by blood *in vivo*. Only one result disagrees with this conclusion. Despite the avid removal of 5-HT by rat lungs *in vitro*, Freer and Stewart (1972) were unable to demonstrate inactivation of 5-HT *in vivo* in rat lungs by comparing the effects of intravenous and intra-arterial injections. Both routes elicited the same systemic pressor response. Such a result is difficult to interpret for substances such as 5-HT, which are known to excite reflexes in the heart and the lungs; in addition, spasmogens released by 5-HT from the lungs (as discussed later) may be affecting the results.

The liver, which receives only a portion of the cardiac output, inactivates 5-HT to rather less an extent than do the lungs. Circulating platelets can only remove 5-HT from the blood by a relatively slow process (Vane, 1969). It must be concluded, therefore, that the major site of inactivation of 5-HT in the body is the lungs and not the liver or platelets. Predominantly right-sided heart lesions associated with carcinoid tumour may be linked with the pulmonary removal of 5-HT (Gobel et al., 1955) and there is evidence that the removal mechanism in man may sometimes fail (Davis, 1968).

The process in the lungs responsible for the uptake and metabolism of 5-HT shows some structural specificity. Although Alabaster (1971) showed that tryptamine was also metabolized by rat lung to a degree of 60–70% in one passage, the uptake process does not extend to other amines; for instance, histamine is not inactivated in heart-lung (Steggeda et al., 1935) or perfused lung (Eiseman et al., 1964) preparations from dogs. Heart–lung–liver preparations of cats rapidly eliminated histamine from the blood but heart–lung preparations alone did not (Lilja and Lindell, 1961). Alabaster (1971) found little or no inactivation of histamine in rat isolated lungs. Alabaster and Bakhle (1970a) also concluded that the uptake process for 5-HT was different from that for norepinephrine.

On which cells does the dramatic removal of 5-HT depend? Storage may be associated with reticuloendothelial cells, for Gershon and Ross (1966a,b) found that after infusions of labeled precursor, some 5-HT was localized in reticuloendothelial cells in the spleen, liver, and lungs; however, these cells do not contain monoamine-oxidase (Gershon, personal communication). Another possible site of uptake is the blood platelet. These cells can take up 5-HT (Stacey, 1961), the uptake can be blocked by amitriptyline-like drugs (Todrick and Tate, 1969), and they are present in lung capillaries in large numbers (Kaufman et al., 1965). However, 5-HT taken up by platelets is found in intracellular storage organelles (Born, 1963; Tranza et al., 1966) and although platelets will oxidize exogenous 5-HT the amount of metabolism is small. Alabaster and Bakhle (1970a) recovered most of the radioactivity in the perfusate after infusions of labeled 5-HT within 40–60 min as the metabolite 5-hydroxyindoleacetic acid, so it seems that platelets are unlikely to be involved. Unpublished results of Alabaster et al., in which the disposition of labeled 5-HT in rat lung was studied by autoradiography, suggest that the pulmonary arteriole is the site of uptake and metabolism. In this respect it would be worthwhile coupling 5-HT to a large molecule such as horseradish peroxidase (Richardson and Beaulnes, 1971) to determine whether removal and metabolism of this large coupled molecule still takes place in the lungs.

Catecholamines

Epinephrine and norepinephrine have a half-life in the circulation of the cat of less than 20 sec (Ferreira and Vane, 1967a) so that they must be substantially removed from the blood in one circulation (20–30 sec; Spector, 1956). In 1905, Elliot showed that epinephrine did not disappear in the lungs but did so in other vascular beds. Ginn and Vane (1968) found that although infusions of epinephrine passed through the pulmonary circulation without loss, up to 30% of an infusion of norepinephrine disappeared in the lungs of the cat. Dog isolated lungs removed norepinephrine from the perfusing blood (Eiseman et al., 1964). Labeled norepinephrine infused into saline-perfused rat lungs was concentrated by the lung tissues by a process which was saturable. Of the radioactivity retained in the lungs, 20% was unchanged norepinephrine (Hughes et al., 1969).

Boileau et al. (1971,1972) showed that pulmonary inactivation of epinephrine and dopamine was negligible in several species, including man, but that there was up to 35% inactivation of norepinephrine in the lungs of rats, cats, rabbits, dogs, and man. They also found that the inactivation process could be saturated by high infusion rates of norepinephrine. Gillis et al. (1972) estimated pulmonary extraction of norepinephrine in patients before and after cardiopulmonary bypass. There was a mean extraction of 23% norepinephrine and this increased immediately after bypass. The increase was substantially more than that seen with 5-HT so that after bypass, 50% of the norepinephrine disappeared. Alabaster and Bakhle (1973) studied removal of norepinephrine from the perfusion fluid on passage through the pulmonary circulation of rat isolated lungs. The proportion removed (40%) tended to decrease with increased concentration, suggesting a saturable process. The removal was inhibited by cocaine but not by metaraminol, normetanephrine, phenoxybenzamine, or 5-HT. They concluded that the uptake process for norepinephrine in the lungs was unlike either the neuronal uptake process (uptake 1) or the extraneuronal uptake (uptake 2) described for other tissues. Because there was no competition for uptake between 5-HT and norepinephrine in the lungs, Alabaster and Bakhle (1973) concluded that the amines have different uptake sites although they share an uptake mechanism with certain common characteristics and which may be unique to the pulmonary circulation. Gillis and Iwasawa (personal communication) chemically destroyed sympathetic nerve endings with 6-hydroxydopamine and found uptake of 5-HT and norepinephrine in lung tissue to be unchanged. Radioautography and fluorescence microscopy localized the norepinephrine in endothelial cells of capillaries and postcapillary venules.

From all these results two interesting conclusions can be drawn. First, if a mixture of epinephrine and norepinephrine is released from the adrenal medulla, preferential removal of some of the norepinephrine in the lung will increase the proportion of epinephrine in the mixture which reaches the arterial circulation. Measurements of catecholamine content in adrenal venous blood will, therefore, give different proportions of epinephrine and norepinephrine from measurements in arterial blood. Indeed, norepinephrine may have little significance as a circulating hormone.

Secondly, drugs which interfere with uptake or storage of norepinephrine may potentiate the effects of norepinephrine on the cardiovascular system, not only by preventing uptake in peripheral tissues but also by interfering with uptake in the lungs, thereby allowing more of the injected norepinephrine to reach the arterial circulation. Such an effect has been shown with desmethylimipramine (Eble et al., 1971).

Acetylcholine

The actions of acetylcholine are usually terminated by acetylcholinesterase close to the site of its release from nerve endings. Cholinesterases in the blood are also highly active and can reduce the concentration of acetylcholine in blood to less than half in two seconds (Vane, 1969). In addition to these inactivating mechanisms Eiseman et al. (1964) found that dog isolated lungs perfused with a dextran saline solution rapidly inactivated large amounts of acetylcholine. Thus, there are several mechanisms which, by rapid metabolism, protect the arterial circulation from high concentrations of acetylcholine.

INACTIVATION OF PEPTIDES

Bradykinin

Bradykinin is fairly rapidly destroyed in blood and has a half-life in the blood stream of the rat or dog of about 17 sec (McCarthy et al., 1965; Ferreira and Vane, 1967b,c). Thus, bradykinin formed in or injected into venous blood is likely to reach the pulmonary circulation. Ferriera and Vane (1967c) showed that the lungs avidly removed bradykinin, about 80% disappearing in one passage through cat lungs. Pulmonary inactivation of bradykinin has since been confirmed in several species, including rat, guinea pig, dog, and sheep (Biron, 1968; Stewart, 1968; Pojda and Vane, 1971; Alabaster and Bakhle, 1972a; Hébert et al., 1972). Cell-free extracts of lung tissue readily inactivate bradykinin (Bakhle, 1968) and Ryan et al. (1968, 1969) showed that bradykinin was inactivated in the pulmonary circulation of rats by enzymic hydrolysis of peptide bonds. Radioactive bradykinin was perfused through blood-free lungs *in situ* and the inactive compounds in the perfusate were identified as peptide fragments of bradykinin. There was no retention of radioactivity by the lungs. The circulation time was identical with that of blue dextran, indicating that bradykinin only equilibrates with the pulmonary extracellular space. They concluded that the enzymes responsible for degradation of bradykinin in the lung are bound on or near the vascular endothelial cells.

Other Peptides

The selectivity of the pulmonary inactivation mechanism is strikingly demonstrated by the way in which the lungs inactivate bradykinin but allow other peptides to pass through without change. Angiotensin II is unaffected by passage through the pulmonary circulation, in all species so far studied (Goffinet and Mulrow, 1965; Hodge et al., 1967; Biron et al., 1968; Bakhle et al., 1969; Biron et al., 1969; Leary and Ledingham, 1969; Biron and Campeau, 1971) including rats, dogs, guinea pigs, cats, and man. Similarly, vasopressin survives passage through the pulmonary circulation of rats, rabbits, cats, dogs, and man (Biron and Boileau, 1969; Gilmore and Vane, 1970; Crexells et al., 1972). Oxytocin also survives unchanged (Biron and Boileau, 1969; Vane and Williams, 1970). Little is known of the way in which the lung treats fibrinopeptides although Bailey et al. (1967) suggested that the lung may be an active site for fibrinopeptide metabolism. Similarly, it is not known whether the lungs have any effects on the activity of cholecystokinin, gastrin, pancreozymin, glucagon, and other peptide hormones of gastrointestinal origin.

INACTIVATION OF PROSTAGLANDINS

Like the regions of the body from which they so often emanate, prostaglandins are interesting more and more experimentalists. Their functions have recently been reviewed by Weeks (1972) and by Hinman (1972). Ferreira and Vane (1967d) showed that up to 95% of prostaglandin E_1, E_2, or $F_{2\alpha}$ was removed in one passage through the pulmonary circulation. The enzyme prostaglandin 15-dehydrogenase which inactivates prostaglandins can be extracted from homogenized lungs (Ånggård and Samuelsson, 1964, 1966, 1967) and the removal process in perfused lungs is enzymic (Piper et al., 1970). In the ewe (Horton et al., 1965), as well as in dogs (Carlson and Orö, 1966), and cats and rabbits (Ferreira and Vane, 1967d), the hypotensive effects of prostaglandins of the E and F series are greater with intra-aortic than with intravenous injections. Their removal in the pulmonary circulation, therefore, takes place in all species so far studied. McGiff et al. (1969) confirmed that prostaglandins E_1 and E_2 were removed by dog lung in vivo and further showed that prostaglandins A_1 and A_2 survived the passage through lungs without change. Thus, within this very closely related group of substances, lung enzymes can distinguish among the individual members. Gibson et al. (1972) compared the removal of prostaglandin $F_{2\alpha}$ in the lungs of dog and sheep. They found that 92% of infused prostaglandin $F_{2\alpha}$ was inactivated or extracted by lung tissue and that in the dog, but not the sheep, the removal was reduced to 84% by intravenous administration of a large dose of aspirin.

Activation or Release of Substances by the Lungs

Although this review deals with detoxication mechanisms, it should be remembered that the lungs may also contribute vasoactive substances to the arterial circulation. Ng and Vane (1967 and 1968) first showed that the inactive decapeptide angiotensin I was converted to the most potent pressor substance known, angiotensin II, by a converting enzyme fixed in lung tissue. This has since been amply confirmed (Vane, 1974) although there is still some contention as to the relative physiological importance of converting enzyme in lung as against other tissue enzymes. It is now becoming clear that, as suggested by Ng and Vane (1968), the same enzyme in the lung can inactivate bradykinin and activate angiotensin I. In isolated perfused lungs of guinea pigs the converting enzyme and kininase activities are indistinguishable (Alabaster and Bakhle, 1972b). Although Scholz and Biron (1969) do not believe that one enzyme serves both functions, the substrate specificity of an enzyme can only effectively be established on homogeneous forms of the protein. Cushman and Cheung (1972) were the first to purify lung converting enzyme to homogeneity. Others (Yang et al., 1971; Elisseeva et al., 1971) have purified plasma and kidney enzymes in a similar way. In each instance, it is clear that converting enzyme also inactivates bradykinin. Thus, one enzyme can remove from the blood the potent vasodilator bradykinin and add the potent vasoconstrictor angiotensin I. However, evidence is lacking as to whether the kininase activity of converting enzyme is physiologically important, for there is at least one other kininase in lung tissue (Ryan et al., 1968).

Other vasoactive substances can also be liberated into the blood stream from lung tissue, not only during the anaphylactic response (Piper and Vane, 1969), but also after other types of pathological, chemical, mechanical, or even physiological stimulation (Piper and Vane, 1971). Moore et al. (1963) showed that 5-HT released histamine from perfused from perfused lungs. Tyramine and 5-HT will also induce release of a mixture of spasmogens from isolated lungs (Alabaster and Bakhle, 1970b; Bakhle and Smith, 1972), as will bradykinin (Piper and Vane, 1969). Of the substances released from lungs, only histamine is stored in the lung tissue; the rest, which includes slow reacting substance in anaphylaxis (SRS-A), rabbit aorta contracting substance (RCS), and prostaglandin E_2 and $F_{2\alpha}$ are synthesized and released at the time of stimulation.

These results suggest that not only do the lungs have a metabolic function but also an endocrine one.

CONCLUSIONS

1. Three types of chemical structures have been considered in detail: amines, peptides and prostaglandins. In each of these groups there are substances which are almost completely inactivated or removed as they pass through the pulmonary circulation and others which are unaffected.

2. For each class of substances the final removal mechanism has been shown to be enzymic, although for amines, the primary mechanism is uptake. Much of the evidence which is accumulating suggests that the endothelial cells of the arterioles, capillaries, and postcapillary venules are important sites for metabolism of vasoactive substances.

3. The selectivity of the removal processes associated with the pulmonary circulation led to the postulate (Vane, 1969) that vasoactive hormones can be divided into two types, "local" and "circulating" hormones. The local hormones (acetylcholine, bradykinin, 5-HT, prostaglandin E_2 and $F_{2\alpha}$) are those which are effectively removed by the lungs and if they have a physiological function it is probably localized at or near the site of release. Venous blood may be full of noxious, as yet unidentified, chemicals released from peripheral vascular beds, but which are removed by the lungs before they can affect the arterial circulation. The circulating hormones are those which pass through the lungs either unchanged (epinephrine, histamine, vasopressin, oxytocin, prostaglandin A_2) or with an actual increase in activity (angiotensin I to II).

4. The inactivation mechanism of the lungs may sometimes be bypassed or overwhelmed. For instance, there may be continuous formation of bradykinin by a circulating enzyme such as kallikrein or release of 5-HT from platelets. The release of substances by the lungs themselves is also an important consideration. These results led to the suggestion that defects in the protective function of the pulmonary circulation may lead to disease states (Vane, 1969). From such considerations, Sandler (1972) has suggested that migraine may be a pulmonary disease. Another way in which the pulmonary protective action may be overwhelmed would be giving enough substance intravenously so that the small percentage which is left still has an effect on the arterial circulation. This, presumably, is the basis of the abortifacient action of prostaglandins given intravenously to women (Karim, 1972).

5. When compounds are tested for their effects on blood pressure the possibility of pulmonary removal or activation should be considered. This is especially relevant to the testing of an homologous series, for the structure–activity relationship associated with the removal in the lungs may be quite different from that associated with activity on receptors. Com-

pounds may be rejected in the belief that they are inactive at receptors, when the apparent inactivity is due to pulmonary removal.

6. The selective removal of some substances by the pulmonary circulation and others by peripheral vascular beds (Vane, 1969) means that venous and arterial concentrations of any one substance will be substantially different. For example, the concentration of norepinephrine in peripheral venous blood will give little indication of the concentration in arterial blood since it would be the sum of the small fraction of the arterial concentration which passes through the peripheral vascular beds added to that which may be escaping from nerve endings. Indeed, even the concentration of norepinephrine in central venous blood (which includes the adrenal medullary secretion) will be different from that in arterial blood because of uptake in the lungs. This example illustrates the importance of stating which blood concentration is being measured and of choosing a site for sampling blood which will have relevance to the problem under investigation.

7. Many of the naturally occurring substances which have been discussed are active on venous vasculature, on pulmonary vasculature and on airways resistance. Another interpretation of the results is that those substances which are inactivated by the lungs have a selective hormonal function on the smooth muscle in the venous or pulmonary circulation. The general description of a substance as a hormone may, therefore, have to be further qualified to "local," "venous," "pulmonary," or "arterial," depending on the site of their release or formation and on the target organ.

8. The analogy between the respiratory and metabolic functions of the lungs with which this article started can be extended. Just as they protect the arterial circulation by removing the waste product, carbon dioxide, so do they remove several vasoactive hormones. Similarly, just as the respiratory function of the lungs adds the vital oxygen to the blood passing through them, so their metabolic activity adds angiotensin II and possibly other vasoactive substances as well.

REFERENCES

Alabaster, V. A., 1971, Ph.D. thesis. London University.
Alabaster, V. A., and Bakhle, Y. S., 1970*a*, *Brit. J. Pharmacol.* **40**: 468.
Alabaster, V. A., and Bakhle, Y. S., 1970*b*, *Brit. J. Pharmacol.* **40**: 582P.
Alabaster, V. A., and Bakhle, Y. S., 1972*a*, *Brit. J. Pharmacol.* **45**: 299.
Alabaster, V. A., and Bakhle, Y. S., 1972*b*, *Circulation Res.* **31**:Supp II, 72.
Alabaster, V. A., and Bakhle, Y. S., 1973, *Brit. J. Pharmacol.* **47**: 325.
Änggård, E., and Samuelsson, B., 1964, *J. Biol. Chem.* **239**: 4097.
Änggård, E., and Samuelsson, B., 1966, *Arkiv Kemi* **25**: 293.
Änggård, E., and Samuelsson, B., 1967, *Proceedings of the 2nd Nobel Symposium Stockholm*, p. 97, Interscience, New York.

Bailey, T., Clements, J. A., and Osbahr, A. J., 1967, *Circulation Res.* **21**: 469.
Bakhle, Y. S., 1968, *Nature (London)* **220**: 919.
Bakhle, Y. S., Reynard, A. M., and Vane, J. R., 1969, *Nature (London)* **222**: 956.
Bakhle, Y. S., and Smith, T. W., 1972, *Brit. J. Pharmacol.* **46**: 543P.
Biron, P., 1968, *Rev. Can. Biol.* **27**: 75.
Biron, P., and Boileau, J. C., 1969, *Can. J. Physiol. Pharmacol.* **47**: 713.
Biron, P., and Campeau, L., 1971, *Rev. Can. Biol.* **30**: 27.
Biron, P., Campeau, L., and David, P., 1969, *Am. J. Cardiol.* **24**: 544.
Biron, P., Meyer, P., and Panisset, J. C., 1968, *Can. J. Physiol. Pharmacol.* **46**: 175.
Boileau, J. C., Campeau, L., and Biron P., 1971, *Rev. Can. Biol.* **30**: 281.
Boileau, J. C., Campeau, L., and Biron, P., 1972, *Rev. Can. Biol.* **31**: 185.
Boileau, J. C., Crexells, C., and Biron, P., 1972, *Rev. Can. Biol.* **31**: 69.
Born, G. V. R., 1963, in: *The Scientific Basis of Medicine Ann Rev.*, p. 269, Athlone Press, London.
Carlson, L. A., and Orö, L., 1966, *Acta Physiol. Scand.* **67**: 89.
Crexells, C., Bourassa, M. G., and Biron, P., 1972, *J. Clin. Endocrinol.* **34**: 592.
Cushman, D. W., and Cheung, H. S., 1972, in: *Hypertension 72* (Genest, J. and Koiw, E., ed.), p. 532, Springer-Verlag, New York.
Davis, R. B., 1968, in: *Advances in Pharmacology* (Garattini, S., Shore, P. A., Costa, E., and Sandler, M., eds.) Vol. 6 , p. 146, Academic Press, New York.
Davis, R. B., and Wang, Y., 1965, *Proc. Soc. Exp. Biol. Med.* **118**: 799.
Eble, J. N., Gowdey, C. W., and Vane, J. R., 1971, *Nature (London)* **231**: 181.
Eiseman, B., Bryant, L., and Waltuch, T., 1964, *J. Thorac. Cardiovasc. Surg.* **48**: 798.
Eliseeva, Y. E., Orekhovich, V. N., Pavlikhina, L. V., and Alexeenko, L. P., 1971, *Clin. Chim. Acta* **31**: 413.
Elliot, T. R., 1905, *J. Physiol. London* **32**: 401.
Ferreira, S. H., and Vane, J. R., 1967a, *Nature (London)* **215**: 1237.
Ferreira, S. H., and Vane, J. R. 1967b, *Brit. J. Pharmacol.* **29**: 367.
Ferreira, S. H., and Vane, J. R., 1967c, *Brit. J. Pharmacol.* **30**: 417.
Ferreira, S. H., and Vane, J. R., 1967d, *Nature (London)* **216**: 868.
Freer, R. J., and Stewart, J. M., 1972, *Federation Proc.* **31**: 512 Abs.
Gaddum, J. H., 1953, *Brit. J. Pharmacol.* **8**: 321.
Gaddum, J. H., Hebb, C. O., Silver, A., and Swan, A. A. B., 1953, *Quart. J. Exp. Physiol.* **38**: 255.
Gershon, M. D., and Ross, L. L., 1966a, *J. Physiol. London*, **186**: 451.
Gershon, M. D., and Ross, L. L., 1966b, *J. Physiol. London* **186**: 477.
Gibson, E. C., Hodge, R. L., Jackson, H. R., Katic, F. P., and Stevens, A. M., 1972, *Australian Physiol. & Pharmacol. Soc.*
Gilmore, N. J., and Vane, J. R., 1970, *Brit. J. Pharmacol.* **38**: 633.
Gillis, C. N., 1971, *Experientia* **27**: 1317.
Gillis, C. N., Greene, N. M., Cronau, L. H., and Hammond, G. L., 1972, *Circulation Res.* **30**: 666.
Gillis, C. N., and Iwasawa, Y., 1972, *Federation Proc.* **31**: 599 Abs.
Ginn, R. W., and Vane, J. R., 1968, *Nature (London)* **219**: 740.
Gobel, A. J., Hay, D. R., and Sandler, M., 1955, *Lancet* **2**: 1016.
Goffinet, J. A., and Mulrow, P. J., 1965, *Clin. Res.* **11**: 408.
Gruby, L. A., Rowlands, C., Varley, B. Q., and Wyllie, J. H., 1971, *Brit. J. Surg.* **58**: 525.
Hébert, F., Fouron, J. C., Boileau, J. C., and Biron, P., 1972, *Am. J. Physiol.* **223**: 20.
Heinemann, H. O., and Fishman, A. P., 1969, *Physiol. Rev.* **49**: 1.
Hinman, J. W., 1972, *Ann. Rev. Biochem.* **41**: 161.

Hodge, R. L., Ng, K. K. F., and Vane, J. R., 1967, *Nature (London)* **215**: 138.
Horton, E. W., Main, I. H. M., and Thompson, C. J., 1965, *J. Physiol. London* **180**: 514.
Hughes, J. R., Gillis, C. N., and Bloom. F. E., 1969, *J. Pharmacol. Exp. Therap.* **169**: 237.
Junod, A. F., 1971, *Federation Proc.* **30**: 671 Abs.
Karim, S. M. M., 1972, *The Prostaglandins*, MTP, Oxford.
Kaufman, R. M., Airo, R., Pollock, S., and Crosby, W. H., 1965, *Blood* **26**: 720.
Leary, W. P. P., and Ledingham, J. G., 1969, *Nature (London)* **222**: 959.
Lilja, B., and Lindell, S. E., 1961, *Brit. J. Pharmacol.* **16**: 203.
McCarthy, D. A., Potter, D. E., and Nicolaides, E. D., 1965, *J. Pharmacol. Exp. Therap.* **148**: 117.
McGiff, J. C., Terragno, N. A., Strand, J. C., Lee, J. B., Lonigro, A. J., and Ng, K. K. F., 1969, *Nature (London)* **223**: 742.
Moore, T. C., Normell, L., and Eiseman, B., 1963, *Arch. Surg. (Chicago)* **87**: 103.
Ng, K. K. F., and Vane, J. R., 1967, *Nature (London)* **216**: 762.
Ng, K. K. F., and Vane, J. R., 1968, *Nature (London)* **218**: 144.
Piper, P. J., and Vane, J. R., 1969, *Nature (London)* **223**: 29.
Piper, P. J., and Vane, J. R., 1971, *Ann. N. Y. Acad. Sci.* **180**: 363.
Piper, P. J., Vane, J. R., and Wyllie, J. H., 1970, *Nature (London)* **225**: 600.
Pojda, S., and Vane, J. R., 1971, *Brit. J. Pharmacol.* **42**: 558.
Rapport, M. M., Greene, A. A., and Page, I. H., 1948a, *Science* **108**: 329.
Rapport, M. M., Greene, A. A., and Page, I. H., 1948b, *J. Biol. Chem.* **176**: 1243.
Richardson, J. B., and Beaulnes, A., 1971, *J. Cell. Biol.* **51**: 419.
Ryan, J. W., Roblero, J., and Stewart, J. M., 1968, *Biochem. J.* **110**: 795.
Ryan, J. W., Roblero, J., and Stewart, J. M., 1969, *Pharm. Res. Comm.* **1**: 192.
Said, S. I., 1968, *New Engl. J. Med.* **279**: 3.
Sandler, M., 1972, *Lancet* **1**: 618.
Scholz, H. W., and Biron, P., 1969, *Rev. Can. Biol.* **28**: 197.
Spector, W. S., 1956, *Handbook of Biological Data*, p. 285, Saunders, Philadelphia.
Stacey, R. S., 1961, *Brit. J. Pharmacol.* **16**: 284.
Starling, E. H., and Verney, E. D., 1925, *Proc. Roy. Soc. B* **97**: 321.
Steggeda, F. R., Essex, H. E., and Mann, F. C., 1935, *Am. J. Physiol.* **112**: 70.
Stewart, J. M., 1968, *Federation Proc.* **27**: 534.
Thomas, D. P., and Vane, J. R., 1967, *Nature* **216**: 335.
Todrick, A., and Tait, C., 1969, *J. Pharm. Pharmacol.* **21**: 751.
Tranza, J. P., DaPrada, M., and Pletscher, A., 1966, *Nature (London)* **212**: 1574.
Vane, J. R., 1964, *Brit. J. Pharmacol.* **23**: 360.
Vane, J. R., 1968, in: *Importance of Fundamental Principles in Drug Evaluation* (Tedeschi, D. H., and Tedeschi, R. E., eds.), p. 217, Raven Press, New York.
Vane, J. R., 1969, *Brit. J. Pharmacol.* **35**: 209.
Vane, J. R., 1974, in: *Angiotensin* (Bumpus, M., and Page, I. H., eds.), Springer-Verlag, New York.
Vane, J. R., and Williams K. I., 1970, *Brit J. Pharmacol.* **38**: 444P.
Weeks, J. R., 1972, *Ann. Rev. Pharmacol.* **12**: 317.
Yang, H. Y. T., Erdös, E. G., and Levin, Y., 1971, *J. Pharmacol. Exp. Therap.* **177**: 291.

DISCUSSION SUMMARY

Garrett inquired whether the saturability of the lung detoxification processes and their substrate dependence were tested. Vane replied that only at several hundredfold higher than physiological concentrations is the process saturable. Brown described certain recent studies by T. Gram and J. Fouts comparing drug metabolism in rat lung and liver microsomes in which lung microsomes were more active toward some substrates. Lemberger and Conney mentioned that tetrahydrocannabinol and benzpyrene are metabolized to some extent in the lung. Conney stated that he had examined human lungs containing tumors for benzpyrene hydroxylase activity and observed no detectable activity. Perhaps these individuals lost the activity of this enzyme because of the malignancy; or, alternatively, as mentioned by La Du, they developed tumors because of lowered or absent activity of the enzyme. A further complication concerning pulmonary drug metabolism was introduced by Gillette, who stressed the extremely heterogeneous nature of pulmonary tissue which is composed of many histologically distinguishable types of cells, with different localization of enzyme systems.

The Importance of Tissue Distribution in Pharmacokinetics

James R. Gillette

Laboratory of Chemical Pharmacology
National Heart and Lung Institute
National Institutes of Health, Bethesda, Maryland

In evoking pharmacological and toxicological responses, drugs generally combine either reversibly or irreversibly with action sites on intrastitial macromolecules or organelles, and thereby cause alterations of physicochemical or biochemical processes in the living animal. These alterations can be evoked by a number of mechanisms. Drugs can either mimic or block the action of normally occurring substances by combining with receptor sites. Drugs can alter the localization of normally occurring substances by interfering with transport mechanisms or changing the number of storage sites. Drugs can change the concentrations of normally occurring substances in tissues by reacting with them directly or by altering the activities of enzymes that catalyze their formation or destruction.

Regardless of the mechanism of drug action, the drug must first reach its site of action in adequate concentrations to produce its effect. With reversibly acting drugs, the amount of drug combined with the action site is dependent on the concentration of unbound drug in the fluid immediately surrounding the action site, the so-called biophase. Unfortunately, the concentration of unbound drug at these sites is seldom known. Most estimates of the concentration of drug at action sites are based on the concentration of unbound drug in blood plasma, the physiological medium of exchange between all tissues. In making these estimates, the investigator assumes that the unbound concentrations of the drug in the plasma and at the locus of action are the same. But this assumption is invalid in a number of instances. Polar compounds slowly transverse membranes such as the blood–brain barrier; thus the levels of quaternary ammonium compounds and sulfonic acid derivatives can be considerably lower in brain than in plasma. Some compounds can be metabolized so rapidly in plasma that their rates of diffusion from their receptor sites determine their duration of action; for example, the pharmacological effects of succinylcholine can still be observed even after the drug has been virtually cleared from plasma (Kalow, 1962). Other polar compounds can be concentrated in tissues by active transport systems; for example, the levels of certain amino acids can be greater within cells than in interstitial fluid.

On the other hand, lipid-soluble compounds readily pass through lipoid membrane barriers and can be concentrated only slightly or not at all by active transport systems; thus, within a short time after the administration of a lipid-soluble compound, its free concentration at the locus of action becomes virtually identical to its free concentration in plasma. Since the pH is usually slightly lower within cells than it is in plasma, however, the unbound concentrations of lipid-soluble weak acids and bases in cells differ slightly from those in plasma (Waddell and Butler, 1959). For example, the concentration of phenobarbital is slightly lower in brain than in plasma (Waddell and Butler, 1957). Moreover, hyperventilation of the lungs or breathing atmospheres containing CO_2 can alter the distribution of phenobarbital by changing the pH of the blood plasma.

The distribution of most drugs, however, is governed by their reversible combinations with proteins and other constituents in blood and tissues. The concentration of unbound drug, therefore, can be considerably lower than either the total plasma level or the total tissue level of the drug. In fact, determination of the tissue to plasma level ratios of the drugs frequently gives a wrong impression of the extent of binding, because drugs are usually bound to both tissue and plasma proteins.

Some drugs are strongly bound to tissue even though the tissue to plasma ratios are low. For example, calculations made from the results of Burns *et al.* (1953) showed that about 98% of the phenylbutazone in plasma is bound to proteins and that about 95% of the drug in liver and kidney is bound. If Burns *et al.* (1953) had determined only the tissue to plasma ratios of the drug they might have concluded that the drug was not appreciably bound since these ratios approached values that might be expected with drugs that are distributed with body water.

On the other hand, a drug can be highly bound to plasma proteins even when the tissue to plasma ratios are high. For example, Dingell *et al.* (1964) found that 90 min after the intravenous administration of imipramine (20 mg/kg) to rabbits, the drug levels were about 12 µg/g in brain and 0.6 µg/

ml in plasma. However, at least 97% of the imipramine in brain and 82% of the drug in plasma were bound, indicating that the concentrations of unbound imipramine in these tissues were less than 0.15 µg/ml ($5 \times 10^{-7} M$, a value that is considerably lower than the concentration which at that time had been assumed to occur *in vivo*.

BINDING OF DRUGS IN PLASMA

Although drugs can bind to various proteins in blood, probably the most important protein is serum albumin. Among the compounds bound to this protein are tetracyclines, digitoxin, salicylates, sulfonamide, phenylbutazone, barbiturates, acid dyes, fatty acids, vitamin C, uric acid, histamine, bilirubin, and tryptophan. Even though albumin has a net negative charge at the *p*H of blood, *p*H 7.4, it binds both positively and negatively charged molecules. Studies with purified albumin preparations have revealed, however, that the number of sites available for drug binding depends on the drug. Some drugs are bound to a single high affinity site and several low affinity sites, whereas others are bound to virtually an infinite number of low affinity sites. For this reason, certain drugs, such as phenylbutazone, can saturate their high affinity sites at plasma levels obtained in therapy (Burns *et al.*, 1953), whereas others, such as imipramine, do not saturate their binding sites with therapeutic levels of the drug even though they are highly bound in plasma (Sasame and Gillette, unpublished results).

The sites that avidly bind one drug may be different from those that avidly bind another. For this reason, not all highly bound anionic drugs can displace one another from serum albumin. For example, campothecin can be displaced from serum albumin by phenylbutazone, but not by dicoumarol even though all three drugs are highly bound to the protein (Guarino *et al.*, 1973). Similarly, indomethacin can be displaced from serum albumin by salicylic acid, but not by phenylbutazone or by probenecid (Yesair *et al.*, 1970). For this reason, it is frequently impossible to predict *a priori* whether two different compounds will compete for the same binding site on serum albumin.

Although drugs in plasma are bound mainly to albumin, they may also be bound to other proteins in plasma. Indeed, some plasma proteins have such a high affinity for certain endogenous substances that they are thought to act as special transport systems for these substances in blood. For example, corticosterone, testosterone, estrogen, and thyroxine are probably bound to specialized proteins. Thus, substances that resemble these hormones may also be bound to a certain extent by these proteins. In addition, some drugs may be bound to antibodies in the gamma globulin fraction. For example, treatment of rabbits with morphine attached covalently to albumin, evokes the formation of antibodies that avidly bind morphine and a number of its analogs (Spector and Parkey, 1970; Spector, 1971). Indeed, as drugs become more and more potent in the future, the use of antisera as drug antidotes may become increasingly more important. In fact, antibodies are now being used as antidotes for extraordinarily potent toxicants, such as botulinus toxin.

Although most studies on the binding of drugs to proteins have been carried out with highly purified preparations of serum proteins, we must remember that blood contains many substances that are avidly bound to serum proteins and thereby affect the binding of drugs. For example, fatty acids are known to affect the binding of phenylbutazone and warfarin to serum albumin (Solomon *et al.*, 1968) and bilirubin affects the binding of certain sulfa drugs, such as sulfaphenazole (Chignell *et al.*, 1971*b*).

Several studies have shown that the plasma concentrations of unbound drugs frequently are higher in neonates than in adults. Although these studies raised the possibility that the serum proteins in neonates differ markedly from those in adults, it now seems likely that the differences in the binding of drugs are mainly due to unusually high concentrations of bilirubin and other endogenous substances in neonatal blood. In accord with this view, Chignell *et al.* (1971*b*) found that the binding of sulfaphenazole to neonatal serum differed markedly from that to adult serum. But after treating the sera with charcoal to remove substances, such as fatty acids and bilirubin, the binding of the drug to neonatal and adult sera was virtually identical. These findings raise the possibility that the binding of drugs to plasma may be markedly altered in patients suffering from diseases in which the plasma levels of avidly bound endogenous substances are markedly altered.

Species differences in the binding of drugs are due not only to the total concentrations and relative proportions of the various classes of proteins, but also to the composition and conformation of albumins. For example, the serum albumins from man, monkey, rabbit, and guinea pig bind salicylate more avidly than do those of rat and dog (Kucera and Bullock, 1969). Moreover, studies of the fluorescence characteristics of warfarin–albumin complexes have revealed that the serum albumins from rats, dogs, and cattle induce a greater blue shift in the fluorescence emission maximum of warfarin than do those from other species, including humans, horses, and rabbits. Thus, there are species differences in the distance between the binding site of the drug and the tryptophan groups in the albumin molecule (Chignell, 1972).

In some instances, the administration of a drug can alter the binding of another in unusual ways. For example, Dollery *et al.* (1961) found that chlorothiazide caused a fourfold increase in the binding of the ganglionic blocking agent, pempidine, possibly by forming an ion-pair complex that is more highly bound than is pempidine itself. On the other hand, some drugs can react covalently with serum albumin and thereby cause conformational changes that affect the binding of other drugs. For example, when aspirin is incubated with serum albumin, the acetyl group of aspirin becomes covalently attached to lysine in albumin. The acetylated albumin thus formed has a higher affinity for phenylbutazone and a lower affinity for flufenamic acid (Chignell and Starkweather, 1971a).

After considering these studies, we can understand how the binding of drugs to various proteins in plasma can manifest complex kinetic relationships that can be made even more complex by the prior or simultaneous administration of other drugs or by changes in the plasma levels of endogenous substances.

BINDING OF DRUGS TO TISSUES

Although the binding of drugs to serum proteins may be complex, the binding of drugs to tissue components is even more so. Not only do tissues have many more different kinds of proteins than plasma, but they also contain many other substances that are able to combine with drugs.

Many drugs, whose structures are planar, combine with DNA by intercalation between the base-pairs of the double helix. Indeed, the acridine dyes probably exert their antibacterial action by intercalation with the DNA of bacteria (Lerman, 1961). Moreover, chlorpromazine and some antimalarial drugs are thought to cause mutagenic effects in certain bacteria by an intercalation mechanism (B. Ames and M. Legator, personal communication). To what extent these substances cause mutagenic effects in animals, however, needs to be clarified.

Some planar aromatic drugs are also bound to melanin granules in eyes and skin. Indeed, there is evidence that the retinopathies caused by chloroquine and phenothiazines may be due to their accumulations in the melanin-containing tissues of the eye (Potts, 1964; Bernstein et al., 1963). Moreover, the ^{125}I analogue of chloroquine accumulates in melanomas and thus can be used to detect the presence of this kind of tumor (Beierwaltes et al., 1968).

The kinetics of the binding of drugs to melanin granules, however, is complex. V. Horak and J. R. Gillette (unpublished results) found that various quinoline derivatives rapidly combine with quinonoid groups on the surface of melanin granules, but slowly diffuse through pores of the granules and combine with the quinonoid groups within the particles. Similarly, Ti^{+3} rapidly reduces the surface quinonoid groups of the melanin particles and slowly reduces the interior quinonoid groups (Horak and Gillette, 1971).

The combination of high affinity of the granules for planar aromatic drugs and the slow diffusion of the drugs into and out of the melanin granules accounts for the extraordinarily long lifetime of the drugs in these particles. Indeed, small amounts of chloroquine can be detected in patients many years after they have stopped taking the drug (Bernstein et al., 1963).

Lipid soluble drugs can become localized in adipose tissue according to their fat/water partition coefficients. For example, it is well known that chlorinated hydrocarbon insecticides including DDT, heptachlor, and aldrin become localized in fat (Robinson et al., 1965). Similarly, large portions of dibenzyline and thiopental are ultimately localized in fat (Brodie et al., 1952; 1954). Since the blood supply to fat is very low, the equilibrium between blood and fat occurs slowly and thus the fat to plasma ratios reach maximal values long after they do in other tissues. Thus, although thiopental is metabolized slowly, it is an ultrashort-acting barbiturate because it rapidly leaves the brain and plasma and enters first the intermediately perfused tissues such as muscle and then the adipose tissue. In fact, when thiopental is given repeatedly, the plasma levels of thiopental can remain above the threshold level required for anesthesia after the redistribution phases are complete. When that occurs the anesthetic effects of thiopental can persist for an exceedingly long time.

Localization of drugs in fat can cause unusual effects. For example, individuals attempting suicide by taking large doses of thiopental may awaken as the plasma and brain levels have been decreased during extracorporeal dialysis. But after the dialysis is stopped, the plasma levels of the drug rise above threshold levels as the thiopental in fat redistributes and the patient returns to sleep. Moreover, inducers of liver microsomal enzymes localized in fat of animals may become mobilized on starvation and thereby enhance their inducing effects (Hart and Fouts, 1965).

Some lipid soluble compounds are so tightly bound to other tissues that their accumulation in adipose tissue may be negligible. For example, imipramine is about as lipid soluble as thiopental, but very little of it becomes localized in fat (Dingell et al., 1964). Since imipramine contains a polycyclic ring that is only slightly puckered, we thought that the binding of imipramine to tissues might be due to intercalation with DNA or RNA. However, studies on the intracellular distribution of bound imipramine revealed that imipramine was preferentially bound to all the particulate organelles and not just to the nuclei (Dingell and Gillette, unpublished results). Moreover, our studies showed that imipramine was bound to a greater extent by smooth-surfaced microsomes, which are devoid of ribosomes, than by rough-surfaced microsomes (Table I). These findings

TABLE I
Binding of Imipramine by Smooth and Rough Microsomes from Rabbit Liver (5 mg protein/15 ml)

	Imipramine added, μmoles	% Drug bound	RNA/Protein
Smooth microsomes	0.6	53	0.026
	1.2	50	
Rough microsomes	0.6	42	0.188
	1.2	39	

(unpublished results) suggested to Dr. H. Sasame and me that imipramine might be bound mainly to phospholipids in the intracellular organelles and plasma membranes. In support of this view, the binding of imipramine to phospholipids isolated from liver microsomes accounted for nearly all of the binding to microsomes (Table II).

Several drugs persist in lungs long after they have left the other organs in the body. Intravenously administered drugs that are soluble in acid or alkali but insoluble at body pH can localize in lungs because they precipitate in the blood and their crystals become lodged in the capillary bed of the lungs. But many drugs accumulate in lungs even when they are administered orally or intraperitoneally. Since intravascular crystallization would not be expected to occur under these conditions, it seems likely that the lungs either contain unique components that bind the drugs or have unique characteristics that permit such unusual localization of the drugs. Studies with homogenates, however, have usually failed to reveal any differences between lung and other tissues in the binding of drugs. For example, imipramine is as highly bound by homogenates of liver as it is by homogenates of lung (Dingell and Gillette, unpublished results). Similarly, norchlorcyclazine is bound by liver and lung homogenates to about the

TABLE II
Binding of Imipramine to Rabbit Liver Microsomes and to Microsomal Lipid in 33 mM Na Phosphate Buffer, pH 7.4

Lipid concentration, mg/ml	% Imipramine (0.1 mM) Bound microsomes	microsomal lipid
0.137	34.3	29.8
0.273	57.0	49.3
0.546	78.8	69.5
1.09	81.7	83.5
1.64	90.7	88.1

same extent even though the drug accumulates to a greater extent in lungs of dogs *in vivo* (Kuntzman *et al.*, 1967). Thus, the mechanism for the accumulation of drugs in lungs remains obscure.

GENERAL CONSIDERATIONS OF DRUG LOCALIZATION

Studies on the relative concentrations of bound and unbound drugs in the various tissues can lead to deceptive impressions. For example, in man the plasma volume represents only about 3.0 liters and the extravascular albumin has a volume of distribution of another 2.5 liters. Thus, the amount of drug that is bound to plasma albumin may represent only a small fraction of the total amount of drug in the body. Indeed, if 90% of the drug in plasma were bound and if the drug were bound only to serum albumin, the amount of bound drug would be only about 50% of the total amount of drug in the body (Table III). Similarly, the amounts of drug bound to liver, lungs and other relatively small organs may also represent only a small percentage of the total amount of drug in the body even when the percent of binding in any given tissue appears to be high. Clearly, therefore, the bound portion of the total amount of drug will be significant only when the degree of binding is very high (for example, more than 90% in plasma) or the volume of the tissues containing the binding sites represents a significant proportion of the volume of the body (for example, skeletal muscle or fat).

The relationship between the degree of binding of drugs to various tissues and the concentration of unbound drug in the body becomes

TABLE III

Relationship between the Proportion of Binding to Plasma Protein and Binding of Total Drug in the Body[a]

Plasma albumin, % bound	Muscle, % bound	Total drug in body, % bound
50	0	9.9
90	0	49.6
99	0	91.5
0	50	37.5
0	90	84.4
0	99	98.4
50	50	41.5
90	90	86.5
99	99	98.5

[a] Volume of plasma albumin 5.5 liters, volume of muscle, 30 liters; volume of body water, 50 liters.

particularly important in determining whether the displacement of one drug by another from binding sites has biological significance. Indeed, if 90% of a drug were bound to plasma albumin and if it were completely displaced by another drug, the concentration of free drug would only be doubled at most (Gillette, 1968). However, a similar increase in the unbound concentration would be expected to occur when the dose of the drug was doubled. Moreover, the plasma levels of drugs in man can vary as much as 50-fold in patients receiving the same dose of drug. Thus, the displacement of drugs from plasma proteins usually plays an insignificant role in affecting the pharmacologic action of drugs in man except when the drug is bound more than 90% or when the drug is unusually toxic.

Although it is well known that the binding of drugs to plasma proteins and to other tissues can profoundly affect the biological half-life of drugs, the ways in which drug binding can affect the rates of elimination of drugs are only vaguely understood by many pharmacologists, particularly those who are not well trained in mathematics. Even though most pharmacologists are aware of the basic concepts of a one-compartment system, they are frequently baffled by the mathematics of multiple-compartment systems. Because of this general lack of understanding, it might be useful to review some of the basic aspects of the two-compartment model.

Pharmacologists usually recognize that after intravenous administration, drug levels in plasma are initially high and rapidly decline biphasically and in some cases polyphasically. The early phases are associated mainly with the distribution of the drug into tissues, and the last phase is associated with the elimination of the drug after the distribution phases have been completed. However, the term "biological half-life" when applied to such polyphasic systems is not always understood.

Let us consider a two-compartment system in which the drug is instantaneously introduced into the central compartment, passes into and out of the side compartment by first-order processes, and is eliminated only from the central compartment by a first-order process, which may be by a combination of excretion and metabolism. This model cannot be used when the levels of drug in the body reach concentrations that saturate binding sites or enzymes and transport systems that catalyze the uptake of the drug into tissues or its elimination from the body. However, the model may still be useful when the concentrations of the saturated binding sites are much smaller than the lowest concentration of drug measured in plasma. In this two-compartment system, k_1 is the rate constant for the passage of the drug from the central compartment (A) to the body compartment (B), k_2 is the rate constant for the passage of the drug from the body compartment (B) into the central compartment (A), and k_3 is the rate constant of elimination as shown in Fig. 1. Inspection of the equations shown in Fig. 2 for the

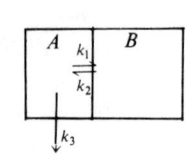

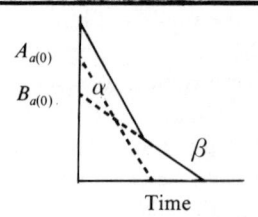

Definitions (for Figs. 1-6)

- A = The central compartment of a two-compartment system. The drug is rapidly injected into this compartment.
- B = The peripheral compartment of a two-compartment system.
- k_1 = The first-order rate constant for the passage of the drug from compartment A to compartment B.
- k_2 = The first-order rate constant for the passage of the drug from compartment B to compartment A.
- k_3 = The first-order rate constant of elimination of the drug from compartment A.
- Q_0 = The amount of drug that is rapidly injected into compartment A.
- Q_a = The amount of drug in compartment A at any given time after injection of the drug.
- Q_b = The amount of drug in compartment B at any given time after injection of the drug. Initially $Q_b = 0$.
- Q_{tot} = The total amount of drug in the system at any given time. $Q_{tot} = Q_a + Q_b$.
- V_a = The volume of compartment A.
- C_a = The concentration of drug in compartment A at any given time. C_a usually is the plasma concentration.
- β = The rate constant for the second phase of the biphasic decline in the level of C_a and Q_b. When the values of C_a are plotted on semilogarithmic graph paper against time, β may be estimated from the slope of the second phase, according to the equation $\beta = 2.303$ slope, or from the half-time of the second phase, according to the relationship $\beta = 0.693/t_{1/2}$.
- $B_{a(0)}$ = The intercept obtained by extrapolating the straight line associated with β back to time zero.
- β-phase = The second phase of the biphasic decline of C_a. It is described by the equation $B_a = B_{a(0)} \exp(-\beta t)$.
- α = The rate constant for the first phase of the biphasic decline of C_a and Q_b. After the straight line of the β-phase is extrapolated back to time zero, the extrapolated values are subtracted from the observed values of C_a and the resultant values are plotted on semilogarithmic graph paper. α may be estimated from the slope or the half-time of the secondary plot as described for β.
- $A_{a(0)}$ = The intercept obtained after extrapolating the secondary plot back to time zero.
- α-phase = The first phase of the biphasic decline of C_a. It is described by the equation $A_a = A_{a(0)} \exp(-\alpha t)$.

Fig. 1. Illustration of two-compartment model and definitions.

Compartment A

$$C_a = \frac{Q_0}{V_a}\left[\left(\frac{\alpha - k_2}{\alpha - \beta}\right)\exp(-\alpha t) + \left(\frac{k_2 - \beta}{\alpha - \beta}\right)\exp(-\beta t)\right]$$

$$C_a = [A_{a(0)}\exp(-\alpha t)] + [B_{a(0)}\exp(-\beta t)]$$

Compartment B

$$Q_b = \frac{Q_0 k_1}{\alpha - \beta}[\exp(-\beta t) - \exp(-\alpha t)]$$

Total Amount in Body

$$Q_{tot} = Q_0\left[\left(\frac{\alpha - k_1 - k_2}{\alpha - \beta}\right)\exp(-\alpha t) + \left(\frac{k_1 + k_2 - \beta}{\alpha - \beta}\right)\exp(-\beta t)\right]$$

$$Q_{tot} = A_{tot(0)}\exp(-\alpha t) + B_{tot(0)}\exp(-\beta t)$$

Fig. 2. Equations for the two-compartment system illustrated in Fig. 1.

amounts of drug in the central and body compartments reveals that both equations contain the exponentials, $\exp(-\alpha t)$. and $\exp(-\beta t)$ Thus, the equation for the amount of drug in the total system also contains both the exponentials. For this reason the amounts of drug in the central compartment and the total system both decline biphasically. After the exponential $\exp(-\alpha t)$ declines to a negligible value, that is, after the distribution phase has been completed, changes in the amount of drug in the total system as well as changes in the amount of drug in the central compartment are governed by the exponential $\exp(-\beta t)$. It should be clear, therefore, that after the distribution is completed the biological half-life of the drug is inversely related to β and not to the rate constant of elimination (k_3). Moreover, the half-time of the β-phase can be determined directly by plotting on semilogarithmic paper the concentrations of the drug found at various times in the central compartment. Thus, the pharmacologist who wishes to know only the biological half-life of a drug in the body, doesn't need to calculate the values of k_1, k_2, or k_3.

In the past, most pharmacologists have assumed that the metabolism of drugs can be adequately explained by a one-compartment system in which $C_a = $ (Dose/Volume of distribution) $\exp(-\beta t)$. They have usually ignored the α-phase after intravenous administration of a drug and frequently have waited for the distribution phases to be completed before assaying the drug in plasma. They thus have assumed that $A_{tot(0)}$ in Fig. 2

equals zero and that $B_{tot(0)}$ equals the dose. However, during the distribution phase, the levels of the drug in compartment (A) are higher than they would be if the drug were instantaneously distributed into both compartments, and thus the amount of drug eliminated during the early phases is at least slightly greater than would be predicted by the second or β-phase alone. Indeed, when the rate constant of elimination is very high, most of the drug may be metabolized during the first phase. Thus it becomes necessary to estimate the amount of drug metabolized during the early phase that is not predicted by the β-phase. In experiments with small and inexpensive animals, such as rats and mice, the total metabolism during both phases may be determined by homogenizing the animals and measuring the amount of drug in the body at various times after its intravenous administration. After plotting the data on semilogarithmic graph paper and extrapolating the straight line of the last phase back to the intercept $(B_{tot(0)})$, the extra amount of drug metabolized during the early phases (y) can be estimated from the value for $B_{tot(0)}$ and the dose by the equation, $y = $ Dose $- B_{tot(0)}$. With drugs that are eliminated largely unchanged, but allowed to accumulate in the urinary bladder (and with human patients and large animals), however, other ways must be used to estimate the importance of the elimination of the drug during the early phase. One way is to plot on semilogarithmic graph paper the plasma levels of the drug measured at various times after intravenous administration of the drug and to extrapolate the straight-line plot back to the intercept at time zero, which provides

$$k_1 = (\alpha + \beta) - (k_2 + k_3)$$

$$k_2 = \frac{A_{a(0)}\beta + B_{a(0)}\alpha}{A_{a(0)} + B_{a(0)}}$$

$$k_3 = \frac{\alpha\beta}{k_2}$$

$$B_{tot(0)} = \frac{Q_0(k_1 + k_2 - \beta)}{\alpha - \beta}$$

These equations have been derived from the following equations:

$$\alpha = \tfrac{1}{2}\{k_1 + k_2 + k_3 + [(k_1 + k_2 + k_3)^2 - 4k_2 k_3]^{1/2}\}$$

$$\beta = \tfrac{1}{2}\{k_1 + k_2 + k_3 - [(k_1 + k_2 + k_3)^2 - 4k_2 k_3]^{1/2}\}$$

$$\alpha + \beta = k_1 + k_2 + k_3$$

$$\alpha - \beta = \{(k_1 + k_2 + k_3)^2 - 4k_2 k_3\}^{1/2}$$

$$\alpha\beta = k_2 k_3$$

Fig. 3. Equations for calculating k_1, k_2, k_3 and $B_{tot(0)}$.

$$A_{a(0)} = \frac{Q_0}{V_a}\left(\frac{\alpha - k_2}{\alpha - \beta}\right) \quad \text{See Figure 2.}$$

$$B_{a(0)} = \frac{Q_0}{V_a}\left(\frac{k_2 - \beta}{\alpha - \beta}\right) \quad \text{See Figure 2.}$$

$$(A_{a(0)}/\alpha) + (B_{a(0)}/\beta) = \frac{Q_0}{V_a k_3}$$

$$X = \frac{B_{a(0)}/\beta}{(A_{a(0)}/\alpha) + (B_{a(0)}/\beta)}$$

$$X = \frac{[(k_2 - \beta)/(\alpha - \beta)]/\beta}{1/k_3} = \frac{(k_2 - \beta)k_3}{(\alpha - \beta)\beta} = \frac{k_2 k_3 - k_3 \beta}{(\alpha - \beta)\beta}$$

But $k_2 k_3 = \alpha\beta$ and $k_3 = (\alpha + \beta) - (k_1 + k_2)$:

$$X = \frac{\alpha\beta - k_3\beta}{(\alpha - \beta)\beta} = \frac{\alpha - k_3}{\alpha - \beta} = \frac{\alpha - [(\alpha + \beta) - (k_1 + k_2)]}{\alpha - \beta} = \frac{k_1 + k_2 - \beta}{\alpha - \beta}$$

But

$$B_{\text{tot}(0)}/Q_0 = \frac{k_1 + k_2 - \beta}{\alpha - \beta} = X$$

Fig. 4. Derivation of X.

the value for $B_{a(0)}$, then to subtract the extrapolated values from the observed plasma levels and plot these resultant values on semilogarithmic graph paper. The intercept of this secondary plot provides the value for $A_{a(0)}$ and the slope is $\alpha/2.303$. The secondary plot is frequently called the α-phase. From the values for $A_{a(0)}$, α, $B_{a(0)}$, and β, the rate constants, k_1, k_2, and k_3 can be calculated according to the equations shown in Fig. 3 and substituted directly into the equation for $B_{\text{tot}(0)}$. However, as shown in Fig. 4, I have devised an easier way to estimate $B_{\text{tot}(0)}$, which I call the "Partition of Areas." In this method the dose is multiplied by X, where X equals $(B_{a(0)}/\beta)/[(A_{a(0)}/\alpha) + (B_{a(0)}/\beta)]$. Since all the data required to evaluate X are readily obtained from the plot of the drug levels in the central compartment, i.e., blood plasma, there is no need to evaluate k_1, k_2, or k_3 in order to calculate the value of X. Thus after the distribution phase is completed, the equation for the total amount of drug present in the two-compartment system degenerates to the following equation:

$$Q_{\text{tot}} = B_{\text{tot}(0)} \exp(-\beta t) = X \cdot \text{Dose} \cdot \exp(-\beta t)$$

and $y = \text{Dose} \cdot (1 - X)$

When X approaches 1.0, the elimination of a drug can be adequately described by a one-compartment system, the kinetics of which are much easier to understand than are the kinetics of polyphasic systems. Thus, it is frequently desirable to determine the value of X and to use the degenerate form of the equation for Q_{tot} given above.

Another concept that is frequently misunderstood is that of the volume of distribution. As originally defined, the volume of distribution of a substance is the total amount of substance in the body divided by the concentration at equilibrium in the reference compartment, which is usually the plasma or central compartment. According to this definition the volume of distribution, $V_{d(eq)}$, can be evaluated only when there is no net transfer of the substance from one compartment to another. Thus, the formula for determining the volume of distribution of a drug in a two-compartment system is as follows:

$$V_{d(eq)} = Q_{tot}/C_{a(eq)} = V_a[1 + (k_1/k_2)]$$

However, this definition of the volume of distribution has a physiological meaning only when the drug is either not excreted or is infused into the central compartment at the same rate that it is eliminated from the central compartment. In the latter case, we also have to assume that the drug is not eliminated from the body by being directly metabolized in or excreted from the peripheral compartment.

If the "volume of distribution" were restricted to this definition, however, it would be virtually useless to the pharmacologist. The pharmacologist wants to be able to calculate the clearance of drug from the body. But the clearance of the drug obviously would be zero if the drug were not eliminated from the body and, in any event, would best be calculated by dividing the rate of infusion (k_0) by the plasma level at steady-state ($C_{a(ss)}$). In no case does he need to calculate the volume of distribution.

After a drug is rapidly injected into the central compartment of a two-compartment system, however, its clearance can be calculated from the following equation:

$$\text{Clearance} = \beta V_{d(k)}$$

But the kinetic volume of distribution ($V_{d(k)}$)* used in this equation differs from the volume of distribution obtained at equilibrium. After the distribution phase is completed, the total amount of drug in the body and in the plasma still declines according to the following equations:

$$Q_{(tot)} = Q_0(k_1 + k_2 - \beta)\exp(-\beta t)/(\alpha - \beta)$$

$$C_a = (Q_0/V_a)(k_2 - \beta)\exp(-\beta t)/(\alpha - \beta)$$

*The kinetic volume of distribution has also been called $V_{d(area)}$ by Riegelman et al. (1968), $V_{d(\beta)}$ by Gibaldi et al., (1969) and both $V_{dist(slope)}$ and $V_{dist(remainder)}$ by Riggs (1963).

Thus, the kinetic volume of distribution is given by

$$V_{d(k)} = Q_{(tot)}/C_a = V_a(k_1 + k_2 - \beta)/(k_2 - \beta) = V_a[1 + k_1/(k_2 - \beta)]$$

For this reason, the kinetic volume of distribution is defined as the total amount of drug in the body at any given time after the distribution phase is completed divided by the plasma concentration at that time. It should be noted, however, that the equation for $V_{d(k)}$ contains β and, thus, when $V_{d(k)}$ markedly differs from $V_{d(eq)}$, $V_{d(k)}$ can be affected by factors which change the half-life of the drug.

With small animals, such as rats and mice, $V_{d(k)}$ can be determined directly by sampling the plasma and homogenizing the animals at various times after the intravenous administration of the drug and substituting these values into the equation $V_{d(k)} = Q_{tot}/C_a$.

At first, the ratio will be small, but it will increase to a constant value as the distribution phase is completed. With larger animals and with human patients, however, the $V_{d(k)}$ of the drug after intravenous administration is frequently estimated by plotting the plasma levels measured at various times on semilogarithmic graph paper, determining the value of $B_{a(0)}$ and then dividing $B_{a(0)}$ into the amount of drug administered. As has been pointed out above, however, the total amount of drug in the body predicted by $B_{a(0)}$ is less than the total dose. Thus, a more precise value for $V_{d(k)}$ can be obtained by the equation

$$V_{d(k)} = X \cdot \text{Dose}/B_{a(0)}$$

in which X again equals $(B_{b(0)}/\beta)/[(A_{a(0)}/\alpha) + (B_{a(0)}/\beta)]$.

The equations for X, $V_{d(k)}$, and clearance can be simplified when the investigator is interested in knowing X without calculating the values of α and β, or when he is interested in knowing the $V_{d(k)}$ without calculating the value of X, or when he is interested in knowing the clearance without calculating the $V_{d(k)}$. As shown in Fig. 5, all three values can be calculated directly from the dose, the half-lives of the α and β-phases, and the values of $A_{a(0)}$ and $B_{a(0)}$. It might also be of interest to the nonmathematician that the denominator $(A_{a(0)}/\alpha) + (B_{a(0)}/\beta)$ in these equations equals the area under the entire curve when the plasma levels are plotted on arithmetic graph paper and $B_{a(0)}/\beta$ equals the area of the β-phase. Moreover, when the time-interval between data points is constant, the total area can be estimated from the trapezoidal rule (Selby, 1970), which is given in the following equation:

$$\text{Area} = \text{Time interval} \left(\tfrac{1}{2}C_{a(0)} + C_{a(1)} + C_{a(2)} + C_{a(n-1)} + \tfrac{1}{2}C_{a(n)}\right)$$

$$X = \frac{B_{a(0)}/\beta}{(A_{a(0)}/\alpha) + (B_{a(0)}/\beta)}$$

But $\alpha = 0.693/t_{1/2}$ of α-phase

and $\beta = 0.693/t_{1/2}$ of β-phase

$$X = \frac{B_{a(0)}(t_{1/2} \text{ of } \beta\text{-phase})}{A_{a(0)}(t_{1/2} \text{ of } \alpha\text{-phase}) + B_{a(0)}(t_{1/2} \text{ of } \beta\text{-phase})}$$

$$V_{d(k)} = X \text{ Dose}/B_{a(0)}$$

$$V_{d(k)} = \frac{\text{Dose}}{\beta[(A_{a(0)}/\alpha) + (B_{a(0)}/\beta)]}$$

$$V_{d(k)} = \frac{\text{Dose }(t_{1/2} \text{ of } \beta\text{-phase})}{A_{a(0)}(t_{1/2} \text{ of } \alpha\text{-phase}) + B_{a(0)}(t_{1/2} \text{ of } \beta\text{-phase})}$$

$$\text{Clearance} = \beta V_{d(k)}$$

$$\text{Clearance} = \frac{\text{Dose}}{(A_{a(0)}/\alpha) + (B_{a(0)}/\beta)}$$

$$\text{Clearance} = \frac{0.693 \text{ Dose}}{A_{a(0)}(t_{1/2} \text{ of } \alpha\text{-phase}) + B_{a(0)}(t_{1/2} \text{ of } \beta\text{-phase})}$$

Fig. 5. Alternative equations for determining X, $V_{d(k)}$ and clearance.

When the rate constant of elimination (k_3) is much smaller than k_2, it can be shown that the $V_{d(k)}$ is virtually identical to $V_{d(eq)}$ and that X nearly equals 1.0. For this reason the distinction between $V_{d(k)}$ and $V_{d(eq)}$ and the value of X becomes important only when the clearance of a drug is rapid. It would be a mistake, however, to assume that the clearance of a drug is always slow when β is small. In fact, a drug that is highly bound to extravascular tissues may have a biological half-life of several hours or days even when its metabolism is limited mainly by the rate of blood flow through the liver. To illustrate the relationship between tissue binding and so-called first-pass kinetics, I have assumed that a drug is completely cleared from blood as it passes through the liver. Under these conditions the biological half-life can be calculated from: $t_{1/2} = 0.693 V_{d(k)}/$ Blood flow rate through the liver. As shown in Table IV, the minimum half-life of a drug that is eliminated solely by the liver and that has a $V_{d(k)}/$ kg of 20 liters/kg in man would be about 10 hr. Moreover, if 50% of the drug were cleared

TABLE IV
Relationships between $V_d(k)$, Liver Plasma Flow, Extraction Ratios, and $t_{1/2}^a$

| $V_d(k)$, liters | $V_{d(k)}$/kg, liters/kg | \multicolumn{4}{c}{Extraction ratios ($t_{1/2}$ in hr)} |
		100%	50%	25%	10%
5.0	0.071	0.036	0.072	0.14	0.36
15	0.214	0.11	0.22	0.44	1.1
50	0.71	0.36	0.72	1.4	3.6
70	1.0	0.5	1.0	2.0	5
140	2.0	1.0	2.0	4.0	10
280	4.0	2.0	4.0	8.0	20
700	10.0	5.0	10.0	20.0	50
1400	20.0	10.0	20.0	40.0	100
2800	40.0	20.0	40.0	80.0	200

[a] For these calculations, it was assumed the blood flow rate was 1.6 liters/min in a 70-kg man, which is equivalent to 96.0 liters/hr and to 1.37 liters per kg/hr.

the biological half-life would be about 20 hr. In this connection it is noteworthy that Dr. Sjoqvist (1973) has reported at this symposium that the relationship between the half-life and the volume of distribution of nortriptyline in some patients is consistent with the view that its metabolism is limited mainly by the blood flow rate through the liver. As he has pointed out, the rate of metabolism of the drug in these patients would be expected to be significantly changed by drugs or diseases that change hepatic blood flow, but not by drugs that induce the liver enzymes which catalyze the metabolism of the drug. For these reasons, it is important to determine the extraction ratio, which is defined as follows:

Extraction ratio = Clearance/Blood flow rate through the organ

Although the binding of drugs to extravascular organs almost invariably increases the biological half-life of drugs, their binding to plasma proteins has diverse effects depending on the mechanism of elimination and the extraction ratio. For example, binding to plasma proteins lowers the unbound concentration of the drugs and thereby tends to decrease the clearance of polar drugs by glomerular filtration and by inefficient transport systems in kidney. Also, there is a decrease in the clearance of lipid soluble drugs that diffuse rapidly from the glomerular filtrate back into blood. Similarly, the binding of drugs to plasma proteins would also decrease the metabolism of drugs by relatively inactive enzyme systems in liver. But when the clearance of a drug by an organ approaches the blood flow rate through the organ, the binding to plasma proteins and even to blood cells may enhance the elimination of the drug. Thus, when the extraction ratio of a drug is not known, it is virtually impossible to predict whether substances that displace a drug from plasma proteins will decelerate or accelerate the elimination of the drug.

Occasionally, a drug is localized so extensively in tissues or is eliminated from the body so rapidly that its plasma level falls rapidly below concentrations that can be detected by our present-day analytical methods. Under these conditions only the α-phase is observed. Continuous infusion experiments, however, can be useful in determining whether the rapid decline in the plasma levels is due mainly to distribution or to elimination. Therefore, it is useful to compare kinetics of intravenous administration with the kinetics of continuous infusion into the central compartment of a two-compartment system. During the infusion the plasma levels of a drug increase rapidly at first, then more slowly until an asymptote is reached at a steady-state ($C_{a(ss)}$). The equation in Fig. 6 predicts that subtracting the

$$C_a \text{ (infusion)} = \frac{k_0}{V_a \alpha \beta} \left\{ k_2 - \left[\frac{(\alpha - k_2)\beta}{\alpha - \beta} \right] \exp(-\alpha t) - \left[\frac{(k_2 - \beta)\alpha}{\alpha - \beta} \right] \exp(-\beta t) \right\}$$

$$A_a \text{ (infusion)} = \frac{k_0}{V_a \alpha \beta} \left[\frac{(\alpha - k_2)\beta}{\alpha - \beta} \right] = \frac{k_0}{V_a k_2 k_3} \left[\frac{k_2 k_3 - k_2 \beta}{\alpha - \beta} \right] = \frac{k_0}{V_a k_3} \left[\frac{k_3 - \beta}{\alpha - \beta} \right]$$

$$= \frac{k_0[\alpha + \beta - (k_1 + k_2) - \beta]}{V_a k_3 (\alpha - \beta)} = \frac{k_0[\alpha - (k_1 + k_2)]}{V_a k_3 (\alpha - \beta)}$$

$$B_a \text{ (infusion)} = \left[\frac{k_0}{V_a \alpha \beta} \right] \left[\frac{(k_2 - \beta)\alpha}{\alpha - \beta} \right] = \frac{k_0}{V_a k_2 k_3} \left[\frac{k_2 \alpha - k_2 k_3}{\alpha - \beta} \right] = \frac{k_0 (\alpha - k_3)}{V_a k_3 (\alpha - \beta)}$$

$$= \frac{k_0\{\alpha - [(\alpha + \beta) - (k_1 + k_2)]\}}{V_a k_3 (\alpha - \beta)} = \frac{k_0(k_1 + k_2 - \beta)}{V_a k_3 (\alpha - \beta)}$$

At steady state:

$$C_{a(ss)} = \frac{k_0 k_2}{V_a \alpha \beta} = \frac{k_0 k_2}{V_a k_2 k_3} = \frac{k_0}{V_a k_3}$$

$$C_{a(ss)} = A_a \text{ (infusion)} + B_a \text{ (infusion)}$$

$$C_{a(ss)} - C_a \text{(infusion)} = [A_a(\text{infusion})\exp(-\alpha t)] + [B_a \text{ (infusion) } \exp(-\beta t)]$$

$$Q_b \text{ (infusion)} = \frac{k_0}{\alpha \beta} \left\{ k_1 - \left(\frac{[k_1 \alpha \exp(-\beta t)] - [k_1 \beta \exp(-\alpha t)]}{\alpha - \beta} \right) \right\}$$

At steady state:

$$Q_b \text{ (infusion)} = \frac{k_0 k_1}{\alpha \beta} = \frac{k_0 k_1}{k_2 k_3}$$

In these equations k_0 is the rate of infusion.

Fig. 6. Equations for the two-compartment system illustrated in Fig. 1 during constant infusion of the drug into compartment A.

$$C_a \text{ (postinfusion)} = \frac{[\alpha Q_{a(0)} - k_2(Q_{a(0)} + Q_{b(0)})]\exp(-\alpha t)}{V_a(\alpha - \beta)}$$
$$+ \frac{[k_2(Q_{a(0)} + Q_{b(0)}) - \beta Q_{a(0)}]\exp(-\beta t)}{V_a(\alpha - \beta)}$$

At $C_{a(ss)}$

$$Q_{a(0)} = \frac{k_0}{V_a k_3} \quad \text{and} \quad Q_{b(0)} = \frac{k_0 k_1}{V_a k_2 k_3}$$

$$A_a \text{ (postinfusion)} = \frac{\alpha Q_{a(0)} - k_2(Q_{a(0)} + Q_{b(0)})}{V_a(\alpha - \beta)} = \frac{k_0}{V_a k_3}\left(\frac{\alpha - k_1 - k_2}{\alpha - \beta}\right)$$

$$B_a \text{ (postinfusion)} = \frac{k_2(Q_{a(0)} + Q_{b(0)}) - \beta Q_{a(0)}}{V_a(\alpha - \beta)} = \frac{k_0}{V_a k_3}\left(\frac{k_1 + k_2 - \beta}{\alpha - \beta}\right)$$

Fig. 7. Equations for the two-compartment system illustrated in Fig. 1 after constant infusion into compartment A has been stopped.

plasma levels obtained at various times before the steady state has been reached from the steady-state level, and plotting the resultant values against time on semilogarithmic graph paper will give a plot that is biphasic. But it frequently may appear to be monophasic when the clearance of the drug is slow. When the clearance is rapid the plot will be biphasic and β can be calculated from the half-time of the β-phase. Moreover, the intercept obtained by extrapolating the straight line of the β-phase back to time zero gives B_a (infusion), which equals $k_0(k_2 - \beta)/[(\alpha - \beta)\beta V_a]$.

If the infusion of the drug is stopped after a steady-state plasma level has been obtained, the plasma level will fall biphasically as predicted by the equation shown in Fig. 7, but frequently may appear to be monophasic. Extrapolation of the straight line of the β-phase to time zero gives B_a (postinfusion), which is identical to B_a (infusion); compare B_a (infusion) in Fig. 6 with B_a (postinfusion) in Fig. 7.

The values of B_a (infusion) and B_a (postinfusion) are proportional to the $B_{a(0)}/\beta$ obtained after rapid intravenous administration of the drug; compare $B_{a(0)}/\beta$ in Fig. 4 with B_a (infusion) in Fig. 6 and B_a (postinfusion) in Fig. 7. Hence the data obtained during and after infusion can be used to predict not only the values of α and β but also the value of X that should be obtained after rapid intravenous injection. Note that X can be calculated by dividing either B_a (infusion) or B_a (postinfusion) by the steady-state concentration, $C_{a(ss)}$, in plasma.

It is noteworthy that both kinds of volume of distribution occur during an infusion experiment; the equilibrium volume of distribution ($V_{d_{(eq)}}$) will occur at steady state and the kinetic volume of distribution ($V_{d(k)}$) will occur after infusion is stopped and the first phase of plasma level decline has been completed. Moreover, at the steady state, the clearance of the drug may be calculated by dividing the rate of infusion by $C_{a(ss)}$.

Since the plasma levels of tracer doses of radiolabeled corticosterone decline rapidly after intravenous administration to rats (Fig. 8), it occurred to Bogdanski et al. (1971) in our laboratory, that the rate of disappearance of the radiolabeled material might not provide accurate values for the turnover of the steroid in the animals. For this reason they compared the rates at which radiolabeled corticosterone disappeared from rat plasma after intravenous injection and after continuous infusion. Their results showed that the half-life of the radiolabeled steroid associated with the β-phase after infusion was about double the half-life of the radiolabeled steroid after intravenous administration or during infusion (Figs. 8 and 9).

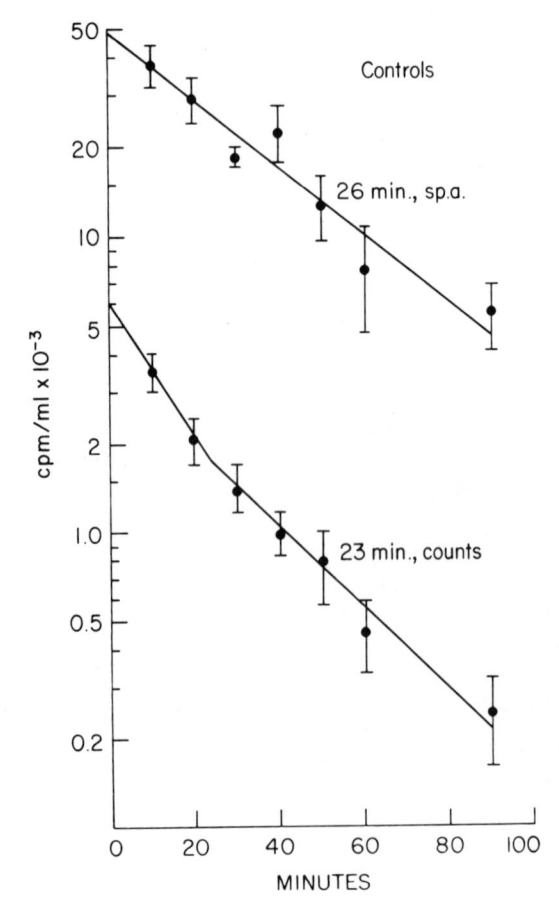

Fig. 8. Disappearance of ^{3}H-corticosterone from the blood of untreated rats after a single, rapid injection. Rats were anesthetized with 40 mg/kg of Na$^+$-pentobarbital and 200 mg/kg of Na$^+$-barbital, i.p. Sixty minutes later, the animals were given an i.v. injection of 0.2 µg/kg of ^{3}H-corticosterone. Blood was collected from decapitated rats, and the plasma was extracted with chloroform. Corticosterone contained in an aliquot of each of the chloroform extracts was assayed fluorimetrically. A second aliquot was transferred to a counting vial, evaporated under a stream of air and assayed by scintillation counting. The upper curve represents the specific activity of plasma corticosterone according to the ratio: counts per minute per milliliter of plasma/micrograms per milliliter of plasma. The lower curve plots the actual counts per minute per milliliter of plasma. Each point on the curve is an average ± S.E. of the ^{3}H-corticosterone levels in the blood of 4 rats, $n = 29$ (Bogdanski et al., 1971).

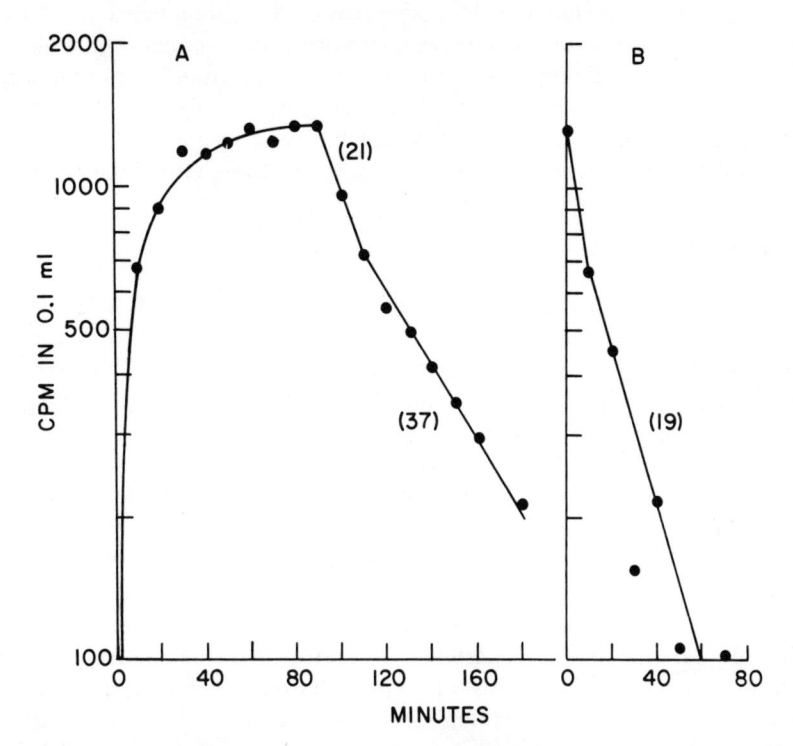

Fig. 9 (A) Infusion of ^{3}H-corticosterone at the steady-state. Anesthetized rats were infused with up to 0.21 μg of ^{3}H-corticosterone/hr, i.v., for 60 to 90 min at which time the infusion was stopped. Samples of blood (0.1 ml) were drawn from the common carotid artery at 10-min intervals during the infusion and for 90 min afterward. To avoid excessive withdrawal of blood, samples were collected during the first 60 min of infusion in half the animals, and during the interval 60 to 90 min in the other half. Data from 14 rats are represented and are normalized to adjust for different doses. (B) Logarithmic plot of $(C_{a(ss)} - C_a)$ during the infusion, where $C_{a(ss)}$ is the steady-state concentration of ^{3}H-corticosterone in counts per minute per milliliter and C_a is the concentration at various time intervals after the start of infusions A (Bogdanski et al., 1971).

Nevertheless, the rapid disappearance of the intravenous dose was only partly caused by rapid metabolism of the steroid, since the intercepts of the β-phases obtained during and after the infusion were approximately 75% of the steady-state level. These data suggest that the α-phase obtained after intravenous administration could account for only about 25% of the metabolism of the radiolabeled corticosterone.

Although the authors were unable to account for the apparent differences in the β-values obtained during and after infusion, it seems possible that a part of the difference might be due to a time-dependent change in the dissociation constants of the complexes of the radiolabeled corticosterone and plasma substances, such as transcortin. In this regard, it should be pointed out that although the bound forms of most substances equilibrate almost instantaneously with their free forms, many substances are bound slowly. For example, the binding of colchicine to microtubular protein is slow and requires several minutes to complete (Zweig and Chignell, 1973).

CONCLUSION

In this paper I have summarized various mechanisms of drug distribution. Among these are differences between intracellular and extracellular pH, active transport systems for drugs, distribution of drugs between fat and water in adipose tissues, and the reversible binding of drugs to phospholipids and to various macromolecules including proteins, nucleic acids, and melanin. These mechanisms usually tend to decrease the concentrations of unbound drugs at their sites of action, but not to the extent that might be expected from binding studies carried out *in vitro*. I have also discussed the effects of drug distribution in altering the biological half-lives of drugs in the body and the interrelationships between the kinetic volumes of distribution of drugs and blood flow rates through the organs that eliminate the drugs. Hopefully, I have dispelled some of the confusion that has arisen in the minds of many pharmacologists in relating the changes in blood levels, which occur during drug disposition, to the mathematics used in multicompartment systems.

REFERENCES

Beierwaltes, W. H., Lieberman, L. M., Varma, V. M., and Counsell, R. E., 1968, *J. Am. Med. Assoc.* **206**: 97.
Bernstein, H., Zvaifler, N., Rubin, M., and Mansour, A. M., 1963, *Invest. Ophthalmol.* **2**: 384.
Bogdanski, D. F., Blaszkowski, T. P., and Brodie, B. B., 1971, *J. Pharm. Exp. Therap.* **179**: 372.
Brodie, B. B., Bermsteom, E., and Mark, L. C., 1952, *J. Pharmacol. Exp. Therap.* **105**: 421.
Brodie, B. B., Aronow, L., and Axelrod, J., 1954, *J. Pharmacol. Exp. Therap.* **111**: 21.
Burns, J. J., Rose, R. K., Chenkin, T., Goldman, A., Schulert, A., and Brodie, B. B., 1953, *J. Pharmacol. Exp. Therap.* **109**: 346.
Chignell, C. F. and Starkweather, D. K., 1971a, *Molecular Pharmacology* **7**: 229.
Chignell, C. F., Vesell, E. S., Starkweather, D. K., and Berlin, C. M., 1971b, *Clin. Pharm. Therap.* **12**: 897.
Chignell, C. F., 1972, in: *Methods in Pharmacology*, Vol. 2, p. 39, Physical Methods (Chignell, C. F., ed.) Appleton-Century-Crofts, New York.
Dingell, J. V., Sulser, F., and Gillette, J. R., 1964, *J. Pharmacol. Exp. Therap.* **143**: 14.
Dollery, C. T., Emslie-Smith, D., and Muggleton, D. F., 1961, *Brit. J. Pharmacol.* **17**: 488.
Gibaldi, M., Nagashima, R., and Levy, G., 1969, *J. Pharm. Sci.* **58**: 193–197.

Gillette, J. R., 1968, in: *Importance of Fundamental Principles in Drug Evaluation*, p. 69 (Tedeschi, D. H., and Tedeschi, R. E., eds.) Proceedings of a Symposium Organized by the Section on Pharmacology and Biochemistry Acad. of Pharmaceutical Sciences, American Pharmaceutical Assn., New York, Raven Press.

Guarino, A. M., Anderson, J. B., Starkweather, D. K., and Chignell, C. F., 1973, *Cancer Chemotherapy Rep.* **57**: 125.

Hart, L. G., and Fouts, J. R., 1965, *Arch. Exp. Pathol. Pharmacol.* **249**: 486.

Horak, V., and Gillette, J. R., 1971, *Molecular Pharmacology* **7**: 429.

Kalow, W., 1962, in: *Symposium on Factors Controlling Duration of Action*, Vol. 6, p. 137, (Brodie, B. B., and Erdos, E. G., eds.) Proceedings of the First International Pharmacology Meeting, Pergamon Press, New York.

Kucera, J. L., and Bullock, F. J., 1969, *J. Pharm. Pharmacol.* **21**: 293.

Kuntzman, R. Tsai, I., and Burns, J. J., 1962, *J. Pharmacol. Exp. Therap.* **158**: 332.

Lerman, L., 1961, *J. Mol. Biol.* **3**: 18.

Potts, A. M., 1962, *Invest. Ophthalmol.* **1**: 522.

Riegelman, S., Loo, J., and Rowland, M., 1968, *J. Pharm. Sci.* **128**: 123.

Riggs, D. S., 1963, in: *The Mathematical Approach to Physiological Problems*, Williams and Wilkins, Baltimore, Md. 221–214.

Robinson, J., Richardson, A., Hunter, C. G., Crabtree, A. N., and Rees, H. J., 1965, *Brit. J. Ind. Med.* **22**: 220.

Selby, S. M., 1970, in: *Handbook of Tables for Mathematics*, 4th ed., p. 14, (Selby, S. M., ed.) The Chemical Rubber Co., Cleveland, Ohio.

Solomon, H. M., Schrogie, J. J., and Williams, D., 1968, *Biochem. Pharmacol.* **17**: 143.

Spector, S., and Parker, C. W., 1970, *Science* **168**: 1347.

Spector, S., 1971, *J. Pharmacol. Exp. Therap.* **178**: 253.

Waddell, W. J., and Butler, T. C., 1957, *J. Clin. Invest.* **36**: 1217.

Waddell, W. J., and Butler, T. C., 1959, *J. Clin. Invest.* **38**: 720.

Yesair, D. W., Remington, L., Callahan, M., and Kensler, C. J., 1970, *Biochem. Pharmacol.* **19**: 1591.

Zweig, M. H., and Chignell, C. F., 1973, *Biochem. Pharmacol.*, **22**: 2141.

Physiological and Physical Factors Governing The Initial Stages of Drug Distribution

Seymour S. Kety
Department of Psychiatry
Massachusetts General Hospital
Boston, Massachusetts

The distribution of a drug, like that of any molecular species introduced into the organism, depends upon a complex series of physical and chemical processes which are often interrelated. These processes take up and dilute the substance at its site of entry, carry it to the various body tissues, permit it to diffuse or actively transport it across several membranes, and determine its accumulation and disposition by the tissues. More specifically, the concentration of a substance thus introduced depends, over time, on the history of its concentration in the arterial blood, the rate at which blood passes through each tissue, the physical processes occurring there (e.g., diffusion and solubility), and the chemical processes of active transport, binding, and metabolism. My interest in these processes began nearly 30 years ago and arose, not so much from a desire to understand the distribution of drugs, as from an interest in deriving from the distribution of a suitable tracer, a measurement of the physiological functions involved. The problem was to describe the tissue distribution of such a foreign substance in terms of physiological parameters rather than empirical constants and precisely enough to derive the physiological function from the distribution.

GENERAL PRINCIPLES OF BLOOD/TISSUE DISTRIBUTION

Because the organism is not homogeneous but is heterogeneous in the extreme, even to differences between individual cells and the intracellular components, mathematical treatment of this process can become hopelessly complex on the one hand or oversimplified on the other. Often, however, special properties of the substance in question make some of the processes involved the limiting ones, reducing others to an insignificant role. This has permitted certain mathematical generalizations to be derived which hold reasonably well for the classes of substances to which they pertain.

Substances which are poorly diffusible across capillary membranes will show a distribution in which diffusion is the limiting factor (Teorell, 1937) with the result that the effect of blood flow is negligible and mathematical treatment is correspondingly simplified. In the case of substances which are readily diffusible, however, their loss from the capillary in one circulation through a tissue is so great that the rate of their replenishment by the blood flow becomes an important factor. It is still possible to incorporate this variable along with diffusion and solubility into a mathematical treatment which describes the behavior of substances which are not appreciably metabolized as well as the initial distribution of those which undergo chemical change within the tissue.

An important class of freely diffusible substances which are metabolically inert are the volatile anesthetics. It is not surprising that their uptake and distribution has been the subject of a number of mathematical models.

It is possible to show (Kety, 1951) that during the inhalation of a constant concentration of a gaseous substance, the arterial concentration of the substance will rise rapidly along a curve for the first few minutes. The rise will then be more leisurely, until eventually, after many hours, the inspired partial pressure of gas will be achieved throughout the tissues of the body. The early rise is dependent upon pulmonary ventilation and circulation and is very strongly influenced by the solubility of the gas in blood. To such an extent is this so that the difference in the times of induction or recovery of anesthesia from the different volatile anesthetics can be explained in terms of this solubility (Fig. 1). The more leisurely approach to equilibrium depends upon the concentration of the gas in the mixed venous blood returning to the heart which in turn is affected by the mass, blood flow, diffusion, and solubility of the gas in the various tissues of the body. The curves shown in Fig. 1 are based upon the simplifying assumption that all the peripheral tissues constitute a single compartment.

The early stages in the accumulation of a substance in a particular tissue, where active transport and metabolism are not involved or can be neglected (the case for a number of drugs in addition to the volatile anesthetics), depend upon the history of the arterial curve and these physical factors.

The relationships following can be derived: if C_a, C_v, and C_i represent,

% OF INSPIRED TENSION

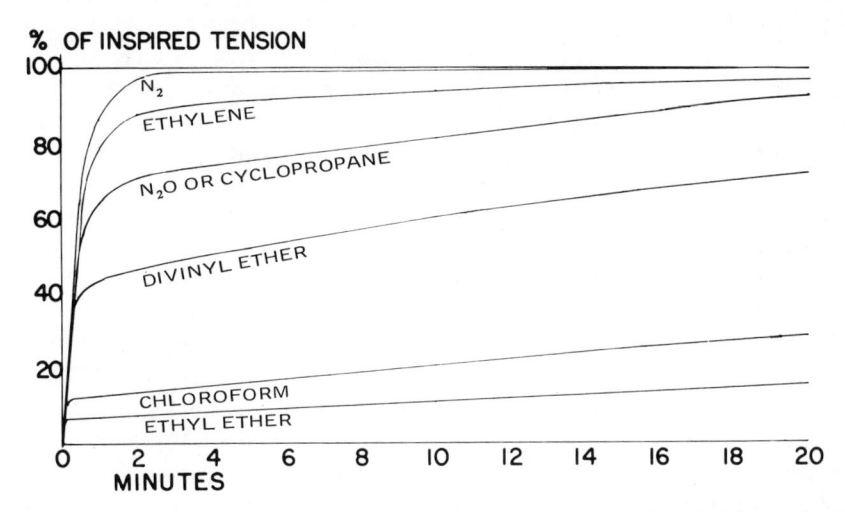

Fig. 1. The uptake of various volatile anesthetics at the lung as described by a simple mathematical model. Cardiac output, pulmonary ventilation, and parameters for the peripheral tissues are held constant and the differences described result from the different solubilities of the agents in blood (from Kety, 1951).

respectively, the arterial concentration going to, the venous concentration exiting from, and the average concentration within the tissue; λ, the tissue/blood partition coefficient for the substance; D, the diffusion coefficient per unit area across the capillary membrane; S the capillary surface; and F the volume flow of blood for a representative portion of the tissue. The assumption is made that there is some mean tissue concentration of gas (C_i) which remains constant during the passage of blood from the arterial to the venous end of the capillary. Since the capillary volume represents less than 5% of the volume of most tissues, marked changes in the blood concentration along the capillary would be reflected in only a slight change in mean tissue concentration. It can then be shown (Kety, 1951):

$$C_a - C_v = m_i(C_a - C_i/\lambda) \qquad (1)$$

where $m = 1 - \exp(-DS/F)$.

It is apparent that when DS/F becomes sufficiently large, m becomes equal to unity. This is essentially the case in many tissues for lipid soluble substances which can diffuse through the entire capillary surface. In the case of the brain, substances with molecular weights as different as hydrogen (Fieschi et al., 1965) and trifluoro-iodo-methane (Kety, 1960) are, by virtue of their lipid solubility and the vascularity of the tissue, taken up without diffusion limitations, since similar values can be computed for regional cerebral blood flow using either one of them and treating m as unity. On the other hand, when DS/F is small, i.e., for substances with low diffusion coefficients or tissues with an unfavorable ratio of capillary surface to blood flow, diffusion becomes a limiting factor. Renkin (1959) has found the expression above useful in describing the behavior of such substances in particular tissues.

The relationship between tissue blood flow and the accumulation of a nonmetabolized substance can be derived as follows (Kety, 1951):

On the basis of the principle of material conservation of which the Fick principle is the physiological statement, the amount (Q_i) of any substance taken up by an individual tissue per unit of time is equal to the quantity brought to the tissue by the arterial blood minus the quantity carried away in the venous blood (neglecting lymphatic and certain specialized modes of efflux, i.e., cerebrospinal fluid, which are generally negligible):

$$\frac{dQ_i}{dt} = F_i(C_a - C_v) \qquad (2)$$

assuming that arterial inflow equals venous outflow equals F_i, and defining a tissue to include its contained blood which usually constitutes only a few percent of its total volume (V_i). Since C_i equals Q_i/V_i, appropriate substitution in and rearrangement of Eqs. (1) and (2) yields

$$\frac{dC_i}{dt} = \frac{m_i F_i}{V_i \lambda} \cdot (\lambda C_a - C_i) \qquad (3)$$

which has the following solutions for the concentration of the particular substance in a single tissue.

If the arterial concentration is constant,

$$C_i = \lambda C_a [1 - \exp(-k_i t)] \qquad (4)$$

If the arterial concentration is negligible (i.e., removal from a tissue),

$$C_i - C_{i_0} \cdot \exp(-k_i t) \qquad (5)$$

where $k_i = m_i F_i / V_i \lambda$. These equations hold for the simplest case, i.e., a tissue homogeneous with respect to blood flow. Where the tissue in question is heterogeneous, i.e., made up of different regions with significantly different perfusion rates, the expression becomes a series of exponential terms, each term pertaining to a homogeneous component.

Where the arterial concentration is variable with time, as is the case with most drugs, the concentration in the tissue depends upon these factors and the history of the arterial curve as follows:

$$C_i(T) = \lambda k_i \cdot \exp(-k_i T) \int_0^T C_a \cdot \exp(k_i t)\,dt \tag{6}$$

From these expressions certain generalizations are evident. Thus, where sufficient time has elapsed, the distribution of a nonmetabolized substance in the various tissues is dependent neither upon diffusion nor blood flow, but simply upon its partition coefficient between tissue and blood. In the early stages of uptake, the accumulation of a substance in a particular tissue will depend upon blood flow in that tissue for substances which are freely diffusible and diffusion processes in the tissue where the substance is poorly diffusible or upon a combination of the two for many substances. In the case of substances which are freely diffusible and tissues with an adequate capillary density, the process is so dependent upon tissue blood flow that the accumulation in a tissue of such substances has been used effectively as a measure of local cerebral blood flow (Kety, 1960; Sokoloff, 1961; Reivich et al., 1969). Removal of freely diffusible substances from tissue as described in Eq. (5) has been used as a measure of blood flow in muscle (Kety, 1949; Lindbjerg, 1969), brain (Lassen and Ingvar, 1961; Fieschi et al., 1965; Nilsson, 1965) as well as in kidney, skin, and other tissues (Aukland et al., 1964; Lindbjerg, 1969).

Scherrer-Etienne and Posternak (1963) have demonstrated autoradiographically the uptake by the brain of ethanol and of pentobarbital (Fig. 2)

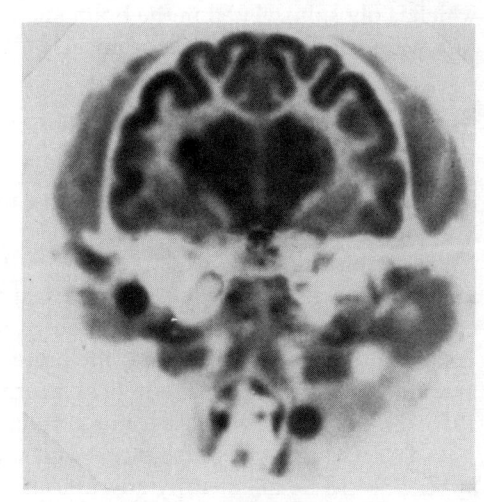

Fig. 2. Autoradiogram of a section of the cat brain showing the distribution one minute after the onset of an infusion of ^{14}C-pentobarbital. The density in the various regions is described by Eq. (6) and is largely influenced by the regional blood flow (from Scherrer-Etienne and Posternak, 1963).

which appears to support the theoretical model of the uptake of diffusible, poorly metabolized substances described above.

The foregoing treatments have been based upon the assumption of negligible metabolic conversion of the substance in question, which holds for inert gases, many anesthetics, and some other substances. For most drugs, however, metabolic conversion is a complicating factor in describing their distribution in various tissues, although the degree to which it affects the models above is variable.

If the rate of metabolism is slow in comparison to the rate of distribution, the latter will still be limited by diffusion and tissue blood flow and will be reasonably well described by the equations above, especially in the early phases of distribution.

If metabolic conversion is limited to certain tissues and does not occur in the tissue under consideration, the distribution in that tissue will follow the description for nonmetabolized substances. Therefore, the effect of metabolism will be merely to alter the arterial concentration curve or to add to the arterial blood certain metabolic products which may be important pharmacologically, but can be treated as separate molecular species. Many drugs which affect the central nervous system are not metabolized there. Antipyrine, which is metabolized largely in the liver and not at all in the brain, follows Eq. (6) quite reliably in its uptake by the central nervous system.

Where a drug is metabolized in the tissue under consideration and sufficiently rapidly to affect its distribution there, it is possible to take this into account by introducing a term for its metabolic removal into Eq. (2). Reivich (1972) describes such an analysis for the uptake of a substance which is phosphorylated in the brain and similar reasoning could be applied to a wide variety of other substances.

BLOOD–BRAIN BARRIER

The brain is protected and enveloped by a system of membranes and extravascular fluid which often prevents and usually complicates the accumulation of administered substances within it. The blood–brain barrier is an empirical term which describes the interference which is often imposed. It was discovered nearly a century ago when it was found that certain dyes, administered intravenously, stained most of the tissues of the body but did not penetrate into the brain substance. Since that time a vast amount of empirical and theoretical information has accumulated (Davson, 1956; Lajtha, 1962) which permits certain generalizations.

A large class of substances which are lipid soluble and nonpolar appear not to be affected by any unusual barriers in their accumulation in brain tissue from the blood. This includes most gases, the volatile anesthetics, and a variety of other substances such as antipyrine, the barbiturates, and probably many other drugs which produce rapid effects upon the central nervous system. Another class of substances includes those that are strongly polar such as sodium, potassium, and other cations; chloride, sulfate, phosphate, and other anions; most amines; and many of the drugs which have markedly delayed or absent central nervous effects. Such substances do not appear in brain tissue in the early phases of their presence in the blood although they may accumulate later but at a slow rate. Their delayed appearance in the brain can probably be accounted for by a rather roundabout path which they have to traverse into the cerebrospinal fluid and thence by the relatively slow circulation of that fluid into the extracellular spaces of the brain. The cerebrospinal fluid is formed, for the most part, within the cerebral ventricles by what has some of the characteristics of a selective filtration process at the choroid plexus. On its way through the ventricles and over the convexity of the brain, this fluid may be altered in composition by exchange with the adjacent brain tissues through the endothelial linings of the ventricle and the pia of the cortex. It is also likely that this fluid passes down the so-called Virchow–Robin perivascular spaces of the brain which ensheath the larger vessels and in that way may come into more intimate contact with the extracellular fluid surrounding the brain cells. Since the formation and movement of cerebrospinal fluid is relatively slow in comparison to the rapid rate of cerebral blood flow, substances which must be carried to the brain parenchyma by those mechanisms enter and leave the brain at an extremely slow rate (half-lives of several hours) in comparison to those substances which enter the brain through the blood capillaries (half-lives of minutes).

In recent years, a new understanding of the morphological basis of the blood-brain barrier has emerged in the recognition that the capillaries of the brain are different from those in other tissues by virtue of the tight junctions which occur between contiguous endothelial cells presenting a continuous membrane rather than the apertures which usually occur between the endothelial cells and which ordinarily permit the leakage of fairly large molecules. In the following paper, Dr. Stanley Rapaport will describe some of the evidence on which this concept is based as well as promising methods for reversibly altering this barrier.

REFERENCES

Auckland, K., Bower, B. F., and Berliner, R. W., 1964, *Circulation Res.* **14**: 164.
Davson, H., 1956, *Physiology of the Ocular and Cerebrospinal Fluids*, Churchill, London.
Fieschi, C., Bozzao, L., and Agnoli, A., 1965, *Acta Neurol. Scand. Suppl.* **14**: 46.

Kety, S. S., 1949, *Am. Heart J.* **38**: 321.
Kety, S. S., 1951, *Pharmacol. Rev.* **3**: 1.
Kety, S. S., 1960, in: *Methods in Medical Research*, Vol. VIII (H. D. Bruner, ed.), pp. 223 and 228, Year Book Publishers, Chicago.
Lajtha, A., 1937, in: *Neurochemistry* (K. A. C. Elliott, I. H. Page, and J. H. Quastel, eds.), Charles C. Thomas, Springfield, Ill.
Lassen, N., and Ingvar, D. J., 1961, *Experientia* **17**: 42.
Lindbjerg, I. F., 1969, *Xenon-133 in the Study of Peripheral Circulation in Obliterative Arterial Disease*, Munksgaard, Copenhagen.
Nilsson, N. J., 1965, *Acta Neurol. Scand. Suppl.* **14**: 53.
Reivich, M., 1972, in: *Cerebral Blood Flow* (J. S. Mayer and J. P. Shade, eds.), Progress in Brain Research, *35*, Elsevier Publishing Co., Amsterdam.
Reivich, M., Jehle, J., Sokoloff, L., and Kety, S. S., 1968, *J. Appl. Physiol.* **27**: 296.
Renkin, E. M., 1959, *Am. J. Physiol.* **197**: 1205.
Scherrer-Etienne, M., and Posternak, J. M., 1963, *J. Suisse Med.* **93**: 1016.
Sokoloff, L., 1961, in: *Regional Neurochemistry* (S. S. Kety aud J. Elkes, eds.), Pergamon Press, Oxford.
Teorell, T., 1937, *Arch. Intern. Pharmacodyn. Therap.* **57**: 205.

Target Organ Modification In Pharmacology: Reversible Osmotic Opening of the Blood–Brain Barrier by Opening of Tight Junctions

Stanley I. Rapoport

Laboratory of Neurophysiology
National Institute of Mental Health
Bethesda, Maryland

We often consider how to modify the physical-chemical properties of a drug—its distribution, excretion, and metabolism—so as to increase its effective action at the target organ. In this paper I shall discuss how a target organ itself—the brain and blood–brain barrier system—can be modified to facilitate entry of normally excluded drugs. I shall present physiological and morphological evidence that the blood–brain barrier can be opened osmotically in a reversible manner without producing gross neurological damage to the animal.

Exchange of lipid-insoluble solutes between blood and brain is controlled in part by a blood–brain barrier at the capillary endothelium of the cerebrovascular system. This barrier is composed of a continuous sheet of endothelial cells, connected by tight junctions (Fig. 1), and has permeability properties of the endothelial cell membranes (Krogh, 1946). Water and other small molecules can probably pass through these membranes (Solomon, 1968). The absence of large intercellular pores, which are found in capillary endothelium elsewhere in the body (Karnovsky, 1968), makes the barrier restrict passive exchange of lipid insoluble nonelectrolytes and electrolytes. Large solutes such as colloidal lanthanum and peroxidase, when introduced into the vascular system, are restricted from passing through the endothelial cell membranes as well as across the tight junctions

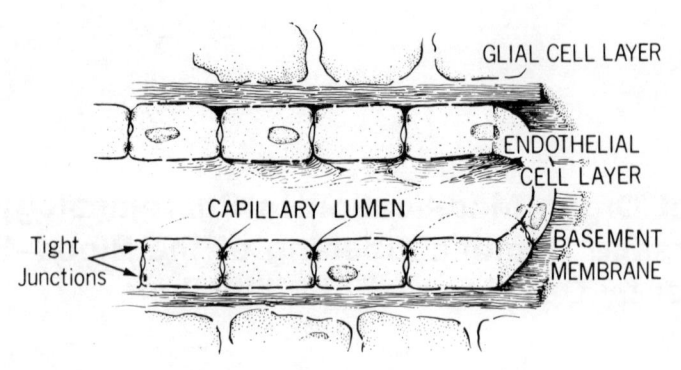

Fig. 1. Diagram of blood–brain barrier at capillary level of brain. A molecule may cross the barrier from blood to brain by passing through the endothelial cell membrane if it is: (1) lipid-soluble so as to pass through the lipid region of the membrane or (2) small enough to pass through an aqueous pore of the membrane (represented as a hiatus in the membrane). It may also cross the barrier by passing through the tight junctions (3) if it is smaller than their equivalent pore diameter. The tight junctions which form continuous belts around endothelial cells (see Fig. 2) are assumed to open when concentrated solutions of electrolytes and lipid insoluble nonelectrolytes osmotically shrink the endothelial cells. The barrier consists of three pathways through which a solute can pass, depending on size and lipid solubility. We exclude in this diagram active transport and facilitated diffusion mechanisms (from Rapoport, 1973; reprinted with permission of C. V. Mosby Company).

(Fig. 2) (Reese and Karnovsky, 1967). Transport of glucose and some amino acids at the vascular capillaries can occur readily by facilitated diffusion (Crone, 1965; Davson, 1967; Oldendorf, 1971).

Urea, mannitol, and other nonelectrolytes have been used to treat brain edema (Davson, 1967). They withdraw water osmotically from the brain because of the partial semipermeability of the barrier cells (Fenstermacher and Johnson, 1966). Morphological evidence that the barrier is composed of cells suggested that high concentrations of these nonelectrolytes, under different experimental conditions, might shrink the endothelia themselves and open the tight junctions (Rapoport, 1970, 1971, 1973).

Early work by Overton (1895) and Collander and Bärlund (1933) (see also Höber, 1945) showed that effectiveness in shrinking plant and animal cells by solutes decreased when solute lipid solubility and cell membrane permeability increased. A lipid-insoluble solute, poorly permeable through the lipoid cell membrane, shrank cells maximally for a given solution osmotic pressure (salts, sucrose, glucose, glycerol). Shrinkage was reversible. More lipid-soluble solutes, which shrank cells less effectively, required higher osmolalities to produce a given degree of shrinkage (urea, lactamide, formamide, acetamide). Very lipid-soluble substances, which easily cross

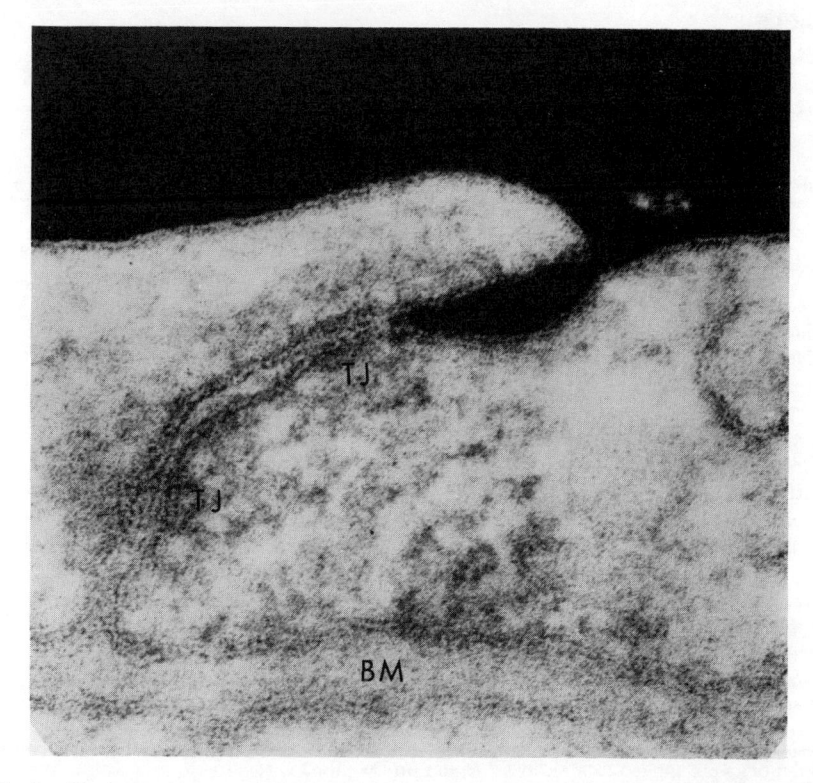

Fig. 2. Blockage of passage of lanthanum from cerebral capillary lumen to neuropil by tight junction between two endothelial cells. Lanthanum fills the capillary lumen (upper dark region), penetrates into the cleft between the endothelial cells, but is prevented from penetrating into the brain by a tight junction (TJ). It has the same distribution as peroxidase. Below the tight junction is a gap, free of lanthanum, which is closed at its other end by another tight junction (TJ). The tight junctions form continuous belts around the cells. BM = basement membrane. Magnification × 100,000 (reduced 45% for reproduction). (From Brightman and Reese, 1969; reprinted with permission of the *Journal of Cell Biology*).

the cell membrane, did not shrink cells at all (ethyl carbamate, ethanol, methanol).

It seemed reasonable to suppose that if the blood–brain barrier acted like a cell layer, as suggested by its morphology (Figs. 1 and 2), lipid-insoluble or slightly lipid-soluble substances might open it reversibly by shrinking barrier cells and opening tight junctions. Furthermore, on the basis of observations on osmotic shrinkage of single cells, threshold osmolalities for a given degree of barrier opening would be expected to increase with increasing lipid solubility of these substances.

TABLE I
Effect of Topically Applied Concentrated Solutions on Blood–Brain Barrier to Evans Blue-Albumin[a]

Substance	Olive oil/water distribution	Reversibility of opening	Threshold at surface osmol	Threshold[c] at barrier site	σ^d
LiCl	[b]	Yes	1.5	0.87	1.1
Na$_2$SO$_4$	[b]	Yes	1.5	0.82	1.2
NaCl	[b]	Yes	1.6	1.0	1.0
Sucrose	[b]	Yes	5.8	1.1	0.91
Glucose	[b]	Yes	3.8	1.0	1.0
Glycerol	0.00007	Yes	5.7	2.1	0.48
Urea	0.00016	Yes	3.0	1.7	0.59
Lactamide	0.0003	Yes	4.6	—	—
Methyl urea	0.00044	Yes	4.3	2.2	0.45
Ethylene glycol	0.0005	No	19.6	—	—
Formamide	0.00083	Yes	4.6	2.9	0.34
Acetamide	0.0009	Yes	6.4	3.5	0.29
Propionamide	0.0037	Yes	6.4	3.2	0.31
		No	8.2		
Cyanamide	0.0045	No	2.5	—	—
Propylene glycol	0.0056	No	27.5	—	—
Methanol	0.008	No	32.7	—	—
Ethanol	0.023	No	12.3	—	—
Methyl carbamate	0.025	No	2.9	—	—
Ethyl carbamate	0.074	No	1.6	—	—

[a] Solutions were applied to a localized region on the rabbit cortex for 10 min with a filter paper pledget. Substances are ranked according to increasing olive oil/water partition, which represents lipid solubility. The barrier to Evans blue closes within 30 min after being opened by reversibly acting solutes. It remains open 30 min after damage by irreversibly acting solutes. Surface thresholds are minimal osmolal concentrations which produced Evans blue extravasation near small veins of pia-arachnoid (Fig. 3). Thresholds at the barrier site and σ were calculated by taking diffusion on the brain surface into account, and are normalized with respect to NaCl values. σ is the reciprocal of the normalized site threshold (from Rapoport et al., 1972b).
[b] Distribution is close to zero.
[c] Thresholds are relative to NaCl threshold at barrier site.
[d] Sigmas are relative to $\sigma_{NaCl} = 1$.

The osmotic pressure π of a nonelectrolyte solution is

$$\pi = RTm' \qquad (1)$$

where R is the gas constant, T the absolute temperature, and m' osmolality (molality x osmotic coefficient). We define effective osmotic pressure for shrinking a cell as

$$\text{Effective osmotic pressure} = \sigma\pi \qquad (2)$$

where σ depends inversely on lipid solubility in a nonlinear way for many cells and cell layers, and on molecular size (Diamond and Wright, 1969).

Earlier work in the rabbit on the blood–brain barrier to HCO_3^- indicated that threshold for barrier opening by NaCl, $NaNO_3$, urea, and ethanol increased with increasing lipid solubility (Rapoport, 1970). Partial barrier opening by each of these agents occurred at a lower osmolality than complete opening, which suggested that opening was a continuous function of osmolality rather than all-or-none.

These observations led to a more extensive study in which reversibility also was measured, as summarized in Table I (Rapoport *et al.*, 1972*b*). Nineteen electrolytes and nonelectrolytes, mostly of mol. wt. < 100, were applied to the pia-arachnoid surface of the rabbit cortex for 10 min.

The intravascular barrier tracer, Evans blue-albumin, measured barrier opening at the pia-arachnoid vessels, which have a continuous endothelial cell layer with tight junctions. Figure 3 shows opening produced by 2

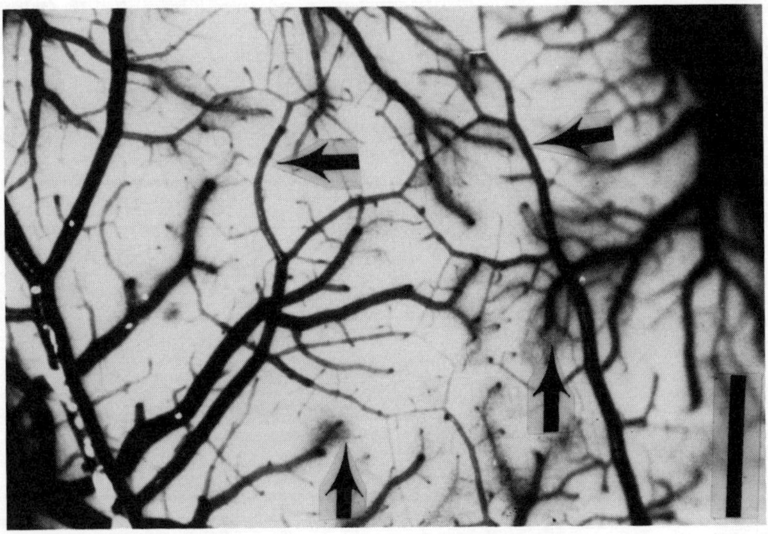

Fig. 3. Opening of blood–brain barrier to intravenous Evans blue following application of 2 osmolal Na_2SO_4 to the pia-arachnoid surface of rabbit brain for 10 min. The smudges represent extravasated dye and are found mainly around small veins (designated by upward arrows). Scale = 1 mm. Arterioles are designated by horizontal arrows (from Rapoport *et al.*, 1972*b*; reprinted with permission of the *American Journal of Physiology*).

osmolal Na_2SO_4. This opening was reversible, since the Evans blue-albumin tracer did not extravasate when injected intravenously one-half hour after application of Na_2SO_4, rather than before application.

Table I gives osmolal thresholds as minimal osmolalities m' needed to produce barrier opening. Substances are ranked according to their olive oil-water distributions (a measure of lipid solubility). Relative thresholds at the barrier site (the endothelial cell layer of the pial vessels) were estimated by taking into account diffusion at the brain surface (Rapoport et al., 1972b). The data support the osmotic model for barrier opening since the electrolytes and relatively lipid insoluble nonelectrolytes opened the barrier reversibly, and thresholds of the reversibly acting agents increased with lipid solubility. The more lipid-soluble solutes acted irreversibly, probably by destroying cell membranes.

By Eqs. (1) and (2),

$$\sigma = \frac{\text{Effective osmotic pressure}}{RTm'} \qquad (3)$$

If each reversibly acting solute opens the barrier when a given effective osmotic pressure is reached, the relative value of σ will be the inverse of relative threshold osmolality, as shown in Table I. The σ decrease as lipid solubility and barrier permeability increase, as predicted by the osmotic

TABLE II
Effect of Internal Carotid Perfusion of 2.2 Molal Urea, 2.5 Molal Lactamide, and 0.9% NaCl on the Blood–Brain Barrier to Evans Blue–Albumin in the Monkey[a]

				Number of animals	
Condition	Flow rate, ml/sec	Solution	No staining	Left hemispheric staining	Normal neurological with staining
Common[b] carotid ligated	0.4–1.7	Urea, 2.2 m	3	9	2
		NaCl, 0.9%	5	1	0
Common[c] carotid not ligated	0.76–0.86	Urea, 2.2 m	2	6	6
		Lactamide, 2.5m	1	6	5
		NaCl, 0.9%	5	1	1

[a] When the common carotid was permanently ligated, left hemispheric staining was easily produced by 30 sec perfusion of urea, but seven of the nine animals with staining had neurological defects such as right-sided weakness. When the common carotid was only temporarily clamped for 20 sec of lingual perfusion (Fig. 6), neurological defects were infrequent after both urea and lactamide perfusion.
[b] Observations from Rapoport et al. (1972a).
[c] Observations from Rapoport and Thompson (1973).

model (Crone, 1965; Katchalsky and Curran, 1965). The σ also decrease as solute size decreases (Diamond and Wright, 1969). The σ for sucrose, glucose, urea, and formamide agree with values determined by another method (Fenstermacher and Johnson, 1966).

We later perfused reversibly acting nonelectrolytes into the internal carotid artery of the rabbit for 30 sec, after ligating the external and common carotids (Steinwall, 1958). Two molal solutions of urea and lactamide were shown to open the barrier reversibly at the capillary endothelium of the homolateral hemisphere, using Evans blue-albumin or sodium fluorescein as barrier tracers (Rapoport et al., 1972b, Rap et al., unpublished). Ethanol and propylene glycol, which act irreversibly at the

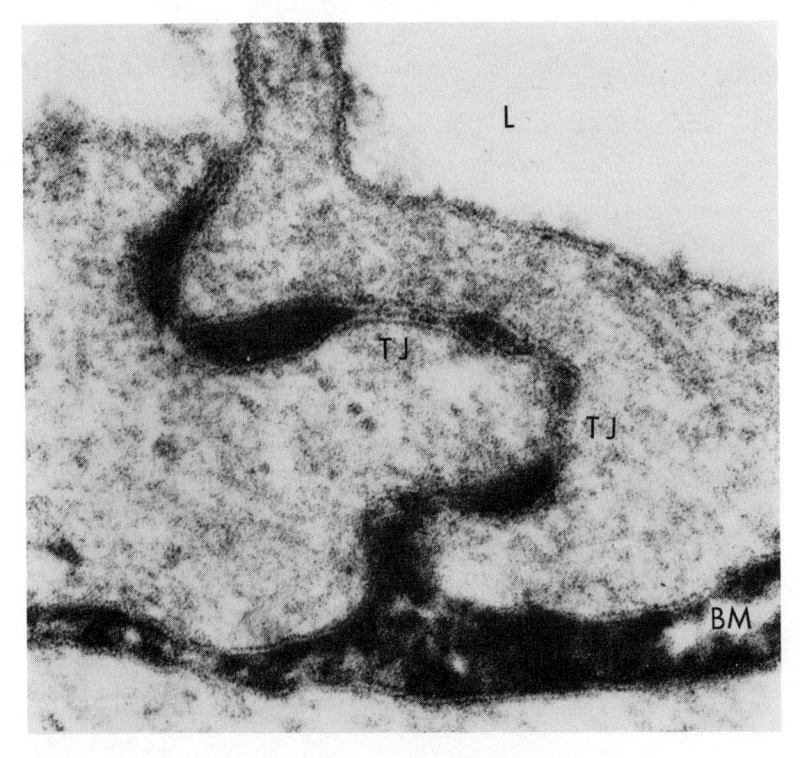

Fig. 4. Opening of the tight junctions between endothelial cells to peroxidase tracer, by intracarotid perfusion of 3 molar urea in the rabbit. Peroxidase was given intravenously 2 min following 30 sec of perfusion of urea solution through the internal carotid artery. It was washed out of the capillary lumen (L) during fixation. Peroxidase is present along the interface between the endothelial cells, in the gaps between the tight junctions (TJ), and in the basement membrane (B.M.). Magnification × 100,000 (reduced 45% for reproduction) (from Brightman et al., 1973).

pia-arachnoid vessel (Table II), also opened the barrier irreversibly at the cortical capillaries (see Fig. 5).

Morphological proof of reversible osmotic opening with internal carotid perfusion was provided by using intravascularly administered horseradish peroxidase as a barrier tracer for electron microscopy (Rapoport et al., 1973; Brightman et al., 1973). Intracarotid 2.5 and 3 molal urea opened the tight junctions of the cerebrovascular endothelium, as predicted by the osmotic model, without damaging endothelial cells (Fig. 4). The tracer was distributed in the extracellular space of the perfused hemisphere.

Following this confirmation, we wanted to know if the barrier could be opened without neurological damage in the Rhesus monkey. We ligated as before the left common and external carotid arteries (Steinwall, 1958), and perfused 2.2 osmol urea into the left internal carotid for 30 sec. The monkeys were permitted to survive for 4 days to 2 weeks (Rapoport et al., 1972a).

While it was possible to open the barrier at the cerebral cortex of the left hemisphere, primarily in the distribution of the middle cerebral artery

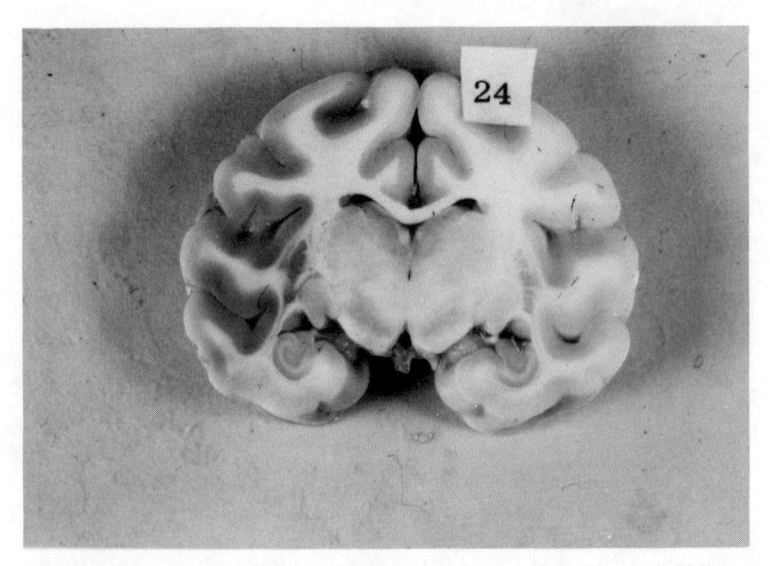

Fig. 5. Coronal section of brain of monkey sacrificed 4 days following internal carotid perfusion of 2.2 molal urea solution. Evans blue dye (dark regions) stains the left hemisphere diffusely, indicating blood–brain barrier breakdown. The monkey was normal neurologically and had no pathological brain lesions (Rapoport et al., 1972a).

(Fig. 5), the incidence of "pure" opening without neurological defects was low. Seven of nine animals in which some left hemispheric staining was produced had associated right-sided weakness and evidence of left hemispheric necrosis (Table II).

With perfusion plus common carotid ligation, the threshold for osmotic opening of the barrier was very close to that for neurotoxicity. It remained possible, however, that permanent unilateral carotid ligation predisposed the brain to homolateral ischemic damage (Levine, 1960). To test this, we used an alternative method of perfusion (Coceani *et al.*, 1966). The lingual artery was catheterized and the distal external carotid and the proximal common carotid were clamped during 20 sec of lingual perfusion (Fig. 6). Since the superior thyroid was ligated, only the internal carotid artery was patent for perfusion of the left hemisphere, and blood flow to the hemisphere could be restored immediately after perfusion by removing the clamps. With temporary carotid clamping, the barrier could be osmotically opened in a majority of animals without producing right-sided weakness or paresis (Table II) (Rapoport and Thompson, 1973).

An interesting side light to these experiments was that the aqueous and vitreous humors of the homolateral eye were stained with Evans blue-

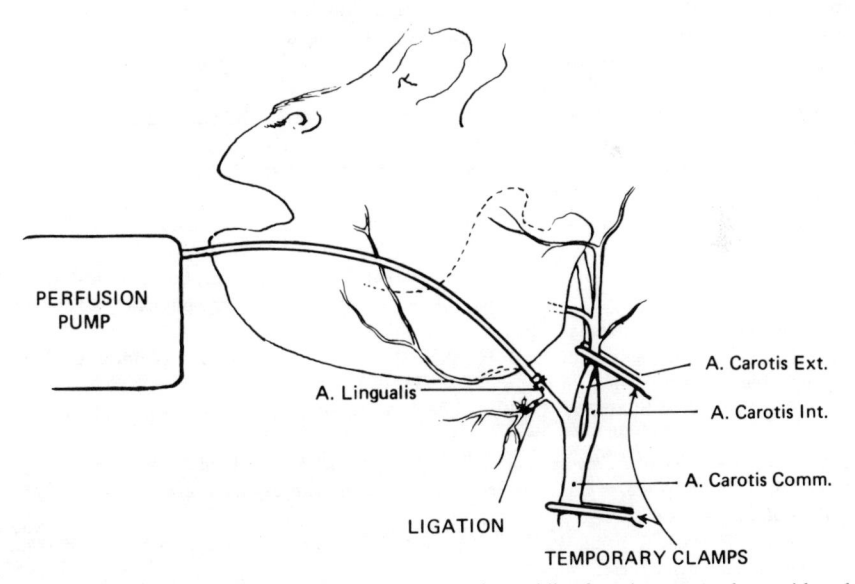

Fig. 6. Perfusion of lingual artery of Rhesus monkey while clamping external carotid and common carotid for 20-sec period of perfusion. (Figure adapted from Hartman and Straus, 1933.)

albumin following hypertonic perfusion. The ophthalmic artery is a branch of the internal carotid. Barriers in the eye, which also depend on tight junctions or continuous vascular endothelium (Kuwabara, 1970), are liable to osmotic action.

In summary: The brain as a pharmacological target organ can be modified to facilitate entry of usually excluded solutes. The blood-brain barrier, which separates brain from blood, is a continuous layer of vascular endothelial cells connected by tight junctions. Concentrated solutions of electrolytes and poorly lipid soluble nonelectrolytes act osmotically on these cells to reversibly open the tight junctions. Osmotic opening can be produced without gross neurotoxicity. However, before osmotic opening can be applied clinically, we must study in more detail brain and eye histology and metabolism, as well as finer neurological functions and behavior.

REFERENCES

Brightman, M. W., Hori, M., Rapoport, S. I., Reese, T. S., and Westergaard, E., 1973 "Osmotic opening of tight junctions in cerebral endothelium," *J. Comp. Neurol.* **152**: 317-326.

Brightman, M. W., and Reese, T. S., 1969, "Junctions between intimately apposed cell membranes in the vertebrate brain," *J. Cell. Biol.* **40**: 648-677.

Broman, T., 1949, *The Permeability of the Cerebrospinal Vessels in Normal and Pathological Conditions*, Munksgaard, Copenhagen.

Coceani, F., Libman, I., and Gloor, P., 1966, "The effect of intracarotid amobarbital injections upon experimentally induced epileptiform activity," *EEG Clin. Neurophysiol.* **20**: 542-558.

Collander, R., and Bärlund, H., 1933, "Permeabilitätsstudien an Chara Ceratophylla," *Acta Botan. Fenn* **11**: 1-20.

Crone, C., 1965, "The permeability of brain capillaries to nonelectrolytes," *Acta Physiol. Scand.* **64**: 407-417.

Davson H., 1967, *Physiology of the Cerebrospinal Fluid*, J & A Churchill, London.

Diamond, J. M., and Wright, E. M., 1969, "Biological membranes: The physical basis of ion and nonelectrolyte selectivity," *Ann. Rev. Physiol.* **31**: 581-646.

Fenstermacher, J. D., and Johnson, J. A., 1966, "Filtration and reflection coefficients of the rabbit blood-brain barrier," *Am. J. Physiol.* **211**: 341-346.

Hartman, C. G., and Straus, W. L., 1933, *The Anatomy of the Rhesus Monkey*, Hafner, New York.

Höber, R., 1945, *Physical Chemistry of Cells and Tissues*, Blakiston, Philadelphia.

Karnovsky, M. J., 1968, "The ultrastructural basis of transcapillary exchanges," *J. Gen. Physiol.* **52**: 64s-95s.

Katchalsky, A., and Curran, P. F., 1965, *Nonequilibrium Thermodymanics in Biophysics*, Harvard University Press, Cambridge.

Krogh, A., 1946, "The active and passive exchanges of inorganic ions through the surfaces of living cells and through living membranes generally," *Proc. Roy. Soc. Ser. B.* **133**: 140-200.

Kuwabara, T., 1970, *Fine Structure of the Eye*, 2nd ed., Harvard Univ. Med. School, Boston.
Levine, S., 1960, "Anoxic-ischemic encephalopathy in rats," *Am. J. Path.* **36**: 1–17.
Oldendorf, W. H., 1971, "Brain uptake of radiolabeled amino acids, amines and hexoses after arterial injection," *Am. J. Physiol.* **221**: 1629–1639.
Overton, E., 1895, "Über die osmotischen Eigenschaften der lebenden Pflanzen and Tierzelle," *Vierteljahresschr. Naturforsch. Ges. Zürich.* **40**: 159–201.
Rapoport, S. I., 1970, "Effect of concentrated solutions on blood–brain barrier," *Am. J. Physiol.* **219**: 270–274.
Rapoport, S. I., 1971, "The cortical acidic response to intravenous $NaHCO_3$ and the nature of blood–brain barrier damage," *Intern. J. Neurosci.* **2**: 1–6.
Rapoport, S. I., 1973, "Evidence for reversible opening of the blood–brain barrier by osmotic shrinkage of the cerebrovascular endothelium and opening of the tight junctions. Relation to carotid arteriography," in: *Small Vessel Angiography. Imaging, Morphology, Physiology and Clinical Applications.* S. K. Hilal, Ed. C. V. Mosby Company, St. Louis.
Rapoport, S. I., Bachman, D. S., and Thompson, H. K., 1972a, "Chronic effects of osmotic opening of the blood–brain barrier in the monkey." *Science* **176**: 1243–1245.
Rapoport, S. I., Brightman, M. W. and Reese, T. S., 1973 "Reversible osmotic opening of the blood–brain barrier by opening tight junctions of cerebrovascular endothelium," *Biophys. Soc. 17th Ann. Meeting Abstr.* **13**: 230a.
Rapoport, S. I., Hori, M., and Klatzo, I., 1972b, "Testing of a hypothesis for osmotic opening of the blood–brain barrier," *Am. J. Physiol.* **223**: 323–331.
Rapoport, S. I. and Thompson, H. K., 1973, Osmotic opening of the blood–brain barrier in the monkey without associated neurological deficits, *Science*, **180**: 971.
Reese, T. S. and Karnovsky, M. J., 1967, "Fine structural localization of a blood–brain barrier to exogenous peroxidase," *J. Cell. Biol.* **34**: 207–217.
Solomon, A. K., 1968, "Characterization of biological membranes by equivalent pores," *J. Gen. Physiol.* **51**: (5, pt. 2) 335s–364s.
Steinwall, O, 1958, "An improved technique for testing the effect of contrast media and other substances on the blood–brain barrier," *Acta Radiol.* **49**: 281–284.

Pharmacogenetics: Single Gene Effects

Bert N. La Du

The Stella and Charles Guttman Laboratories
   for Human Pharmacology and Pharmacogenetics
Department of Pharmacology*
New York University Medical School
New York, New York

Dr. Vesell and I have been asked to review some principles of pharmacogenetics that relate to the pharmacokinetic theme of this conference. We have divided the topic: Dr. Vesell will discuss multiple gene effects and their implications, and I will mention some single gene effects which can modify drug metabolism and drug response in man. We both are studying the way genetic factors account for rather remarkable person-to-person differences in drug responses and pharmacodynamics, and we hope that pharmacokinetic models will be designed that will take into account these genetically determined individual differences.

As Dr. Vesell will discuss in more detail later, we know of a number of adverse drug reactions which occur in people who have an inherited deficiency of certain enzymes which are important in the inactivation of specific drugs. These hereditary conditions are like the inborn errors of metabolism, except the enzymatic deficiencies affect the metabolism of drugs, rather than endogenous compounds of intermediary metabolism. Some examples of genetically determined adverse drug reactions are given in Table I.

Once it has been established that a particular drug metabolism enzyme deficiency is inherited, and individuals with this deficiency will show an adverse drug reaction when given the usual dose of the drug, it would be

*Supported by National Institue of General Medical Sciences Grant 17184.

TABLE I
Some Genetically Determined Types of Adverse Drug Reactions[a]

Types	Examples
1. Acute drug toxicity	Succinylcholine sensitivity
2. Cumulative drug toxicity	Isoniazid polyneuritis
3. Drug-drug interactions	Isoniazid-diphenylhydantoin
4. Side reactions—hemolysis, methemoglobinemia	Acetophenetidin
5. Ineffectiveness of drugs	Allopurinol
6. Resistance to drug effects	Warfarin
7. Unexpected metabolic reactions	Hyperthermia, rigidity from anesthetics
8. Allergic reactions	Penicillin

[a] See La Du (1972); Vesell (1972) for recent general reviews.

important to identify these individuals in order to prevent toxic drug reactions. Genetic analysis of the families with sensitive people should establish whether the drug sensitivity is inherited as a recessive or dominant trait, whether it is inherited as an autosomal or sex-linked condition, and whether carriers of the trait can be identified. The frequency of sensitive individuals in the general population can be estimated if suitable tests can be developed for surveys of sample populations. Sensitivity to succinylcholine, for example, can be analyzed very easily without exposure to the drug by tests on the individual's serum for the level and quality of the cholinesterase (Kalow and Genest, 1957; Harris and Whittaker, 1961). The test identifies the sensitive person, a carrier of the gene for sensivity, and those who have the usual type of cholinesterase. Experience has shown that people with very low levels of serum cholinesterase activity are sensitive to succinylcholine but this genetic combination (inheriting "silent" genes from both parents) occurs very rarely. Most of the sensitive people have inherited a double dose of genes which produce a modified type of serum cholinesterase with reduced affinity for choline ester substrates (Table II). This "atypical" esterase is essentially ineffective in catalyzing the hydrolysis of succinylcholine.

TABLE II
Types of Serum Cholinesterase and Sensitivity to Succinylcholine

Genotype, E_1 locus alleles	Types of enzymes	Prevalence	Response to succinylcholine
$E_1^u E_1^u$	Usual	96:100	Normal
$E_1^A E_1^A$	Atypical (dibucaine resistant)	1:2500	Prolonged
$E_1^F E_1^F$	Fluoride resistant	Very rare	Prolonged
$E_1^S E_1^S$	Silent (no activity)	1:100,000	Prolonged

In the general population about 1:2500 have the atypical serum cholinesterase and 1:25 are heterozygous carriers, with a mixture of normal and atypical esterases in their serum. The latter individuals rarely show succinylcholine sensitivity, so a moderate reduction in the level of the usual type of esterase is still sufficient to hydrolyze circulating succinylcholine very quickly. Sensitivity to succinylcholine is thus inherited as a simple, autosomal recessive trait.

With this background about succinylcholine sensitivity, it is worth making a few remarks about the meaning of risk, or the probability of showing a drug sensitivity when this much is learned about its cause and the inherited trait responsible for it. It may be true that 1:2500 in the general population have atypical serum cholinesterase and a sensitivity to succinylcholine, but the probability of being that one person in 2500 is not really shared equally. If we knew the genotype of the parents of each person in the sample population, our risk figures would be considerably different. If both parents have the usual type of esterase, the offspring should also have the usual kind of esterase and be at no risk; if both parents are heterozygous carriers of the atypical esterase gene, the chances that a child would be sensitive and have atypical esterase are 1:4; and if, by chance, both parents are sensitive, all children would also inherit the sensitivity. The genetic association of a drug reaction with particular genetic markers allows a reclassification of the general population into distinct subpopulations with different risk values. The critical point about this reclassification according to the particular genetic trait is that it is unique; in fact, it is the only basis for making this important distinction. The susceptible group may be indistinguishable from the rest of the population by all other tests.

The same genetic considerations apply to the risk of sensitivity in close relatives of a person known to be sensitive to succinylcholine. Both parents of a person proved to have atypical serum cholinesterase must at least be heterozygous carriers in order to have transmitted the atypical genes. Brothers and sisters of an affected sibling have a 1:4 risk (or higher) of also being sensitive to succinylcholine; not 1:2500.

Perhaps the above examples of Mendelian inheritance are obvious. It appears, however, that better use of population genetic information could be made in predicting risk for drug sensitivities and adverse drug reactions. In a way, present models seem to emphasize mean values with standard deviations to account for variation; but the genetically determined variability is quite different—because of particular genetic traits, individuals fall into distinct groups, with different orders of magnitude in their risk of adverse reactions, rates of drug metabolism, or drug receptor site sensitivities.

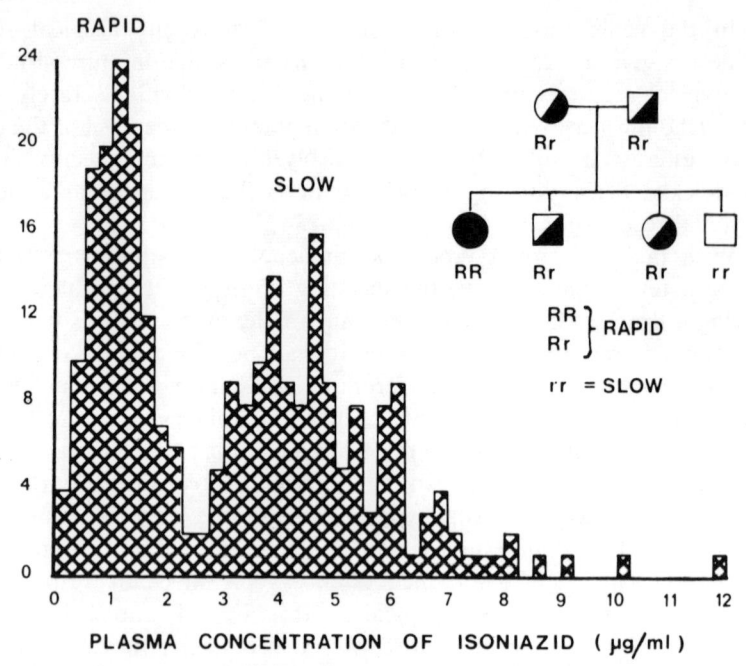

Fig. 1. Plasma concentrations of isoniazid 6 hr after oral administration of the drug to 267 members of 53 families (from Evans et al., 1960).

Another well-known pharmacogenetic condition illustrates some further points that apply to pharmacokinetics. This is the rapid or slow rate of acetylation of isoniazid which is also inherited as an autosomal Mendelian trait (Fig. 1). Slow acetylators are homozygous for a recessive gene, and about half of the population in the United States is in this class (Mitchell et al., 1960). The proportion of slow acetylators varies in different ethnic and geographic areas around the world; only about 5% in the Canadian Eskimos (Armstrong and Peart, 1960), but up to 83% in Egyptians (Hashem et al., 1969). Since differences in gene frequency are not unusual, the risk of drug reactions or the expectations of unusual rates of drug metabolism from experience in one sample population may be inappropriate for individuals or people from another locality.

The differences in rapid and slow acetylators of isoniazid are correlated with the level of liver N-acetyltransferase activity, and a number of other drugs which are inactivated by acetylation seem to depend upon the same liver enzyme as isoniazid. These include sulfamethazine, hydralazine, phenelzine, and diaminodiphenylsulfone (Weber, 1973). Slow acetylators are more likely to develop cumulative toxicity to isoniazid (Devadatta et al.,

1960), toxic symptoms from phenelzine (Evans et al., 1965), and a lupus erythematosus-like reaction from hydralazine (Perry et al., 1967). In addition, very slow acetylators are more likely to show an accumulation of diphenylhydantoin in patients receiving both drugs (Kutt et al., 1966; Brennan et al., 1970). This seems to be due to the inhibition of diphenylhydantoin metabolism (hydroxylation) in liver microsomes by the accumulated isoniazid (Kutt et al., 1968). This is a very instructive model of a drug–drug interaction, based upon a genetic difference in the rate of metabolism of one drug influencing the metabolism of another drug.

It would be useful to know the acetylator phenotype of many patients, but unfortunately there are no simple tests to do this. Isoniazid or sulfamethazine must be given, and either blood concentrations of the drug or the urinary free and acetylated drug must be measured at specific time intervals (Weber, 1973). None of the chemical tests clearly distinguish between homozygous rapid and heterozygous rapid acetylators, although one group [Sunahara et al. (1961)] reports that this is possible using a very sensitive microbiological assay. Human erythrocytes contain an N-acetyltransferase but its acetylation rate of p-amino-benzoic acid (Motulsky, 1964) does not correlate with the liver isoniazid phenotype. Weber and Hearse have made further studies of the acetylation systems in liver and red cells of rabbits and man to compare the properties of these enzymes (Hearse et al., 1970; Hearse and Weber, 1970).

Probably everyone is familiar with the inherited sensitivity to primaquine which is due to a deficiency of red cell glucose-6-phosphate dehydrogenase (Motulsky et al., 1971; Kirkman, 1968). Males are more likely to show the enzymatic deficiency than females since the gene determining the characteristics of the dehydrogenase is carried on the X chromosome (Childs et al., 1958). Over 80 distinct variant forms of the dehydrogenase have been identified (Motulsky et al., 1971) but all of these are not associated with primaquine sensitivity. Only those in which the dehydrogenase activity is reduced to less than about 30% of normal are regularly found to have hemolytic reactions (Kirkman, 1968).

Thus, there are large numbers of genetic variations in the structure and activity of enzymes, only some of which may be associated with disease or adverse drug reactions. The range of rates of drug metabolism in individuals is relatively wide and it is not unusual to observe severalfold or even a tenfold difference in the sample population for metabolic rates or enzyme activities. In the following chapter, Dr. Vesell will expand on the genetic basis for these differences and how these have been shown to be primarily genetic, rather than environmental variations.

The striking examples in pharmacogenetics are those which show marked differences from the normal response, and they generally are rather unusual, if not rare, drug reactions. It is worth noting that genetic factors also account for graded differences in enzyme activities or protein concentration within a continuous spectrum even when the range of activities, if plotted as a frequency distribution histogram, may be normally distributed. Thus a normal distribution in some variable measurement does not necessarily mean that the observed variation is environmental; or if known to be due to genetic factors, that a large number of genes must be involved. A very few genes, perhaps allelic genes, can account for variation which is both continuous and approximates a normal distribution.

Although human red cell acid phosphatase is not known to be associated with any type of drug metabolism or drug reaction, the genetic analysis of the factors which determine the level of activity in each person illustrates these points very well. Harris and co-investigators (Hopkinson *et al.*, 1963; Harris *et al.*, 1968) have established some important findings in respect to the red cell acid phosphatase:

1. The level and type of acid phosphatase in red cells is determined by three allelic genes: A, B, and C.
2. The acid phosphatase activity level differs according to the allele in the ratio A:B:C as 2:3:4 (Spencer *et al.*, 1964).
3. The acid phosphatases from the three alleles have different electrophoretic migration patterns (Fig. 2).

It was the distinctive electrophoretic patterns of the different acid phosphatases that permitted Harris and his group to prove that the three genes (A, B, and C) were allelic and show the corresponding differences in level of activity. Three allelic genes would give six different possible genotypes (AA, AB, AC, BB, BC, and CC).

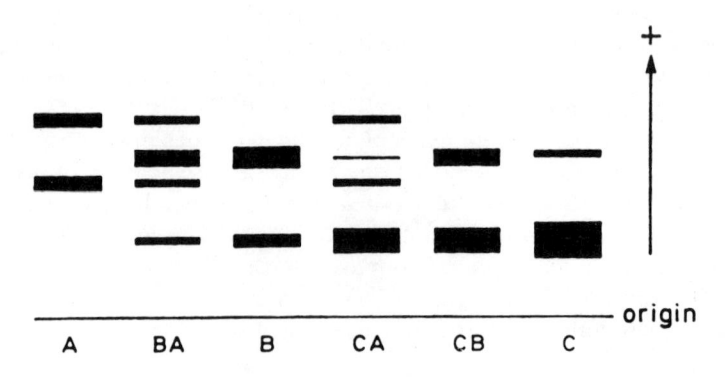

Fig. 2. Electrophoretic patterns of different red cell acid phosphatase phenotypes (from Harris, 1970). For method, see Hopkinson and Harris, 1969.

Pharmacogenetics: Single Gene Effects

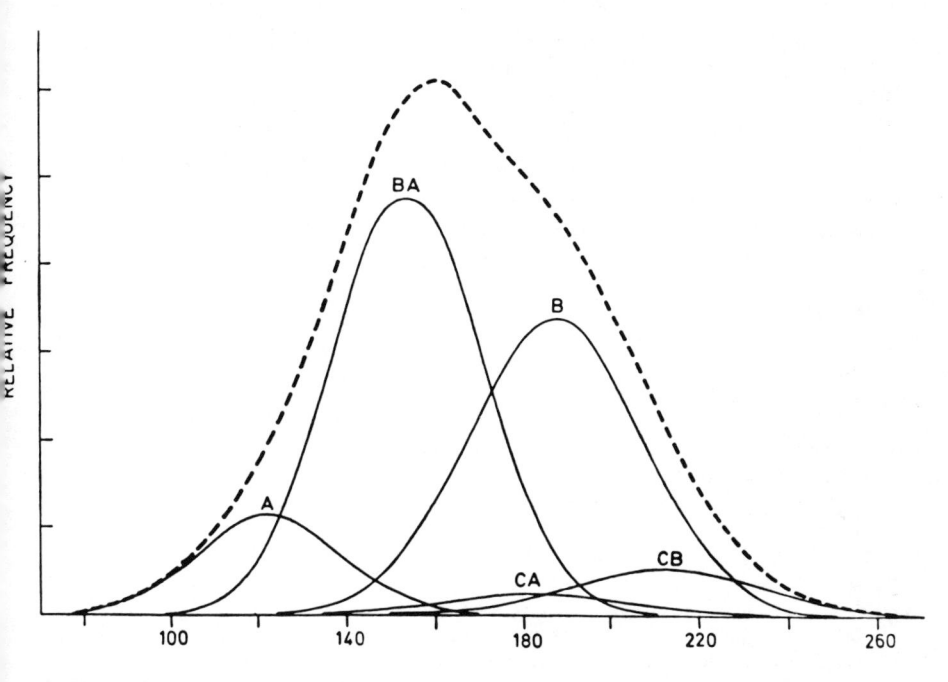

Fig. 3. Distribution of red cell acid phosphatase activity in the general population (from Harris, 1970).

Family studies confirmed that the genotypes of children were those expected and permitted by the assigned genotypes of the parents (Harris et al., 1968).

It can be seen in Fig. 3 that the range of individual values for red cell acid phosphatase in a sample population approximates a normal distribution, but this is really the composite effect from a series of subpopulations corresponding to each of the possible genotypes, and each of the latter has its own mean and standard deviation.

If low red cell acid phosphatase activity were associated with an adverse drug reaction (which it is not), individuals of the AA genotype would be the high risk group, and those of the CC genotype would be at the other end of the scale. By electrophoresis, individuals of the AA genotype could be identified (Fig. 2) (but so could the other genotypes), and knowing the genes are allelic, one could predict from parental typing the probability that the children and relatives would be AA as well.

As more genetic study is made of the enzymes involved in drug metabolism and the proteins concerned with drug responses, we can expect that more examples will be found where single genes that confer selected types of drug sensitivity can be sorted out, even though the gene products may seem to be hidden in a continuous spectrum, as presently measured.

Several other pharmacogenetic conditions could be mentioned; these few examples demonstrate the relationship between distinctive genetic traits and important pharmacokinetic parameters. The difficulties in distinguishing single gene effects are apparent, and the situation is even more complicated when multiple genetic effects are considered.

REFERENCES

Armstrong, A. R., and Peart, H. E., 1960, *Am. Rev. Respirat. Diseases* **81**: 588.
Brennan, R. W., Dehejia, H., Kutt, H., Verebely, K., and McDowell, F., 1970, *Neurology* **20**: 687.
Childs, B., Zinkham, W., Browne, E. A., Kimbro, E. L., and Torbert, J. V., 1958, *Bull. Johns Hopkins Hosp.* **102**: 21.
Devadatta, S., Gangadharam, P. R. J., Andrews, R. H., Fox, W., Ramakrishnan, C. V., Selkon, J. B., and Velu, S., 1960, *Bull. World Health Organ.* **23**: 587.
Evans, D. A. P., Manley, K. A., and McKusick, V. A., 1960, *Brit. Med. J.* **2**: 485.
Evans, K. A. P., Davison, K., and Pratt, R. T. C., 1965, *Clin. Pharmacol. Therap.* **6**: 430.
Harris, H., and Whittaker, M., 1961, *Nature (London)* **191**: 496.
Harris, H., Hopkinson, D. A., Luffman, J. E., and Rapley, S., 1968, In *Hereditary Disorders of Erythrocyte Metabolism* (E. Beutler, ed.), Grune and Stratton, New York.
Harris, H., 1970, *The Principles of Human Biochemical Genetics*, London. Amsterdam-North Holland Publishing Co.
Hashem, N., Khalifa, S., and Nour, A., 1969, *Am. J. Phys. Anthropol.* **31**: 97.
Hearse, D. J., Szabadi, R., and Weber, W. W., 1970, *Pharmacologist* **12**: 274.
Hearse, D. J., and Weber, W. W., 1970, *Fed. Proc.* **29**: 803.
Hopkinson, D. A., Spencer, N., and Harris, H., 1963, *Nature (London)* **199**: 969.
Hopkinson, D. A. and Harris, H., 1969, in: *Biochemical Methods in Red Cell Genetics* (G. Yunis, ed.), Academic Press, New York.
Kalow, W., and Genest, K., 1957, *Can. J. Biochem. Physiol.* **35**: 339.
Kirkman, H. N., 1968, *Ann. N.Y. Acad. Sci.* **151**: 753.
Kutt, H., Winters, W., McDowell, F. H., 1966, *Neurology* **16**: 594.
Kutt, H., Verebely, K., and McDowell, F., 1968, *Neurology* **18**: 706.
La Du, B. N., 1972, *Ann. Rev. Med.* **23**: 453.
Mitchell, R. S., Bell, J. C. and Riemensnider, D. K., 1960, *19th Conf. Chemother. Tuberc. Trans.* **19**: Veterans Admin., Washington, D.C.
Motulsky, A. G., 1964, in: *Progress in Medical Genetics* (Steinberg, A. G., and Bearn, A. G., eds.), Grune and Stratton, New York.
Motulsky, A. G., Yoshida, A., and Stamatoyannopoulos, G., 1971, *Ann. N.Y. Acad. Sci.* **179**: 636.
Perry, H. M., Jr., Sakamoto, A., and Tan, E. M., 1967, *J. Lab. Clin. Med.* **70**: 1020.
Spencer, N., Hopkinson, D. A., and Harris, H., 1964, *Nature (London)* **201**: 299.
Sunahara, S., Urano, M., and Ogawa, M., 1961, *Science* **134**: 1530.
Vesell, E. S., 1972, *New Engl. J. Med.* **287**: 904.
Weber, W. W., 1973, *Acetylation of Drugs in Metabolic Conjugation and Metabolic Hydrolysis*, Vol. III (W. H. Fishman, ed.), Academic Press, New York.

Application of Pharmacokinetic Principles to the Elucidation of Polygenically Controlled Differences in Drug Response

Elliot S. Vesell

Department of Pharmacology
Pennsylvania State University College of Medicine
Milton S. Hershey Medical Center
Hershey, Pennsylvania

The preceding chapter illustrated how pharmacokinetic measurements made in families can be employed to define the Mendelian mode of inheritance of certain primary disorders of drug response. The aberrant drug responses about which Dr. LaDu spoke are transmitted by genes at a single genetic locus; such defects are designated simple single factors. Approximately a dozen examples have been gathered of such simple factors which have as primary effects, adverse reactions to drugs (Kalow, 1962; La Du, 1972; Vesell, 1973) (Table I). Of course, many additional inborn errors of metabolism exhibit abnormal drug response as secondary effects.

Application of pharmacokinetics to the elucidation of differences in drug disposition controlled by genes at multiple loci is more difficult for many reasons. Thus, evidence for the polygenic control of drug disposition is sparse; such data are only available for bishydroxycoumarin, nortriptyline, and phenylbutazone. Even more broadly, polygenic control has been firmly established for very few traits in man. Nonetheless, we believe that genes at multiple loci play important roles in regulating such metrical, quantitative traits as stature (Burt and Howard, 1956), intelligence (Burt and Howard, 1956), blood pressure (Pickering, 1962), and large variations in the elimination rates of certain drugs (Vesell, 1972*a*). Also, multigenic effects have been hypothesized in certain congenital malformations such as

TABLE I
Twelve Pharmacogenetic Conditions with Putative Aberrant Enzyme, Mode of Inheritance, Frequency, and Drugs that Can Elicit the Signs and Symptoms of the Disorder[a]

Name of condition	Aberrant enzyme and location	Mode of inheritance	Frequency	Drugs that produce the abnormal response
Genetic Conditions Probably Transmitted as Single Factors Altering the Way the Body Acts on Drugs (Altered Drug Metabolism)				
1. Acatalasia	Catalase in erythrocytes	Autosomal recessive	Mainly in Japan and Switzerland, reaching 1% in certain small areas of Japan	Hydrogen peroxide
2. Slow inactivation of isoniazid	Isoniazid acetylase in liver	Autosomal recessive	Approximately 50% of U.S.A. population	Isoniazid, sulfamethazine, sulfamaprine, phenelzine, dapsone, hydralazine
3. Suxamethonium sensitivity or atypical pseudocholinesterase	Pseudocholinesterase in plasma	Autosomal recessive	Several aberrant alleles; most common disorder occurs 1 in 2500	Suxamethonium or succinylcholine
4. Diphenylhydantoin toxicity due to deficient parahydroxylation	? Mixed function oxidase in liver microsomes that parahydroxylates diphenylhydantoin	Autosomal or X-linked dominant	Only 1 small pedigree	Diphenylhydantoin
5. Bishydroxycoumarin sensitivity	? Mixed function oxidase in liver microsomes that hydroxylates bishydroxycoumarin	Unknown	Only 1 small pedigree	Bishydroxycoumarin
6. Acetophenetidin-induced methemoglobinemia	? Mixed function oxidase in liver microsomes that deethylates acetophenetidin	Autosomal recessive	Only 1 small pedigree	Acetophenetidin

Genetic Conditions Probably Transmitted as Single Factors Altering the Way Drugs Act on the Body

1. Warfarin resistance	? Altered receptor or enzyme in liver with increased affinity for vitamin K	Autosomal dominant	2 large pedigrees	Warfarin
2. Glucose 6-phosphate dehydrogenase deficiency, favism or drug-induced hemolytic anemia	Glucose 6-phosphate dehydrogenase	X-linked incomplete codominant	Approx. 100,000,000 affected in world; occurs in high frequency where malaria is endemic; 80 biochemically distinct mutations	A variety of analgesics [acetanilide, acetylsalicylic acid, acetophene-tidin (phenacetin), antipyrine, aminopyrine (Pyramidon)], sulfonamides and sulfones [sulfanilamide, sulfapyridine, N_2-acetylsulfanilamide, sulfacetamide sulfisoxazole (Gantrisin), thiazolsulfone, salicylazosulfa-pyridine (Azulfadine), sulfoxone, sulfamethoxypyridazine (Kynex)], antimalarials [primaquine, pamaquine, pentaquine, quinacrine (Atabrine)], non-sulfonamide antibacterial agents [furazolidone, nitro-furantoin (Furadantin), chloramphenicol, p-aminosalicylic acid], and miscellaneous drugs [naphthalene, vitamin K, probenecid, trinitrotoluene, methylene blue, dimercaprol (BAL), phenyl-hydrazine, quinine, quinidine]

TABLE I (continued)

Name of condition	Aberrant enzyme and location	Mode of inheritance	Frequency	Drugs that produce the abnormal response
3. Drug sensitive hemoglobins				
(a) Hemoglobin Zurich	Arginine substitution for histidine at the 63rd position of the β-chain of hemoglobin	Autosomal dominant	2 small pedigrees	Sulfonamides
(b) Hemoglobin H	Hemoglobin composed of 4 β-chains	Autosomal recessive	1 in 300 births in Bangkok	Same drugs as listed above for G-6-PII deficiency
4. Inability to taste phenylthiourea or phenylthiocarbamide	Unknown	Autosomal recessive	Approximately 30% of Caucasians	Drugs containing the $N-C=S$ group such as phenylthiourea, methyl and propylthiouracil
5. Glaucoma due to abnormal response of intraocular pressure to steroids	Unknown	Autosomal recessive	Approximately 5% of U.S.A. population	Corticosteroids
6. Malignant hyperthermia with muscular rigidity	Unknown	Autosomal dominant	Approximately 1 in 20,000 anesthesized patients	Such anesthetics as halothane, succinylcholine, methoxyfluorane, ether and cyclopropane

[a] From Vesell. (1972b).

cleft lip and palate, pyloric stenosis and club foot, and in certain common disorders such as peptic ulcer and diabetes mellitus (Roberts, 1964).

This mode of inheritance is referred to as polygenic or multifactorial. As opposed to inheritance patterns of traits transmitted as single factors, in polygenically controlled traits the multiple genes at several discrete loci each make a quantum contribution. Thus, the final expression in the individual of a polygenically controlled trait is the sum of the contributions from each of these multiple loci. Whereas distribution curves of response for genetic traits inherited as single factors are discontinuous, generally being either bimodal or trimodal, the distribution curves for polygenically controlled traits are continuous, as illustrated in large populations by the bell-shaped Gaussian distribution curves for intelligence quotients and blood pressure. Several hundred disease states inherited as simple single factors have been identified in man and intensively investigated (McKusick, 1971), but much less attention has been devoted to genetic analysis of such prevalent disorders as cancer, arteriosclerosis, and hypertension, which may be to some extent under polygenic control.

Although the Mendelian law of segregation of allelic genes applies to polygenically controlled traits, the genetic analysis of commonly occurring polygenically controlled disease states is technically more difficult than genetic analysis of rare conditions transmitted as simple single factors. This is because in simple single factor inheritance, rare abnormal genes segregate according to Mendelian laws in successive generations in an easily recognizable manner without the complication of the introduction through marriage of similar abnormal genes. Another reason for the absence of extensive genetic analysis of polygenically transmitted disorders is that polygenic control may be expressed only through complex interactions with etiological factors of an entirely environmental nature.

In applying pharmacokinetics to the elucidation of polygenic factors involved in drug disposition, there should be posed three related questions: (1) How extensive is the variation among individuals in rate of plasma clearance of commonly used drugs?; (2) If appreciable variation occurs, what are the relative contributions of genetic and environmental factors to its maintenance?; (3) What role is played by polygenic factors in maintaining this variation?

The magnitude of variations among individuals in the plasma decay of frequently used drugs was discovered in the early 1950's in the laboratory of Bernard B. Brodie. Figure 1 shows the decay rates of phenylbutazone in plasma of six unrelated cirrhotic patients after they received a single intramuscular dose of phenylbutazone (Burns et al., 1953). Figure 2 shows the variation in plasma decay of the anticoagulant ethyl biscoumacetate in eight unrelated normal individuals after a single intravenous dose of this

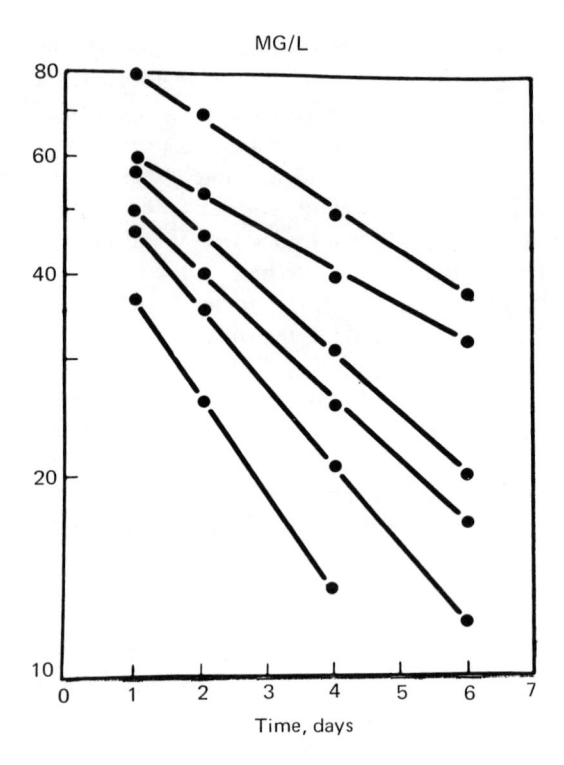

Fig. 1. Decay of phenylbutazone in the plasma of six cirrhotic subjects after a single intramuscular dose of 800 mg. (Reproduced by permission from Burns *et al.*, 1953).

drug (Brodie *et al.*, 1952). The range in plasma half-life among the 12 cirrhotic individuals receiving phenylbutazone in this study was more than threefold; and among the 35 normal subjects after ethyl bicoumacetate the range in half-life was more than twelvefold. Variations among normal individuals in rates of decay of such commonly used drugs as diphenylhydantoin (Kutt *et al.*, 1964), nortriptyline (Alexanderson *et al.*, 1969), procainamide (Koch Weser, 1971), and propranolol (Shand *et al.*, 1970), are as large, and in some cases, larger than the variations observed for phenylbutazone and ethyl biscoumacetate. After an initial period of equilibration, the pharmacokinetics of most of these drugs are characterized by first-order decay curves from which plasma half-lives can be calculated. If a very large dose of drug is given, the drug-metabolizing system becomes saturated and consequently the plasma decay curve is not exponential. Saturation of the enzymatic mechanism for biotransformation of diphenyl-

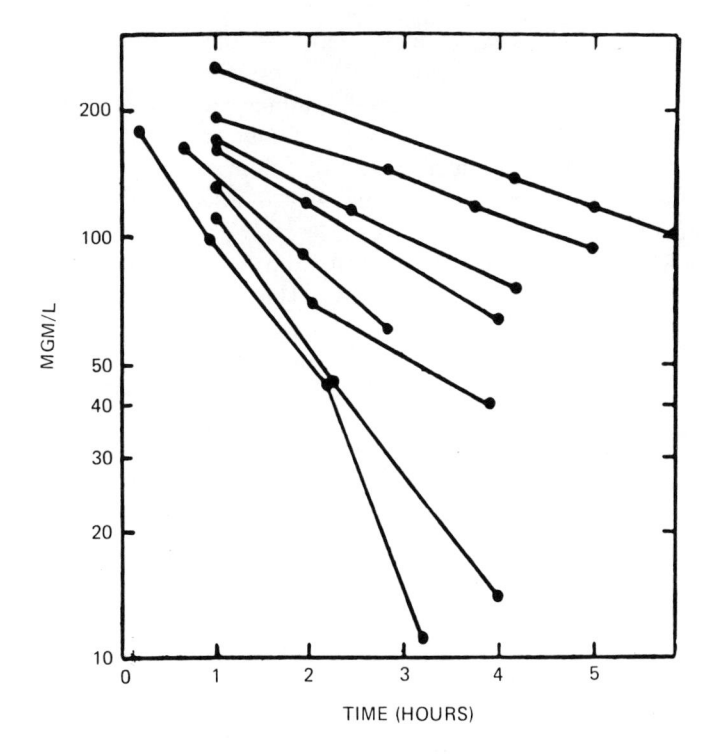

Fig. 2. Decay of ethyl biscoumacetate in the plasma of eight normal volunteers after a single intravenous dose of 20 mg/kg. (Reproduced by permission from Brodie et al., 1952).

hydantoin has recently been offered by Gerber and Wagner (1972) as an explanation for failure to observe an exponential decay of this drug at high concentrations in human plasma (Arnold and Gerber, 1970).

Since variations among normal, unrelated, nonmedicated individuals in rates of drug decay are frequently of a tenfold or greater range, the answer to the first question is that very large differences exist among unrelated, nonmedicated, normal individuals in the disposition of commonly used drugs. This fact is generally appreciated by most pharmacologists and physicians. However, the application of pharmacokinetics to define the relative contributions of genetic and environmental factors to these interindividual differences appears to pose more complex problems. Pharmacologists are familiar with numerous environmental factors, such as exposure to inducing agents, degree of health or illness, and hormonal and nutritional status, known to alter the rates at which humans metabolize certain drugs.

Several drugs such as phenylbutazone enhance their own metabolism (Conney, 1967). In mice, responsiveness to a drug such as hexobarbital differs according to age, sex, litter, painful stimuli, ambient temperature, degree of crowding, time of day of drug administration, and type of bedding (Vesell, 1968). These data suggest that in man a large component in the causation of variations among individuals in drug metabolism would be environmental.

Study of human twins permits separation of the control of a trait into hereditary and environmental components. This method, introduced in

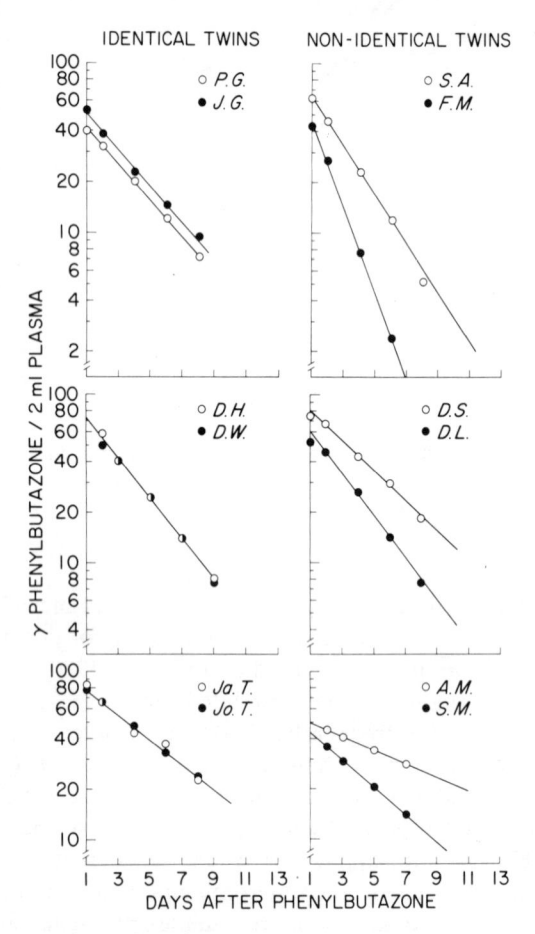

Fig. 3. Decline of phenylbutazone in the plasma of three sets of identical twins (left) and three sets of fraternal twins (right) after a single oral dose of 6 mg/kg. (Reproduced by permission from Vesell and Page, 1968a).

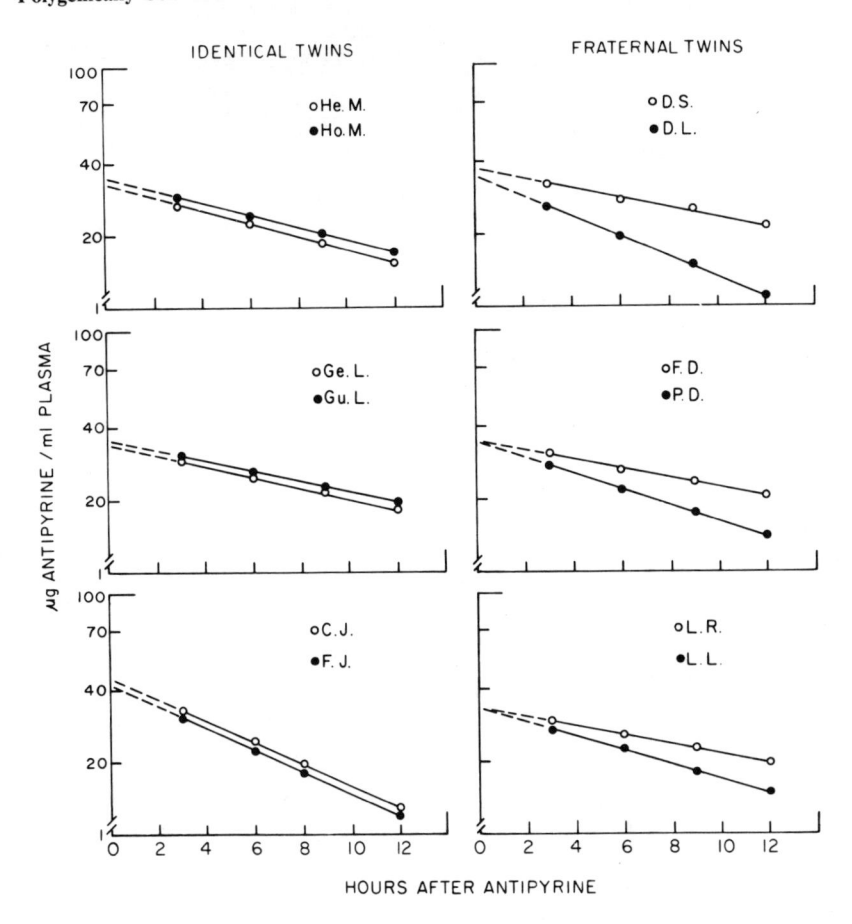

Fig. 4. Decline of antipyrine in the plasma of three sets of identical twins (left) and of three sets of fraternal twins (right) after a single oral dose of 18 mg/kg. (Reproduced by permission from Vesell and Page, 1968b).

1875 by Francis Galton, has the advantage of comparing age and sex-matched individuals and depends on the fact that identical twins have identical genomes, whereas fraternal twins share on the average, only half of their genes. The major assumption implicit in all twin studies is that identical and fraternal twins exist within similar environments. This assumption has been challenged on the grounds that even adult identical twins living in different households tend to create more similar environments for themselves than do fraternal twins under these circumstances. We employed the twin method to identify the relative contribution of genetic and environmental factors to large interindividual differences in rates of

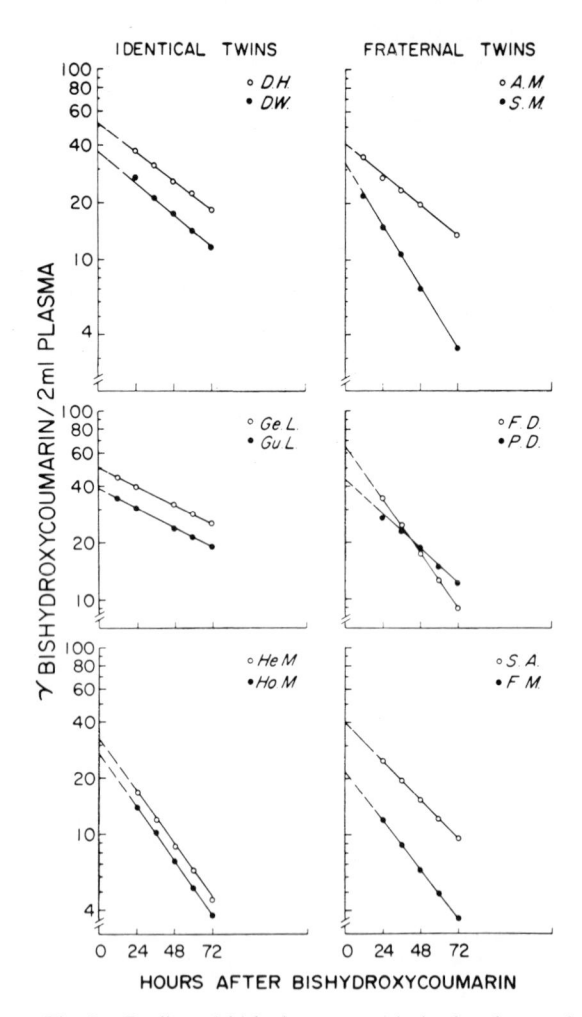

Fig. 5. Decline of bishydroxycoumarin in the plasma of three sets of identical twins (left) and of three sets of fraternal twins (right) after a single oral dose of 4 mg/kg. (Reproduced by permission from Vesell and Page, 1968c).

decay of commonly used drugs. These twins were healthy, adult, nonmedicated twins living in the Washington, D.C. area. Figures 3, 4, and 5 show the decay curves for phenylbutazone (Vesell and Page, 1968a), antipyrine (Vesell and Page, 1968b), and bishydroxycoumarin (Vesell and Page, 1968c), respectively, in three sets of identical and in three sets of fraternal twins. For these drugs, as well as for ethanol (Vesell et al., 1971), halothane

(Cascorbi et al., 1971), and nortriptyline (Alexanderson et al., 1969), large interindividual differences in half-life tend to vanish within a set of identical twins, but tend to be preserved within a set of fraternal twins. Table II shows the collection of data for three drugs investigated in seven sets of identical and seven sets of fraternal twins.

TABLE II
Bishydroxycoumarin, Antipyrine, and Phenylbutazone Half-Lives with Smoking and Coffee History in 28 Twins[a]

Twin	Age, sex	Bishydroxy-coumarin	Antipyrine	Phenyl-butazone	Smoking, packs/day	Coffee, cups/day
Identical Twins						
Ho.M	48, M	25.0 hr	11.3 hr	1.9 days	0.5	2
Ho.M.	48, M	25.0	11.3	2.1	1	3
D.T.	43, F	55.5	10.3	2.8	0	5–6
V.W.	43, F	55.5	9.6	2.9	2	8–10
J.G.	22, M	36.0	11.5	2.8	1	1–2
P.G.	22, M	34.0	11.5	2.8	1	1–2
Ja.T.	44, M	74.0	14.9	4.0	0	6
Ja.T.	44, M	72.0	14.9	4.0	0	2–3
C.J.	55, F	41.0	6.9	3.2	0	2
F.J.	55, F	42.5	7.1	2.9	0	2
Ge.L.	45, M	72.0	12.3	3.9	0	4
Gu.L.	45, M	69.0	12.8	4.1	0	4
D.H.	26, F	46.0	11.0	2.6	0	0–1
D.W.	26, F	44.0	11.0	2.6	0	3–4
Fraternal Twins						
A.M.	21, F	45.0	15.1	7.3	1.5	2
S.M.	21, M	22.0	6.3	3.6	0	0
D.L.	36, F	46.5	7.2	2.3	0	2–3
D.S.	36, F	51.0	15.0	3.3	2	3–4
S.A.	33, F	34.5	5.1	2.1	1	2
F.M.	33, F	27.5	12.5	1.2	0.5	2
Ja.H.	24, F	7.0	12.0	2.6	0	10–15
Je.H.	24, F	19.0	6.0	2.3	1.5	10
F.D.	48, M	24.5	14.7	2.8	0	1
P.D.	48, M	38.0	9.3	3.5	1.5	8
L.D.	21, F	67.0	8.2	2.9	1	6
L.W.	21, F	72.0	6.9	3.0	1	2–3
E.K	31, F	40.5	7.7	1.9	0	0
R.K.	31, M	35.0	7.3	2.1	1	0

[a] The difference between identical and fraternal twins in intrapair variance is significant: $P < 0.005$ ($F = 36.0$, $N_1 = N_2 = 7$). From Vesell and Page (1968c).

A rough estimate of the relative contributions of environmental and genetic factors to the control of a trait can be made by estimating the mean variance within the sets of identical and fraternal twins, according to the following formula for heritability H (Neel and Schull, 1954; Osborne and DeGeorge, 1959):

$$H = \frac{V_F - V_I}{V_F}$$

where V_F is the variance within pairs of fraternal twins and V_I is the variance within pairs of identical twins. This formula yields values from 0 (indicating negligible hereditary and complete environmental control) to 1 (indicating virtually complete hereditary influence). For phenylbutazone, antipyrine, bishydroxycoumarin, and ethanol, values for the contribution of heredity were 0.99, 0.98, 0.97, and 0.99, respectively. Our studies on twins yielded intraclass correlation coefficients close to theoretical expectation solely on the basis of genetic control, according to which fraternal twins, having in common approximately half of their total number of genes, should have a value of 0.5, whereas identical twins should have a value of 1. For rates of metabolism of phenylbutazone, antipyrine, bishydroxycoumarin, and ethanol the intraclass correlation coefficients of identical twins were 0.83, 0.85, 0.85, and 0.82, respectively; and for fraternal twins, 0.33, 0.47, 0.66, and 0.38, respectively. Evidently for these drugs, large interindividual differences in rates of elimination from plasma in nonmedicated, normal subjects are surprisingly free of environmental influence. As shown by repeated half-life determinations, nonmedicated, normal subjects have a remarkably reproducible plasma half-life for these drugs. Since phenylbutazone (Burns *et al.*, 1953) and bishydroxycoumarin (Weiner *et al.*, 1950) are 98% bound to plasma proteins, differences among individuals in plasma elimination rates of these drugs might possibly involve binding of the drugs to albumin. However, antipyrine and ethanol are not appreciably bound to plasma proteins (Soberman *et al.*, 1949). Therefore, it seems reasonable to conclude that for antipyrine and ethanol, if not also for phenylbutazone and bishydroxycoumarin, variations in plasma half-life arise from genetic differences in metabolism rather than in distribution. Appreciable interindividual variations do exist in rates of metabolism of these drugs, as indicated by ranges for the plasma half-lives of ethanol, antipyrine, phenylbutazone, and bishydroxycoumarin of twofold, threefold, sixfold, and tenfold, respectively, among the 28 individuals in our study (Table II).

Since the answer to the second question posed at the start is that large variations among normal individuals in plasma decay of commonly used drugs appear to be controlled predominantly by genetic rather than by environmental factors, the third question concerning the mode of inherit-

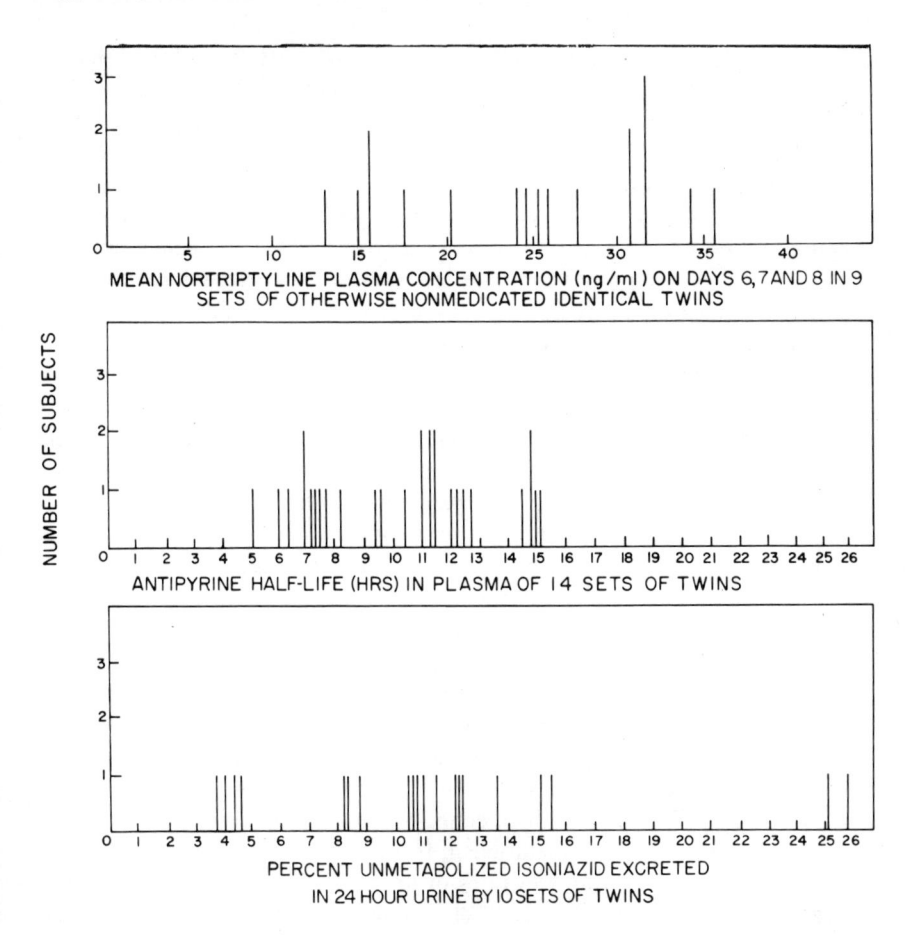

Fig. 6. Plots of the distribution of three different parameters of drug elimination in three different twin studies on isoniazid, antipyrine and nortriptyline.

ance of these genetic factors with particular reference to polygenic effects must now be approached. It is not generally appreciated, even among geneticists, that twin studies can provide important clues toward the elucidation of the mode of inheritance of pharmacogenetic variation. Figure 6 shows a discontinuous distribution curve strongly suggesting single factor inheritance of variations among ten sets of twins in response to isoniazid (Bönicke and Lisboa, 1957). On the other hand, twin studies with other drugs reveal a unimodal distribution of antipyrine half-lives (Vesell and Page, 1968b) and of nortriptyline steady-state blood levels (Alexanderson et al., 1969) consistent with polygenic control of these variations (Fig.

6). A distribution curve based on these twin studies clearly helps to distinguish among the different modes of inheritance of genetically controlled variations in response to drugs.

Twin studies can be a particularly valuable initial step in identifying the relative genetic and environmental contributions to a new trait. As a second step, once an appreciable genetic component is established, the construction of a distribution curve of these twins can provide a useful hint as to whether such variations are transmitted polygenically or as simple single factors. For a rare autosomal recessive trait, a unimodal curve might result if too few individuals are tested, leading to an erroneous interpretation of polygenic control. Twin studies alone cannot conclusively establish the mode of inheritance of a pharmacogenetic entity, but through distribution curves of drug response, twin data can be utilized more than they have been previously. As the third step in the genetic delineation of a new trait, family studies should then be performed selecting individuals at the extremes of this twin distribution curve. At these extremes of the distribution curve pedigrees would be most likely to prove genetically informative.

In the evaluation of variations in drug metabolism, twin studies enjoy several distinct advantages over family studies and have been utilized on rare occasions as subjects for investigations of the genetic component of interindividual variations in drug metabolism (Bönicke and Lisboa, 1957; Kappas and Gallagher, 1960). Twins are by definition age corrected and dizygotic twins can easily be selected from the same sex. As studies in rodents have shown and as studies in man have suggested (O'Malley et al., 1971), rates of drug metabolism change with age and sex. Thus, the genetic analysis of data on drug metabolism from family studies is complicated by incorporation of variations in rates of drug metabolism from differences in age and sex, two factors readily eliminated in twin studies. Furthermore, differences in the environment of children, parents, and grandparents with respect to exposure to certain environmental compounds capable of inducing or inhibiting the hepatic microsomal drug-metabolizing enzymes must be considered as a source of possible variation in family studies. Such environmental influences on drug metabolism arising from common exposure in the same household to inducers or inhibitors of drug-metabolizing enzymes could explain why in one family study (Whittaker and Price Evans, 1970) there was a correlation in phenylbutazone metabolism between husbands and wives before phenobarbital administration.

Nevertheless, the family studies performed using pharmacokinetic measurements tend to support the results of the twin studies in showing predominantly genetic control over large interindividual variations in plasma half-lives of bishydroxycoumarin (Motulsky, 1964) and phenylbutazone (Whittaker and Price Evans, 1970). Furthermore, the results of both these studies suggested polygenic control. Whittaker and Price Evans (1970) obtained a normal distribution of phenylbutazone half-lives in plasma after correcting for height and also after administering a three-day course of phenobarbital to "render the environment more uniform." A significant regression of mean offspring value on midparent value indicated to Whittaker and Price Evans that approximately 65% of the observed phenotypic variance was caused by the additive effects of genes. These results agree closely with those from our earlier study on phenylbutazone metabolism in twins (Vesell and Page, 1968a) if V_D (variance due to the effect of dominant genes) is not neglected in the following formula derived from Falconer (1960):

$$H = \frac{\frac{1}{2}V_A + \frac{3}{4}V_D}{\frac{1}{2}V_A + \frac{3}{4}V_D + V_{Ew}} = \frac{V_F - V_I}{V_F}$$

Whittaker and Price Evans (1970) state that V_D is too small to be significant, although they believe that V_{Ec} is probably large. ($V_E = V_{Ew} + V_{Ec}$ where V_{Ew} and V_{Ec} are the within-twin-pair variance and the common variance between twin pairs, respectively.) Neither V_D nor V_{Ec} were measured in their family study. However, in other studies of polygenically controlled traits in man, V_D has been measured and is not negligible. For example, in their classic study of height and intelligence, Burt and Howard (1956) reported a value of 0.16 and 0.17 for the contributions of V_D to height and intelligence, respectively. If their value of 0.16 for V_D is utilized as an estimate of V_D in calculating the family data of Whittaker and Price Evans, which seems more reasonable than to disregard V_D completely, there is good agreement between the results of the family study of Whittaker and Price Evans ($H = 0.88$) and our twin data on phenylbutazone ($H = 0.75$ or 1.00) (Table III). Since these values are close to the estimate (0.99) based on the formula for heritability that we employ $[H = (V_F - V_I)/V_F]$, differential environmental factors operating between twinships in our investigation appear to be quite small. In another recent study, Åsberg et al. (1971)

TABLE III

Heritability of Variations in Drug Metabolism of Twins Utilizing Different Methods of Data Analysis[a]

	Antipyrine	Phenyl-butazone	Bishydroxy-coumarin	Ethanol	Halothane
$(V_F - V_I)/V_F$	0.98	0.99	0.97	0.98	0.88
r_I	0.85	0.83	0.85	0.82	0.52
r_F	0.47	0.33	0.66	0.38	0.36
$(r_I - r_F)/(1 - r_F)$	0.72	0.75	0.56	0.71	0.25
$2(r_I - r_F)$	0.76	1.00	0.38	0.88	0.32

[a] r = intraclass correlation coefficient. From Vesell (1972a).

investigated two extensive Swedish pedigrees with high steady-state plasma concentrations of nortriptyline; appreciable interindividual differences in the steady-state plasma concentrations of this drug were compatible with a polygenic mode of inheritance. Thus far both the family studies and the twin data have agreed in their conclusions that large differences among healthy, nonmedicated volunteers in rates of drug metabolism are primarily controlled by genetic factors which appear to be polygenic in character. More such studies should be performed to determine how many other drugs resemble bishydroxycoumarin, phenylbutazone, and nortriptyline in exhibiting polygenic control over large variations in rates of elimination and, by contrast, how many drugs are controlled through operation of simple single factors which have been established for the conditions listed in Table I.

Predominantly genetic control of large interindividual variations in phenylbutazone, antipyrine, and bishydroxycoumarin plasma half-lives (Vesell and Page, 1968a, b, and c), indicates that pharmacokinetic parameters closely related to plasma half-life such as apparent volume of distribution, steady-state blood concentration, and drug elimination rate would also be under genetic control. This was later demonstrated to be the case for steady-state blood concentration and apparent volume of distribution of nortriptyline (Alexanderson et al., 1969).

The field of pharmacogenetics is in an early stage of development. Rapid progress is anticipated by the application of pharmacokinetics in systematic studies of drug absorption, distribution, biotransformation, interaction with receptor sites, and excretion. In attempting to estimate rates of drug biotransformation by measuring plasma decay curves, it is important to make sure that the methods employed assay parent drugs rather than metabolites, that the parent drugs are not excreted unchanged in the urine or other biological fluids, that absorption of the drug from its site of administration is complete and does not constitute a rate-limiting process and that tissue binding or sequestration of the drug does not play a significant role in its rate of disappearance from plasma. Stated in more pharmacokinetic terminology, "the parameter which should be taken to represent metabolism rate is the half-life ($t_{1/2} = 0.693/K$) for the metabolism process being studied"; "it is not sufficient to determine the overall rate of drug elimination since variation in the rate of processes in competition with the process of interest may mask or distort variation in rate of the latter" (Nelson, 1963; 1965).

CLINICAL APPLICATIONS

Several practical consequences of these studies merit discussion, although their full clinical exploitation lies far in the future. Firstly, genetic control of large interindividual variations in the plasma decay of commonly used drugs implies reproducibility of the plasma half-lives in healthy, nonmedicated subjects; such reproducibility has been demonstrated for antipyrine, bishydroxycoumarin, nortriptyline, and phenylbutazone. Since the plasma half-life of many commonly used drugs is a genetically controlled, highly reproducible value in nonmedicated normal subjects, these values could be utilized as a basis for drug administration in an individual requiring medication. Large variations among normal people in rates of drug decay indicate that the same dose of a drug should not be administered to all subjects. When the same dose of drug is given, some people will exhibit an ineffective blood concentration of the compound, others will be in the therapeutic range, and still others will be in the toxic range and display adverse reactions.

Secondly, predominantly genetic control over the biotransformation of these drugs offers the opportunity to discover whether within an individual correlations exist in the rates at which chemically unrelated drugs are cleared from plasma. Several studies of this nature have been performed (Vesell and Page, 1968c; Hammer et al., 1969; Davies and Thorgeirsson, 1971), and the results suggest that within an individual rates of clearance of several chemically dissimilar drugs are correlated. These observations raise the possibility that categories of drugs could be constructed such that once the rate of clearance of one member of the category was determined in a patient, the relative rates of clearance of the others could also be ascertained.

These applications are based on determination of the plasma concentrations of various drugs; under certain clinical circumstances such procedures could constitute logistic problems, rendering them impractical when rapid decisions on dosage are required. For this reason, simplified methodologies are currently being sought to classify patients as rapid, intermediate, or slow drug metabolizers. Measurements of rates of urinary excretion of metabolites of salicylates or antipyrine, and determinations of urinary glucaric acid or ratios of cortisol to 6-β-hydroxycortisol have been proposed. At the present time, an individual's capacity to metabolize drugs and the effect of various conditions in altering that basal, genetically determined capacity seem to be best indicated by measurements of the plasma antipyrine half-life. Eventually, measurement of drug-metabolizing enzymes in circulating leukocytes might prove feasible, but such approaches are only in a very preliminary stage of investigation.

This discussion, as well as several others during the course of the conference, has come to focus on the measurement of drug concentrations in various biological fluids as a guide to the more rational administration of therapeutic agents. While most clinical pharmacologists recognize the theoretical advantages of obtaining blood concentrations of drugs as a guide to their more rational administration, several problems have been raised, some of which merit enumeration:

1. Patients take many medications, often at different intervals, making decisions concerning the timing of drug concentration determinations difficult.
2. At home, and even in the hospital, patients can either fail to take prescribed medication or, unsuspected by the physician, they can receive additional drugs capable of exerting profound pharmacokinetic effects on the prescribed agents.
3. Some drugs cannot be assayed conveniently in biological fluids. Furthermore, many assays cannot distinguish between the pharmacologically inert, protein-bound form of the drug and the pharmacologically active free form of the drug.
4. Some drugs reach high tissue concentrations although present in low or undetectable concentrations in biological fluids.
5. For many compounds, sufficient experimental work has not been performed to establish quantitatively clear ranges between ineffective, therapeutic, and toxic drug concentrations in biological fluids.
6. For other drugs there may be appreciable overlap between these three clinically significant regions so that a given blood concentration might be ineffective, therapeutic, or toxic depending on the individual patient.
7. In some patients rapidly changing cardiovascular, renal, and hepatic status might fluctuate so dramatically that meaningful drug concentrations would be difficult to obtain or, even if obtainable, more perplexing than edifying to the physician. Furthermore, it has been too readily assumed that in a variety of disease states receptor sites react with drugs in the same manner as they do under normal physiologic circumstances. Changes in the kinetics of interaction between receptor sites and drugs as a consequence of disease could drastically alter the clinical significance of a given drug blood concentration.
8. Some "hit and run" drugs such as reserpine exert their pharmacological actions long after their plasma concentrations have receded to low levels so that plasma concentrations of these agents could not be a useful guide to their administration.
9. Certain anticoagulants and antihypertensives exert physiologic or biochemical effects on easily measured parameters (prothrombin time and blood pressure, respectively), thereby obviating the necessity of measuring their concentrations in biological fluids.
10. Drugs such as salicylates and certain antibiotics have high therapeutic indices permitting the physician a very wide latitude in

dosage; large amounts of these agents can be administered without fear of toxicity. Therefore, no advantage accrues to the patient from precise quantitative data on the concentrations of these drugs in his biological fluids.

Despite the existence of these strictures on the utility of measurements of drug concentrations in biological fluids, such determinations are gaining an increasingly important role in clinical medicine. The question concerns what agents should be closely monitored in the biological fluids of patients. In general, the ideal compound for such an approach is one possessing a low therapeutic index but with clearly separable ineffective, therapeutic and toxic regions of drug concentration in biological fluids. The agent should be potent, act reversibly at receptor sites, and exhibit large interindividual variations in metabolism so that the same dose could conceivably yield ineffective, therapeutic and toxic blood concentrations in different subjects. Recently, Koch-Weser (1972) has suggested that for digitoxin, digoxin, diphenylhydantoin, lidocaine, lithium, nortriptyline, procainamide, propranolol, quinidine, and salicylates, whose therapeutic serum concentrations he lists, determinations of blood concentration yield significant information helpful to the physician in the management of certain patients. This list and the indications for measuring drug concentrations in biological fluids probably will be expanded in the future, as research in this area of clinical pharmacology is extended. It should be stressed that, like all other clinical chemical determinations, drug concentrations are maximally useful when they are placed in the broad clinical context of a particular patient's problem; taken out of this context, such measurements may prove of limited value or even misleading.

REFERENCES

Alexanderson, B., Price Evans, D. A., and Sjöqvist, F., 1969, *Brit. Med. J.* **4:** 764.
Arnold, K. and Gerber, N., 1970, *Clin. Pharmacol. Therap.* **11:** 121.
Åsberg, M., Price Evans, D. A., and Sjöqvist, F., 1971, *J. Med. Genetics* **8:** 129.
Bönicke, R., and Lisboa, B. P., 1957, *Naturwiss.* **44:** 314.
Brodie, B. B., Weiner, M., Burns, J. J., Simson, G., and Yale, E. K., 1952, *J. Pharmacol. Exp. Therap.* **106:** 453.
Burns, J. J., Rose, R. K., Chenkin, T., Goldman, A., Schulert, A., and Brodie, B. B., 1953, *J. Pharmacol. Exp. Therap.* **109:** 346.
Burt, C., and Howard, M., 1956, *Brit. J. Statistical Psychol.* **8/2:** 95.
Cascorbi, H. F., Vesell, E. S., Blake, D. A., and Hebrich, M., 1971, *Clin. Pharmacol. Therap.* **12:** 50.
Conney, A. H., 1967, *Pharmacol. Rev.* **19:** 317.
Davies, D. S., and Thorgeirsson, S. S., 1971, *Ann. N.Y. Acad. Sci.* **179:** 411.
Falconer, D. S., 1960, in: *Introduction to Quantitative Genetics.* Ronald Press, New York.
Galton, F., 1875, *J. Brit. Anthropol. Inst.* **5:** 391.
Gerber, N., and Wagner, J. G., 1972, *Res. Comm. Chem. Pathol. and Pharmacol.* **3:** 455.

Hammer, W., Mårtens, S., and Sjöqvist, F., 1969, *Clin. Pharmacol. Therap.* **10**: 44.
Kalow, W., 1962, in: *Pharmacogenetics: Heredity and the Response to Drugs*. Saunders, Philadelphia.
Kappas, A., and Gallagher, T. F., 1960, *J. Clin. Invest.* **39**: 620.
Koch-Weser, J., 1971, *Ann. N.Y. Acad. Sci.* **179**: 370.
Koch-Weser, J., 1972, *New Engl. J. Med.* **287**: 227.
Kutt, H., Wolk, M., Scherman, R., McDowell, F., 1964, *Neurology* **14**: 542.
La Du, B. N., 1972, *Ann. Rev. Med.* **23**: 453.
McKusick, V. A., 1971, in: *Mendelian Inheritance in Man, Catalogs of Autosomal Dominant, Autosomal Recessive and X-Linked Phenotypes*. The Johns Hopkins Press, Baltimore.
Motulsky, A., 1964, *Progr. Med. Genet.* **3**: 49.
Neel, J. V., and Schull, W. J., 1954, in: *Human Heredity*. University of Chicago Press, Chicago.
Nelson, E., 1963, *J. Theoret. Biol.* **5**: 493.
Nelson, E., 1965, *Life Sci.* **4**: 949.
O'Malley, K., Crooks, J., Duke, E., Stevenson, I. H., 1971, *Brit. Med. J.* **3**: 607.
Osborne, R. H., and DeGeorge, F. V., 1959, in: *Genetic Basis of Morphological Variation, An Evaluation and Application of the Twin Study Method*. Harvard University Press, Cambridge.
Pickering, G., 1962, *Lancet* **II**: 1402.
Roberts, J. A. F., 1964, *Progr. Med. Genet.* **3**: 178.
Shand, D. G., Nuckolls, E. M., and Oates, J. A., 1970, *Clin. Pharmacol. Therap.* **11**: 112.
Soberman, R., Brodie, B. B., Levy, B. B., Axelrod, J., Hollander, V., and Steele, J. M., 1949, *J. Biol. Chem.* **179**: 31.
Vesell, E. S., 1968, *Pharmacology* **1**: 81.
Vesell, E. S., 1972a, *Federation Proc.* **31**: 1253.
Vesell, E. S., 1972b, *New Engl. J. Med.* **287**: 904.
Vesell, E. S., 1973, in: *Progress in Medical Genetics* (Steinberg, A. G., and Bearn, A. G., eds.) Grune and Stratton, New York.
Vesell, E. S., and Page, J. G., 1968a, *Science* **159**: 1479.
Vesell, E. S., and Page, J. G., 1968b, *Science* **161**: 72.
Vesell, E. S., and Page, J. G., 1968c, *J. Clin. Invest.* **47**: 2657.
Vesell, E. S., Page, J. G., and Passananti, G.T., 1971, *Clin. Pharmacol. Therap.* **12**: 192.
Weiner, M., Shapiro, S., Axelrod, J., Cooper, J. R., Brodie, B. B., 1950, *J. Pharm. Exp. Therap.* **99**: 409.
Whittaker, J. A. and Price Evans, D. A., 1970, *Brit. Med. J.* **4**: 323.

DISCUSSION SUMMARY

Riegelman cautioned about the use of histogram plots of drug half-life against frequency, which often result in a skewed distribution. The appropriate correlation with frequency is not drug half-life in plasma but the overall rate constant of drug elimination. The skewed distribution published by Whittaker and Price Evans for phenylbutazone can be largely removed if, instead of phenylbutazone plasma half-life, the overall rate constants of phenylbutazone are calculated and then plotted against the number of subjects.

Immediate Immunologic Reactions: Noncytolytic Mediator Release and Cytolytic Cell Destruction*

Edward J. Goetzl,[†] Shaun Ruddy,[‡] Daniel J. Stechschulte,[§] and K. Frank Austen

*Department of Medicine, Harvard Medical School
and
Robert B. Brigham Hospital
Boston, Massachusetts*

Two of the principal mechanisms by which immunologic reactions generate chemical mediators of the inflammatory response differ both in their mode of interaction with target cell membranes and in their ultimate effect on these membranes. In the *cytolytic* reaction [Fig. 1(A)] antibodies of certain immunoglobulin classes (IgM or IgG) bind to the target cell via combining sites specific for antigens which are either intrinsic to the cell membrane or have become passively bound to it. A resultant configurational change in the Fc portion of the antibody (Ashman and Metzger, 1971) is associated with the initiation of a sequence of reactions among certain serum proteins, the components of complement,* contained in the surrounding *milieu*. The

---

*Supported by grants AI-07722, AI-10356, and RR-05669 from the National Institutes of Health

[†] Investigator, Howard Hughes Medical Institute

[‡] Recipient of Research Career Development Award AM-70233 from the National Institutes of Health

[§] Former recipient of Research Career Development Award AI-28405 from the National Institutes of Health

*By international agreement (Austen *et al.*, 1968) the components of complement are symbolized by a letter "C" and an arabic number. They react with an erythrocyte (E) coated with antibody (A) in the sequence Cl, C4, C2, C3, C5, C6, C7, C8, and C9. Fragments of components produced during the reaction are suffixed with letters (e.g., C3a, C3b) and the activated form of a component is symbolized by a bar over the number (e.g., $\overline{Cl}$).

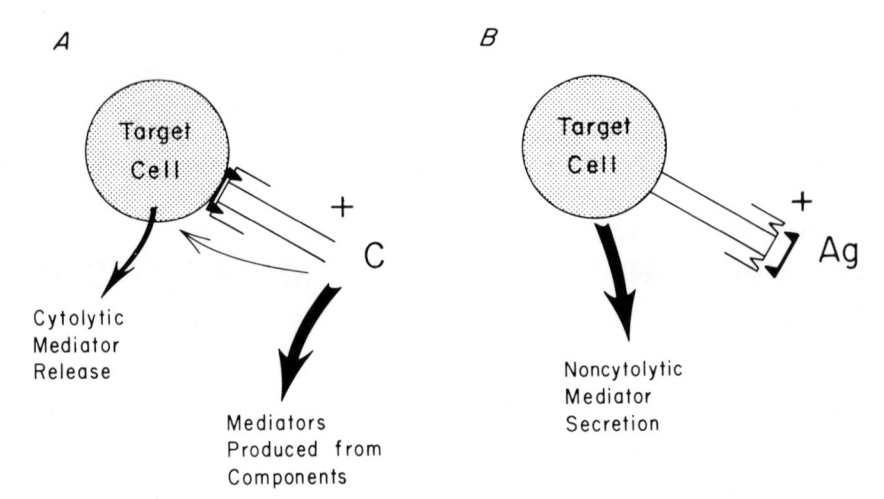

Fig. 1. Release of chemical mediators by cytolytic and noncytolytic immunologic reactions. (A.) The cytolytic reaction is dependent on the complement system (C) which is activated by antibody combining with a cell surface antigen. (B.) The noncytolytic reaction is initiated by antigen (Ag) combining with antibody fixed to a unique cell surface receptor.

physicochemical characteristics and mechanism of interaction of the nine components have recently been reviewed (Muller-Eberhard, 1968; Ruddy, et al., 1972). Chemical mediators of inflammation are generated during the complement reaction sequence *per se*, by the limited proteolysis of the components. These mediators represent both major (e.g., C3b, an enhancer of opsonization) and minor (e.g., C3a, an anaphylatoxin) fragments of component cleavage as well as complexes (e.g., $\overline{C567}$, a chemotactic principle) formed by the interaction of products from different components. If completion of the reaction sequence occurs on a cell membrane, *cytolytic* destruction of the cell results which in some instances, may eventuate in mediator release. In the *cytotropic* reaction (Becker and Austen, 1966), antibody molecules of certain immunoglobulin classes (IgE or IgG) bind via their Fc portions to unique receptors on the membrane of the target cell. The release of mediators from the cell is initiated by the union of antigen with its specific combining site on the antibody, leading to a form of immunologically-induced secretion. It is apparent, then, that although the antigen specificity of different classes of immunoglobulins may be the same, the consequences of their encounter with that antigen may be entirely different because of their different biologic specificity.

COMPLEMENT-INDUCED CYTOLYSIS: THE ONE-HIT MODEL

In immune hemolysis, the system from which most of the information about kinetics of complement-induced membrane damage has been derived, the target cell sheep erythrocyte (E) is coated with rabbit antibody (A), reacted with fresh serum as a source of complement (C), and the extent of hemolysis determined from measurements of hemoglobin released into the supernatant fluid. When the proportion of cells lysed is plotted against the dilution of serum, the result is a typical sigmoidal dose–response, resembling the cumulative normal distribution. Early theories to explain this dose–response either postulated a requirement for cumulative damage on the surface of a single erythrocyte to eventuate in lysis, or focused on the heterogeneity of the erythrocytes in their susceptibility to lysis. The demonstration that the absolute number of erythrocytes lysed by a given amount of complement was independent of the total cell concentration suggested a one-hit reaction mechanism (Mayer, 1961). Subsequent studies have suggested that instability of certain of the erythrocyte-component complexes generated during the reaction sequence accounts for the sigmoidal shape of the dose response for whole complement. Experiments with purified components have demonstrated that the reaction of the cell with any individual component is a one-hit phenomenon.

Since a fruitful interaction with a complement component represents a discrete event occurring randomly in the continuum of membrane surfaces, the Poisson distribution can be used to estimate the true mean number of such interactions per cell surface from the observed amount of lysis (Rapp and Borsos, 1970). In its general form, the distribution gives the probability (P) of observing r events per unit area as

$$P(r) = \frac{Z^r}{r!} e^{-Z} \qquad (1)$$

where Z is the true mean number of events occurring per unit area and e is the natural logarithm base. In the specific case of the cell which survives a hemolytic reaction, i.e., has *no* hits occurring on its surface, $r = 0$, and the equation simplifies

$$P(0) = e^{-Z} \qquad (2)$$

Since, in a reaction in which the proportion of cells lysed is y, the probability of survival of any given erythrocyte is $(1 - y)$, then

$$(1 - y) = e^{-Z} \qquad (3)$$

Taking the logarithm of both sides and rearranging, one solves the equation for Z:

$$Z = -\ln(1 - y) \qquad (4)$$

and a formula for computing the average number of damaged sites (Z)

occurring per erythrocyte from the observed proportion of cells lysed in the reaction mixture (y) is obtained.

An example of how the one-hit model works in practice is given by the effective molecule titration of the ninth component of complement (C9) (Ruddy et al., 1971). The target cell is the erythrocyte coated with antibody and reacted with the first eight complement components (EACl-8). The reaction is as follows:

$$EAC1\text{-}8 + C9 \rightarrow EAC1\text{-}9$$

Conditions are adjusted so that the rate and extent of the reaction are dependent only on the concentration of C9. The kinetics of generation of EACl-9 are shown in Fig. 2. In this experiment EACl-8 at a concentration of 1×10^8/ml were incubated with limited C9 in isotonic Veronal buffered saline at 37°C. At the indicated times, samples were removed, immediately centrifuged, and the proportion of cells already lysed was determined from measurements of hemoglobin in the supernatant. To determine the proportion of cells destined to lyse because of being in the state EACl-9 at the time of the sampling, the cell button was resuspended in buffer and incubated for an additional 180 min at 37°C. From Fig. 2 it is apparent that, although the generation of EACl-9 begins immediately and is maximal within 30 min, the manifestation of membrane damage, i.e., lysis, requires a considerably longer period of time. For this reason, in the effective molecule titration of C9, in which the proportion of cells in the state EACl-9 is inferred from the proportion of lysed cells, an incubation time of 180 min is required.

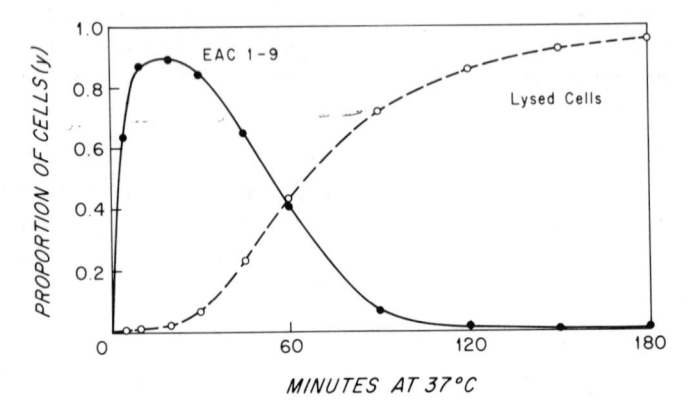

Fig. 2. Kinetics of generation of EACl-9 (●) and of hemolysis (○) by the interaction of EACl-8 and C9 at 37°C.

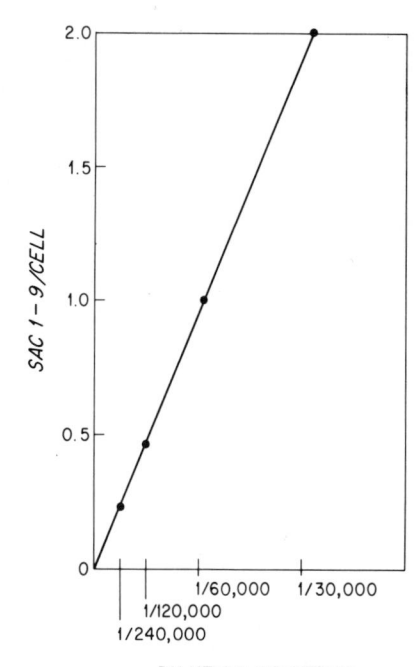

Fig. 3. Titration of C9 activity in normal human serum.

A sample titration curve is shown in Fig. 3 where the average numbers of sites (S) in the state SACl-9, computed by the Poisson distribution, is plotted against the varying inputs of normal human serum used to generate these sites. Conformity with the one-hit model, indicated by a linear curve passing through the origin, is apparent. A dilution of 1/59,000 corresponds to the generation of 1.0 sites per cell in a reaction mixture containing 10^8 cells per ml, so that the number of effective molecules of C9 contained in 1 ml of the serum is 5.9×10^{12}. Studies with purified C9 and estimates of the actual concentration of C9 protein contained in human serum indicate that the C9 reaction has an efficiency close to 1.0 (Hadding and Müller-Eberhard, 1969) so that the estimated number of effective molecules observed from Fig. 3 corresponds quite closely to the actual number of C9 molecules contained in the test sample.

METABOLISM OF COMPLEMENT COMPONENTS

The components of complement, as is the case for other serum proteins, are subject *in vivo* to dynamic equilibria, their serum concentrations reflecting the balance between synthesis and catabolism, and the fraction of the total body pool contained within the plasma space. An

TABLE I
Results of Complement Metabolism Studies of Normal Humans

	C1q	C4	C3	C3	IgG
Serum concentration (μg/ml)	182, 151	210–640[a]	1127–1841	1000–1870	940–1820	6900–17,300
Fractional catabolic rate (percent of plasma pool/hr)	2.8, 2.7	0.9–2.7	1.2–3.4	1.6–2.7	1.1–2.6	0.15–0.41
Synthetic rate (mg/kg/hr)	0.19, 0.18	0.35–1.34	0.87–1.89	0.9–1.42	0.38–1.32	0.47–0.93
Fraction in plasma pool	0.51, 0.75	0.45–0.83	0.43–0.67	0.51–0.83	Not given	~0.45
Number of individuals studied	2	11	10	13	10	23
Reference	Kohler and Müller-Eberhard, 1972	Carpenter et al., 1969	Alper and Rosen, 1967	Petz et al., 1968	Hunsicker et al., 1972	Wochner et al., 1966

[a] Ranges shown are mean ±2 S.D.

approach to the measurement of these parameters has been afforded by the availability of highly purified and radiolabeled complement components. Following injection of these trace-labeled proteins into the plasma space, serial measurements of the disappearance of plasma protein-bound radioactivity and the appearance of free label in the urine provide data from which estimates of the fractional catabolic rates of the injected protein may be derived. Table I gives the ranges of catabolic and synthetic rates and distribution between extravascular and intravascular compartments which have been observed in such studies. The values for catabolic rates, which indicate that almost one-half of the intravascular complement protein is being renewed each day, are among the highest observed for any plasma proteins.

Superimposed on the usual degradative processes which apply to all plasma proteins may be the catabolism of complement components consequent to the activation of the reaction sequence in the "normal" course of body defense or as a result of a disease process. Observed examples of the latter include the increased catabolism of the fourth component and, to a lesser extent, the third component in patients with hereditary angioedema, a disease in which inherited deficiency of a control protein permits the circulation of activated $\overline{C1}$ (Carpenter et al., 1969). Patients with renal allograft rejection, systemic lupus erythematosus, autoimmune hemolytic anemia, and certain kinds of glomerulonephritis may also exhibit hypercatabolism of the third complement component (Alper and Rosen, 1967; Petz et al., 1968; Carpenter et al., 1969; Hunsicker et al., 1972). In patients with rheumatoid arthritis, only modest elevations of the plasma catabolic rate for the third component have been observed, but marked local hypercatabolism within the synovial space has been inferred from studies in which C3 labeled with either ^{125}I or ^{131}I has been simultaneously administered into the plasma and synovial spaces (Ruddy et al., 1971).

NONCYTOLYTIC IMMUNOLOGIC RELEASE OF CHEMICAL MEDIATORS

The attachment of cytotropic antibody molecules to a receptor on target cells, a process termed sensitization, and the subsequent binding of specific antigen to the combining site of these antibodies activates the cells to synthesize and/or secrete their mediators without cell destruction. The antibodies possess a dual specificity, with recognition of cell receptors by the Fc fragment (Ishizaka et al., 1970a and Sullivan et al., 1971) and of antigens by the Fab portion of the molecule (Porter, 1959). *In vitro* models of immunologic mediator release have been developed utilizing fragments of human (Orange et al., 1971a) or guinea pig lung (Baker et al., 1964), mixed human leukocyte suspensions (Levy and Osler, 1967), or mixed rat peritoneal cell suspensions (Becker and Austen, 1966) passively sensitized with antibody-rich serum and challenged with specific antigen. These systems have been employed to identify the class of sensitizing immunoglobulins, characterize the mediators released, and define the biochemical requirements and pharmacologic controls of mediator release. These data have recently been reviewed (Austen and Becker, 1971) and will be summarized to provide background for our present consideration of the kinetics of release of these mediators.

The heat labile immunoglobulin found in sera of allergic humans which can passively sensitize primate lung fragments for the subsequent antigen-induced release of chemical mediators has been firmly established to belong to the IgE class (Ishizaka et al., 1970b). This critical role of IgE antibody in the sensitization of human lung has been proved by the unique ability of anti-IgE antiserum to elicit mediator release *in vitro* from normal human lung apparently carrying autologous IgE on appropriate receptors (Kay and Austen, 1971), and by the suppression of antigen-elicited immune mediator release from human lung either by utilizing IgE myeloma protein specifically to block sensitization of receptors (Orange et al., 1971a) or by treating the atopic sera with anti-IgE selectively to remove IgE antibody before sensitization (Ishizaka et al., 1970b and Orange et al., 1971b).

The known physicochemical characteristics of the three chemical mediators detected in the diffusates of human lung fragments are noted in Table II. Slow reacting substance of anaphylaxis (SRS-A) of human origin profoundly contracts the human bronchiole in the presence of antagonists of other known chemical mediators (Brocklehurst, 1960). Rat and human SRS-A are indistinguishable by physicochemical means (Orange et al., 1973) or pharmacological antagonists (Orange et al., 1971a); and guinea pig, cat, and rat SRS-A cannot be distinguished by resistance to enzymatic digestion (Brocklehurst and Lahiri, 1962; Anggärd et al., 1963; Orange and Austen, 1969). Rat SRS-A has recently been highly purified and clearly shown to be an acidic hydrophilic molecule of 400 mol. wt. able to contract guinea pig ileum in amounts of a nanogram or less (Orange et al., 1973). Eosinophil chemotactic factor of anaphylaxis (ECF-A) is 500–1000 mol. wt. and is specifically chemotactic for homologous eosinophils using an *in vitro* micropore filter technique (Kay et al., 1971). While SRS-A has not been extractable before the immune reaction, both histamine and ECF-A are found preformed in human lung (Stone et al., 1955; Wasserman et al., 1974). Mediators recognized in other model systems include serotonin (Herxheimer, 1955), kinin-forming factors (Jonasson and Becker, 1966),

TABLE II
Chemical Mediators Released Immunologically from Human or Guinea Pig Lung Fragments

Mediator	Chemical structure or characteristics	Quantitative identification
Histamine	β-Imidazolylethylamine MW = 111	Contraction of guinea pig ileum in the presence of atropine
Slow reacting substance of anaphylaxis (SRS-A)	Acidic and hydrophilic MW = 400. High resolution mass spectrometry[a] fails to reveal: amino acids, peptides, prostaglandins	Contraction of guinea pig ileum in presence of antihistamine and atropine
Eosinophil chemotactic factor of anaphylaxis (ECF-A)	Presumptive peptide[b] MW = 500 − 1000	Attraction of eosinophils across millipore membrane

[a] Ethanol extracted diffusate desalted by nonionic chromatography, subjected to base hydrolysis, and fractionated by silicic acid partition chromatography and LH_{20} gel filtration.
[b] Ninhydrin positivity of material isolated from diffusate by G-25 gel filtration and subjected to paper chromatography.

prostaglandins (Piper and Vane, 1969), and a platelet activating factor (Siraganian and Osler, 1971). Mast cells have clearly been demonstrated to be the source of histamine released immunologically from guinea pig lung (Mota and Vugman, 1956) and also possibly from human and other primate lung (Ishizaka et al., 1972). The lung cell source of SRS-A is not known. A recent report demonstrates human basophils to be not only the source of histamine (Valentine et al., 1955), but also one source of ECF-A (Parish, in press).

The biochemical prerequisites for the immunologically-induced secretion of chemical mediators have been extensively reviewed (Austen and Becker, 1971). Immunologic release of histamine from human lung requires the activation of a diisopropylfluorophosphate (DFP) inhibitable serine esterase, the function of a glycolytic pathway as revealed by inhibition with iodoacetate or 2-deoxyglucose when glucose is limited, and calcium ions as indicated by inhibition with ethylenediamine-tetraacetate (EDTA) and reversal upon restoration of free Ca^{++} concentration (Orange et al., 1971b). Examination of the sequential order of various blocking agents has demonstrated that activation of the serine esterase by antigen is preceded and followed by a calcium-dependent step (Kaliner and Austen, 1973).

Studies with human lung fragments have suggested that the target cells involved in the release of mediators possess prototype receptors of the alpha and beta adrenergic and cholinergic types which, when stimulated, modulate the secretory reaction initiated by antigen-IgE interaction (Kaliner et al., 1972). Effective inhibition of release by beta adrenergic agonists was accompanied by an increase in whole tissue levels of cyclic adenosine 3', 5'-monophosphate (cyclic AMP) presumably reflecting a similar rise of cyclic AMP in target cells (Kaliner et al., 1972). Both effects were prevented by the introduction of a beta receptor antagonist. A kinetic relationship existed between the effects of the beta adrenergic agents on the tissue levels of cyclic AMP and the inhibition of mediator release. Phosphodiesterase inhibitors, which prevent the destruction of cyclic AMP, acted synergistically with the beta adrenergic agonists. Inversely, alpha adrenergic agents enhanced both histamine and SRS-A release from sensitized human lung in association with a reduced level of whole tissue cyclic AMP (Kaliner et al., 1972). Cholinergic agents also enhanced the immunologic release of these mediators, but unlike the alpha adrenergic agents their effect was blocked by atropine, unrelated to changes in tissue levels of cyclic AMP, and possibly mediated by increased levels of cyclic guanosine 3', 5'monophosphate (cyclic GMP) (Kaliner et al., 1972). In addition, dibutyryl cyclic AMP yielded a dose-response inhibition of immunologic mediator release from sensitized human lung, whereas 8-bromo-cyclic GMP afforded a dose-related enhancement of release (Orange et al., 1971a; Kaliner et al., 1972).

TIME COURSE OF MEDIATOR RELEASE FROM GUINEA PIG LUNG

Mediator release from guinea pig lung has been studied using a heat stable antibody of the IgG_1 class to sensitize the tissue (Baker et al., 1964). Unlike human IgE, IgG_1 is heat stable, 7S in size, and present in high concentrations in serum. The biochemical requirements for release and the character of the mediators secreted—histamine (Mota and Vugman, 1956), SRS-A (Brocklehurst, 1960; Stechschulte et al., 1967), and ECF-A (Kay et al., 1971)—are the same as those in human lung fragments. Despite the heterogeneity of target cells, sensitizing immunoglobulins, and chemical mediators, an initial effort has been made to study the kinetics of immunologic mediator release from guinea pig lung fragments. A protocol which permitted investigation of the influence of temperature and antigen concentration on the time couse of release of each mediator was as follows. Fragments of perfused lung, prepared as described (Kay et al., 1971) and also as shown schematically in Fig. 4, were obtained from guinea pigs actively immunized with crystalline ovalbumin in $Al(OH)_3$ adjuvant (Le-

Immediate Immunologic Reactions

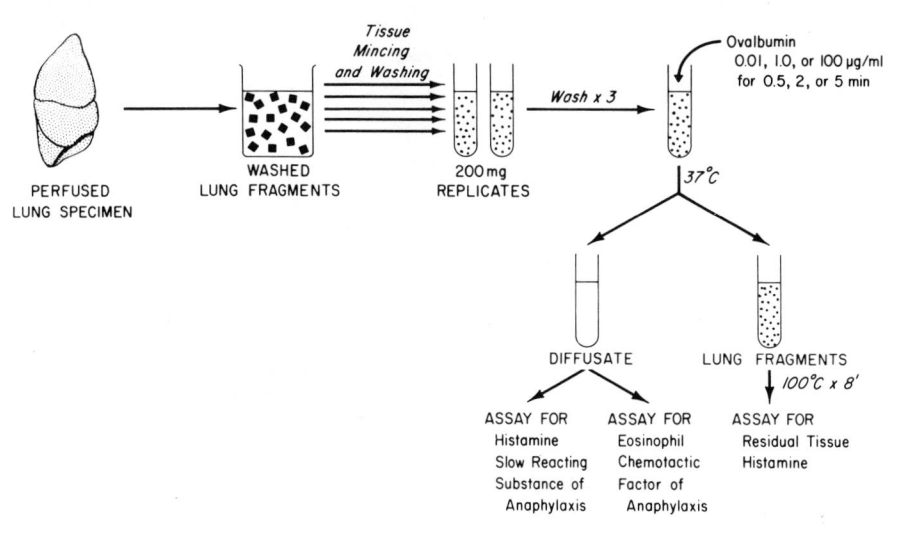

Fig. 4. Preparation of lung tissue from actively sensitized guinea pigs for antigen-induced release of mediators.

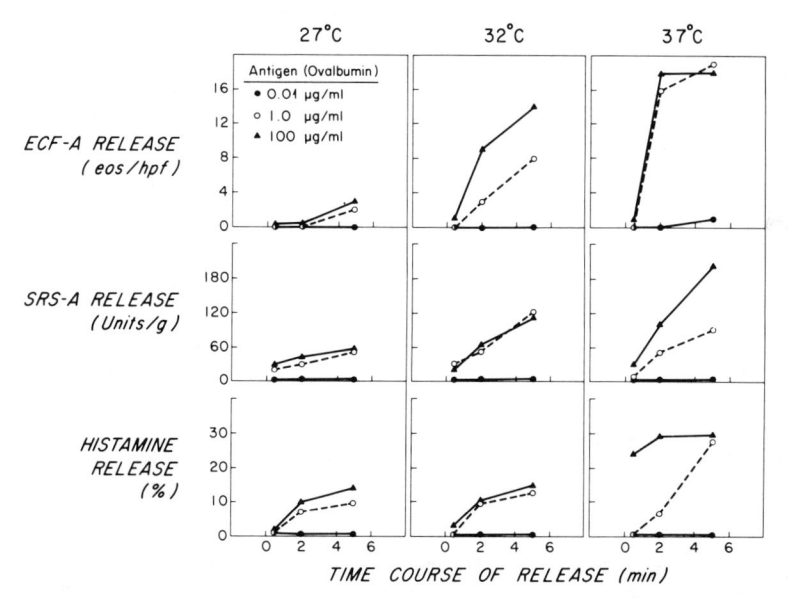

Fig. 5. Release of chemical mediators from actively sensitized guinea pig lung fragments. The time courses of the release reactions were studied at 27, 32, and 37°C with three concentrations of ovalbumin.

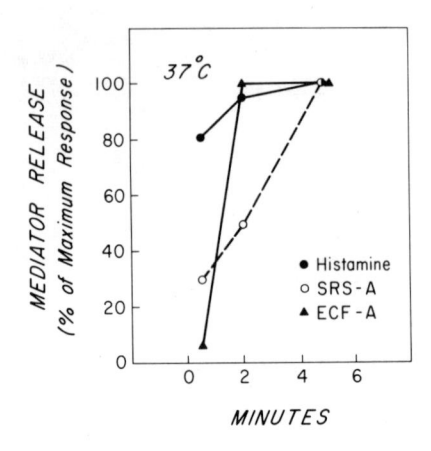

Fig. 6. Kinetics of release of mediators. Incubation temperature was 37°C and ovalbumin concentration was 100 μg/ml. Maximum response was defined as the maximum release of any mediator by 5 min under these conditions.

vine et al., 1971) and were incubated in triplicate at 27, 32, or 37°C with ovalbumin at final concentrations of 0.01, 1.0, or 100 μg/ml. After specified incubation times, the supernatant diffusates were aspirated into clean test tubes, and aliquoted for assays of histamine, SRS-A and ECF-A by standard methods (Orange et al., 1971a; Kay and Austen, 1971). Residual histamine was released by boiling the fragments. As shown in Fig. 5, all three mediators were released most rapidly and in the greatest total amount at 37°C. At 27°C, only a trivial quantity of any mediator was released at

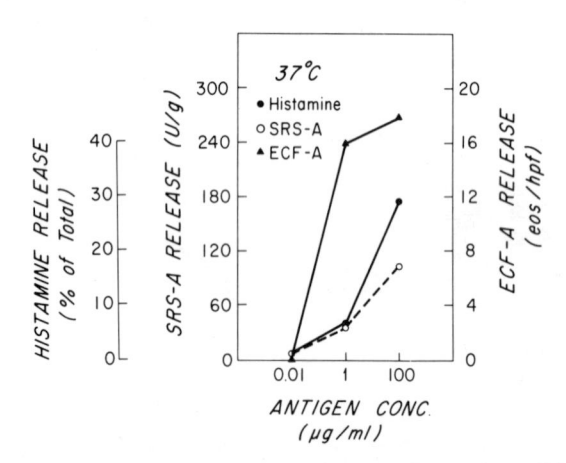

Fig. 7. Antigen concentration-dependence of rate of mediator release. Histamine release is expressed as the percent of total tissue histamine, which equals the sum of released and residual. SRS-A release is given in units of activity by bioassay per gram of lung tissue. ECF-A activity was assessed by the mean number of eosinophils per high-power microscopic field which had migrated through an 8-μ micropore filter.

TABLE III
Kinetic Variables of Mediator Release

Mediator	$^n\text{Ag}^a$	k'^b	k'/maximum[c] release
Histamine	0.60	3.0[d]	0.105
ECF-A	0.40	1.4[e]	0.089
SRS-A	0.22	19.1[f]	0.096

[a] The order of the mediator release reaction with respect to the antigen ovalbumin.
[b] The apparent rate constant of mediator release at 37°C corrected for antigen concentration dependence (see Eq. 7).
[c] Maximum release is defined as the concentration in the diffusate after 5 min incubation at 37°C with ovalbumin concentration 100 μg/ml; ECF-A and histamine release are shown to be at a plateau (Fig. 4), and SRS-A release is also in fact maximal (not shown).
[d] Net percent histamine release—ml/μg ovalbumin-min.
[e] Eosinophils per hpf—ml/μg ovalbumin-min.
[f] Units of SRS-A per gram lung—ml/μg ovalbumin-min.

even the highest ovalbumin concentration. As depicted in Fig. 6, SRS-A was more slowly released than either of the performed mediators, histamine or ECF-A; maximal release of both histamine and ECF-A occurred within 2 min although SRS-A was only at 50% of maximal levels at this time. When the effect of varying antigen concentration was examined (Fig. 7), the rate of mediator release, as reflected by the concentrations in the diffusate at 2 min, rose progressively with increasing antigen dose, although these increments were less for SRS-A than for the two performed mediators.

Assuming that antigen collides with an antibody bound to a membrane receptor on a target cell in a closed ideal gas system to initiate mediator release, one can express the earliest definable rate of mediator release dx/dt in terms of the initial concentrations of reactants:

$$\frac{dx}{dt} = (k[T]^{n_t}[Ab]^{n_{Ab}})[Ag]^{n_{Ag}} \tag{5}$$

where [Ag] is the antigen concentration, [T] is the target cell concentration, [Ab] is the sensitizing antibody concentration, n is the order of the initiating reaction in any reactant and therefore describes the exponential relation between reaction rate and the concentration of any reactant, and k is the rate constant for the reaction.

Assuming that the number of antibody-prepared target cell receptors ([T][Ab]) available to antigen is the same for each concentration of antigen, and using the subscripts 1 and 2 to denote any two concentrations of ovalbumin antigen and the corresponding reaction rates at these concentrations, one can solve for n_{Ag}:

$$n_{Ag} = \frac{\log(dx/dt)_1 - \log(dx/dt)_2}{\log[Ag]_1 - \log[Ag]_2} \tag{6}$$

With the use of reaction rates corresponding to ovalbumin concentrations of 0.01, 1.0, or 100 μg/ml,* the values of n_{Ag} at 37°C have been calculated for each of the mediators as shown in Table III; the SRS-A value is clearly lowest. Assuming that the concentration of target cells and sensitizing antibody are the same for any one mediator, then an apparent rate constant for these conditions, k', can be substituted for $k[T]^{n_t}[Ab]^{n_{Ab}}$; and taking the log of equation (5) and solving for log k',

$$\log k' = \log(dx/dt) - n_{Ag} \log[Ag] \qquad (7)$$

Again by employment of the earliest definable appearance rate of mediator activity in the diffusate at 37°C with ovalbumin concentration 100 μg/ml,* and the derived values of n_{Ag}, k' was calculated for each mediator (Table III). This reflects the rate of mediator release adjusted for the influence of antigen concentration dependence. To allow for comparison among the apparent rates of release of different mediators, the k' for each mediator has been related to the maximum release of that mediator at 37°C (Table III). These relative apparent rates of mediator release are quite similar for the three mediators once the rates have been adjusted for antigen concentration dependence. It is therefore possible to suggest that the intrinsic rate of release for SRS-A at 37°C is equivalent to that of the two preformed mediators, ECF-A and histamine. The rate-limiting reaction for the release of all three mediators may then be similar. However, since a higher antigen concentration is required for optimal SRS-A release, this reaction may require pinocytosis of immune complexes formed at the activating site while histamine and ECF-A release may follow activation of the antibody sensitized target cell by the initial antigen interaction. Since k' is a function of both the true rate constant k and also the density of target cells [T] and their degree of sensitization [Ab], there are other alternative explanations for the similarity of the relative apparent rate constants k'. It is possible that SRS-A, which is not preformed, is intrinsically more slowly released but that more target cells capable of elaborating SRS-A exist in guinea pig lung or that sensitizing antibody has greater affinity for these cell receptors. These preliminary data do not permit an analysis that would discriminate among these possibilities, since actively sensitized whole tissue fragments were employed and only three time points were obtained at two temperatures in each segment of the experiment. Release at 27°C was insufficient for analysis and a higher temperature experiment was not

---

*The following release rates were utilized for the calculation of n_{Ag} and k': histamine and SRS-A rates from 0.5 to 2 min at 1.0 μg ovalbumin/ml, ECF-A rate from 0.5 to 2 min at 0.01 μg and 100 μg ovalbumin/ml, and histamine and SRS-A rates from 0 to 0.5 min at 100 μg ovalbumin/ml.

included because the system is inactivated for immunologic mediator release at 42°C (Schild, 1968). Further analysis will require passive sensitization of tissue with hapten-specific antibody of a single immunoglobulin class and multiple determinations during the early phase of mediator release at additional temperatures between 32° and 37°C.

REFERENCES

Alper, C. A., and Rosen, F. S., 1967, *J. Clin. Invest.* **46:** 2021.
Anggärd, E., Bergquist, U., Hogberg, B., Johansson, K., Thon, L., and Uvnas, B., 1963, *Acta Physiol. Scand.* **59:** 97.
Ashman, R. F., and Metzger, H., 1971, *Immunochem.* **8:** 644.
Austen, K. F., Becker, E. L., Borsos, T., et al., 1968, *Bull. World Health Organ.* **39:** 935.
Austen, K. F., and Becker, E. L., eds., 1971, *Biochemistry of the Acute Allergic Reactions, Second International Symposium.* Blackwell Scientific, Oxford, England.
Baker, A. R., Bloch, K. J., and Austen, K. F., 1964, *J. Immunol.* **93:** 525.
Becker, E. L., and Austen, K. F., 1964, *J. Exp. Med.* **120:** 491.
Becker, E. L., and Austen, K. F., 1966, *J. Exp. Med.* **124:** 379.
Brocklehurst, W. E., 1960, *J. Physiol. (London)* **151:** 416.
Brocklehurst, W. E., and Lahiri, S. C., 1962, *J. Physiol. (London)* **165:** 39P.
Carpenter, C. B., Ruddy, S., Shehadeh, I. H., Müller-Eberhard, H. J., Merrill, J. P., and Austen, K. F., 1969, *J. Clin. Invest.* **48:** 1495.
Hadding, U., and Müller-Eberhard, H. J., 1969, *Immunology* **16:** 719.
Herxheimer, H., 1955, *J. Physiol. (London)* **128:** 435.
Hunsicker, L. G., Ruddy, S., Carpenter, C. B., Schur, P. H., Merrill, J. P., Müller-Eberhard, H. J., and Austen, K. F., 1972, *New Engl. J. Med.* **287:** 835.
Ishizaka, K., Ishizaka, T., and Lee, E. H., 1970a, *Immunochem.* **7:** 687.
Ishizaka, T., Ishizaka, K., Orange, R. P., and Austen, K. F., 1970b, *J. Immunol.* **104:** 335.
Ishizaka, T., Ishizaka, K., and Tonioka, H., 1972, *J. Immunol.* **108:** 513.
Jonasson, O., and Becker, E. L., 1966, *J. Exp. Med.* **123:** 509.
Kaliner, M. A., Orange, R. P., and Austen, K. F., 1972, *J. Exp. Med.* **136:** 556.
Kaliner, M. A., and Austen, K. F., 1973, *J. Exp. Med.* **138:** 1077.
Kay, A. B., Stechschulte, D. J., and Austen, K. F., 1971, *J. Exp. Med.* **133:** 602.
Kay, A. B., and Austen, K. F., 1971, *J. Immunol.* **107:** 889.
Kohler, P. F., and Müller-Eberhard, H. J., 1972, *J. Clin. Invest.* **51:** 868.
Levine, B. B., Chang, H., Jr., and Vaz, N. M., 1971, *J. Immunol.* **106:** 29.
Levy, D. A., and Osler, A. G., 1967, *J. Immunol.* **99:** 1068.
Mayer, M. M., 1961, in: *Experimental Immunochemistry,* p. 133, (Kabat, E. A., and Mayer, M. M., eds.) Charles C. Thomas, Springfield, Ill.
Mota, I., and Vugman, I., 1956, *Nature* **177:** 427.
Müller-Eberhard, H. J., 1968, *Advan. Immunol.* **8:** 1.
Orange, R. P., and Austen, K. F., 1969, In: *Advances in Immunology* Vol. 10, p. 105, (Dixon, F. J., Jr. and Humphrey, J. H., eds.) Academic Press, New York.
Orange, R. P., Austen, W. G., and Austen, K. F., 1971a, In: "Symposium on Immune Complexes and Disease." *J. Exp. Med. (Suppl.)* **134:** 136s.
Orange, R. P., Kaliner, M. A., and Austen, K. F., 1971b, in: *Biochemistry of the Acute Allergic Reactions,* p. 189 (Austen, K. F., and Becker, E. L., eds.) Blackwell Scientific, Oxford, England.
Orange, R. P., Murphy, R. C., Karnovsky, M. L., and Austen, K. F., 1973, *J. Immunol.* **110:** 760.

Parish, W. E., In *Control Mechanisms in Reagin-Mediated Hypersensitivity* (International Symposium) (Goodfriend, L. and Sehon, A., eds.) Montreal (in press).
Petz, L. D., Fink, D. J., Letsky, E. A., Fudenberg, H. H., and Müller-Eberhard, H. J., 1968, *J. Clin. Invest.* **47**: 2469.
Piper, P. J., and Vane, J. R., 1969, *Nature* **223**: 29.
Porter, R. R., 1959, *Biochem J.* **73**: 119.
Rapp, H. J., and Borsos, T., 1970, *Molecular Basis of Complement Action*, Appleton-Century-Croft, New York.
Ruddy, S., Everson, L. K., Schur, P. H., and Austen, K. F., 1971, *J. Exp. Med.* **134**: 259S.
Ruddy, S., Gigli, I., and Austen, K. F., 1972, *New Engl. J. Med.* **287**: 489, 545, 593, 642.
Ruddy, S., Müller-Eberhard, H. J., and Austen, K. F., 1971, *Arth. Rheum* **14**: 410.
Schild, H. O., 1968, In: *Biochemistry of the Acute Allergic Reactions*, p. 99 (Austen, K. F., and Becker, E. L., eds.) Blackwell Scientific, Oxford, England.
Siraganian, R. P., and Osler, A. G., 1971, *J. Immunol.* **106**: 1244.
Stechschulte, D. J., Austen, K. F., and Bloch, K. J., 1967, *J. Exp. Med.* **125**: 127.
Stone, J. L., Merrill, J. M., and Meneely, G. R., 1955, *Federation Proc.* **14**: 147.
Sullivan, A. L., Grimley, P. M., and Metzger, H., 1971, *J. Exp. Med.* **134**: 1403.
Valentine, W. N., Lawrence, J. S., Pearce, M. L., and Beck, W. S., 1955, *Blood* **10**: 154.
Wasserman, S. I., Goetzl, E. J., and Austen, K. F., 1974, *J. Immunol.* **112**: 351.
Wochner, R. D., Drews, G., Strober, W., and Waldmann, T. A., 1966, *J. Clin. Invest.* **45**: 321.

DISCUSSION SUMMARY

Teorell indicated that kinetic analysis of mediator release was based on the same mass action principles as those employed in earlier studies of colloid reactions. Segre recommended application of solid state kinetics to assess antigen–antibody collisions. This suggestion was based on the assumption that IgE antibody is firmly attached to target cell surfaces at the time of collision.

Austen discussed several control mechanisms, aberrations in which could lead to anaphylaxis. These include: (1) genes regulating the immune response; such genes recognize haptenic determinants allowing them to initiate an immune response; (2) factors regulating the serum IgE levels; (3) affinity of IgE antibodies for antigen and target cell surfaces; and (4) modulation of mediator release by prototype adrenergic and cholinergic receptors on target cells. Axelrod amplified this latter point by analogy to denervation models where receptors become more sensitive to circulating mediators, suggesting that the adrenergic receptors on target cells are unmasked by the immune reaction. LaDu suggested that the processes of hapten assimilation and transfer to immunogenic protein carriers, as well as their ability to initiate an immune response, may be under specific genetic control. Ariens noted that mechanisms for the cellular synthesis, storage, and secretion of mediators must be more clearly understood before the above mentioned control mechanisms can be fully appreciated. With regard to the complement system, Teorell pointed out that the analysis of the interaction of target cells with complement components by the one-hit model represents an application of classical collision theory, developed much earlier in connection with studies on the coagulation of colloids. Austen noted that studies of the catabolism of complement proteins *in vivo* involve the kinetics of pharmacologically active molecules produced by the body. Such studies present problems in analysis beyond those generally encountered in more classical investigations of protein metabolism, for example, detection of marked local hypercatabolism associated with inflammatory events in cases where one space (e.g., the joint space in rheumatoid arthritis) is small relative to the total body pool of complement protein.

Pharmacokinetic Studies with Amphetamines: Relationship To Neuropsychiatric Disorders

Lars-M. Gunne and Erik Änggård

Psychiatric Research Center
Ulleråker Hospital
Uppsala, Sweden

In Sweden there has been a long-lasting epidemic of amphetamine abuse. It became evident at the end of the fifties and seems to have culminated around 1969. At that time the approximate number of intravenous abusers of high doses of amphetamine was estimated to be 10,000, the majority of whom lived in, or close to, the capital of Sweden (Inghe, 1969). In this area mainlining amphetamine abusers represented about 0.5% of the total population, corresponding to a similar percentage of heroin addicts in New York City at the same time. Since 1969 we have witnessed a rise in opiate abuse, which has gradually changed the drug scene into a more American-like picture. The present report deals with pharmacokinetic and clinical studies of effects of high amphetamine doses in intravenous abusers. All studies were carried out in a specialized four-bed metabolic unit, where appropriate cases were received during the period of investigation.

SUBJECTIVE EFFECTS OF SINGLE DOSES

Earlier there was anecdotal evidence for a succession of contrasting subjective effects following administration of amphetamine. Davidoff and Reifenstein (1937) noted that the initial state of exhilaration and stimulation was followed by prostration and depression. Rosenberg *et al.* (1963), who were the first to register the amphetamine-induced euphoria, also made the observation that the euphoria, lasting for 8–10 hr, was followed by dysphoria throughout the night. We have attempted to record both the euphoric and dysphoric effects of amphetamine.

Twelve addicts, detoxified 1–2 weeks earlier, volunteered for the study. Two intravenous injections were given at three-day intervals. In randomized order physiological saline or 200 mg of amphetamine sulfate was administered and mood changes were registered on 18 different occasions during 48 hr by means of a 42-item questionnaire, partly obtained from Haertzen *et al.* (1963). Five items were considered to reflect euphoria, since the distribution of positive answers, minus placebo response, corresponded well with the results obtained by a self-rating technique for registration of euphoria (Gunne *et al.*, 1970). The euphoria-sensitive items were: (1) "My thoughts come more easily than usual," (2) "I am in the mood to talk about the feelings I have," (3) "A thrill has gone through me one or more times since I started the test," (4) "I feel less discouraged than usual," and (5) "All sorts of plans are running through my mind."
In addition five dysphoria-sensitive items were introduced: (1) "I am feeling blue," (2) "I feel tense and anxious," (3) "I'd like to have some tranquilizer," (4) "I've noticed that I am easily irritated and upset," and (5) "I feel more moody than usual."

It was found that amphetamine induced a stage of euphoria noticeable for 10–12 hr (with a maximum 15 min after administration of amphetamine), followed by signs of dysphoria which were noticeable early, but

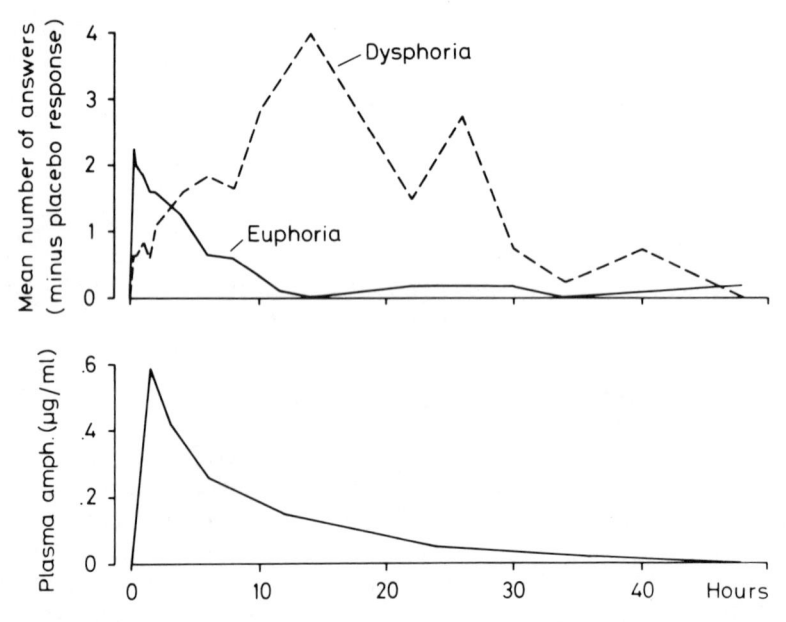

Fig. 1. Time course for the development of euphoric and dysphoric effects and amphetamine blood levels in 12 human subjects following 200 mg of *d,l*-amphetamine sulfate injected intravenously.

reached a maximum at 14 hr after the injection and remained for 48 hr (Fig. 1). Blood levels of amphetamine were measured under the same experimental conditions. All patients participating in these studies were given ammonium chloride, in order to maintain an acidic urine and render the amphetamine elimination reproducible from one experiment to another. It is shown in Fig. 1 that amphetamine is to a large extent eliminated within the 48 hr studied. At the time point (10–12 hr) when the subjectively experienced euphoria disappeared, there were still appreciable amounts of amphetamine in the plasma. Both the euphoric and dysphoric effects should probably be regarded as a direct drug-mediated action.

It is tempting to speculate that this amphetamine-induced dysphoria is a premonitory symptom of an oncoming amphetamine psychosis. Studies by Griffith *et al.* (1970) indicate that there may be a gradual increase of dysphoria during continuous amphetamine administration in volunteering subjects which is followed by a sudden outburst of psychotic manifestations.

EXPERIMENTS WITH AMPHETAMINE BLOCKING AGENTS

Since amphetamine has been shown to be an indirectly acting amine (Hansson, 1967) and exerts its excitatory action only in the presence of releasable catecholamines in the brain, various attempts to block its effects have been directed toward the neuronal catecholamine stores. Reserpine does not inhibit the stimulating action of amphetamine, probably since it does not interfere with the rapid resynthesis of catecholamines. On the contrary, reserpine potentiates amphetamine, possibly by denervation hypersensitivity induced by the pharmacological "sympathectomy" (Stolk and Rech, 1969).

Inhibition of the rate-limiting enzyme tyrosine hydroxylase, on the other hand, was shown by Weissman *et al.* (1966) and Randrup and Munkvad (1966) to eliminate various behavioral effects of amphetamine in rats. A corresponding degree of inhibition of amphetamine-induced excitation and stereotyped behavior had earlier been demonstrated from various neuroleptic drugs, particularly chlorpromazine (Janssen *et al.*, 1965).

In all, 38 subjects (34 males, 4 females), all detoxified amphetamine addicts, participated in the present studies. Five subjects were given various doses of amphetamine *in vivo* (0, 20, 40, 80, and 160 mg of amphetamine sulfate) and rated their feeling of amphetamine-induced "high" by a simple self-rating method (Jönsson *et al.*, 1969). A dose–response relationship was established within this dose range. It was found that α-methyltyrosine (αMT) reduced or eliminated the effect of the highest amphetamine doses

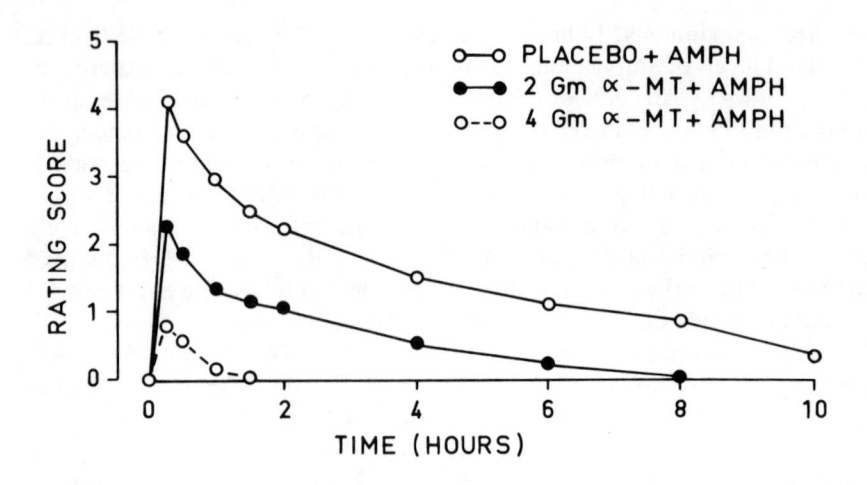

Fig. 2. Blockade of amphetamine euphoria by α-methyltyrosine (α-MT). Self-ratings of the euphoric effect of 200 mg d,l-amphetamine sulfate injected intravenously. Before the amphetamine injection the subjects were pretreated with placebo (o———o), α-MT 0.5 g × 4 (●———●) or 1.0 g × 4 (o– – –o) for one day.

employed in these studies (160–200 mg). Two grams of αMT reduced the self-rated euphoria to about 50% and 4 g almost eliminated the subjective effects of amphetamine (Fig. 2). The duration of this amphetamine blockade was more than 24 hr (Fig. 3), but after 48 hr the effect had disappeared. The daily administration of 4 g/day of αMT rendered the subjects insensitive to the amphetamine blocking effect within a week and withdrawal of αMT after one week gave an enhancement of the amphetamine effect. When αMT was reinstituted 3 days after withdrawal there was another almost complete blockade. For a maximal amphetamine blocking effect

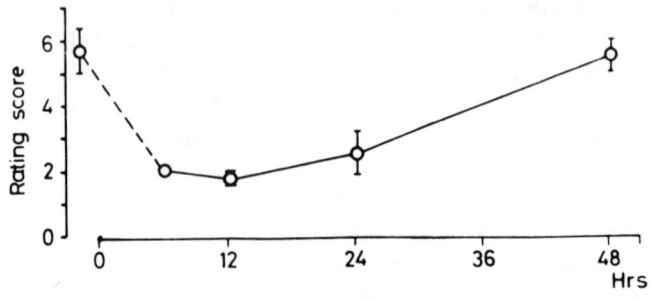

Fig. 3. Duration of the antiamphetamine action of α-methyltyrosine. Maximal self-ratings of amphetamine-induced euphoria (± standard error) before and at different intervals after oral administration of a single dose (4 g) of α-methyltyrosine at zero time.

during long-term administration it should probably be given at 2-day intervals.

Other blockers of the subjective effects of amphetamine were less effective. Some neuroleptics, chlorpromazine and pimozide, gave a reduction corresponding to 2 g αMT, but this effect could not be improved by increased dosage. Chlorpromazine has been used with reported success in the treatment of amphetamine intoxication (Espelin and Done, 1968). Propranolol (a sympathetic β-receptor blocker) and phenoxybenzamine (an α-receptor blocker) were without effect on amphetamine-induced euphoria.

The experiments cited indicate a possible mediation of amphetamine-induced euphoria by catecholamine containing neurons in the brain, but do not clarify which neuron systems are of greatest importance.

Preliminary studies with d- and l-isomers administered in separate experiments, with precautions being taken to maintain an acidic urine, indicate an approximate potency for euphoria induction of 3-4:1 for d vs. l. Such a quotient would favor the view that noradrenaline is of some importance, since d-amphetamine has greater effect on noradrenaline neurons (Taylor and Snyder, 1970), but the fact that part of the euphoria is eliminated by a specific dopamine receptor blocking agent, pimozide, probably points to a certain role also for dopamine in the development of this subjective effect.

PHARMACOKINETIC STUDIES IN AMPHETAMINE-DEPENDENT SUBJECTS

One of the objectives of the present investigation was to obtain data on the fate of amphetamine, specifically in amphetamine-dependent subjects using large intravenous doses and to relate these data to the clinical manifestations of amphetamine abuse, such as paranoid psychosis and development of tolerance.

Nineteen cases were admitted in a state of amphetamine psychosis. They were studied with regard to intensity and duration of the psychotic symptoms, urinary, plasma, and cerebrospinal fluid levels of amphetamine and urinary output of amphetamine metabolites. During the first 24 hr the patient received additional oral doses of 50 mg d,l-amphetamine sulfate every 6 hr. The first dose was added to either 0.2 mC of ^{3}H-labeled or ^{14}C-labeled d,l-amphetamine sulfate. Fifteen subjects received oral ammonium chloride to acidify the urine, whereas four received sodium bicarbonate to produce an alkaline urine. Amphetamine in urine, plasma and cerebrospinal fluid was determined according to Änggård et al. (1970a). Psychological assessment of the psychosis was performed according to Jönsson and Sjöström (1970).

In the subjects having an acidic urine, the psychosis was relatively mild and lasted for about 2 days following the withdrawal of amphetamine (Fig.

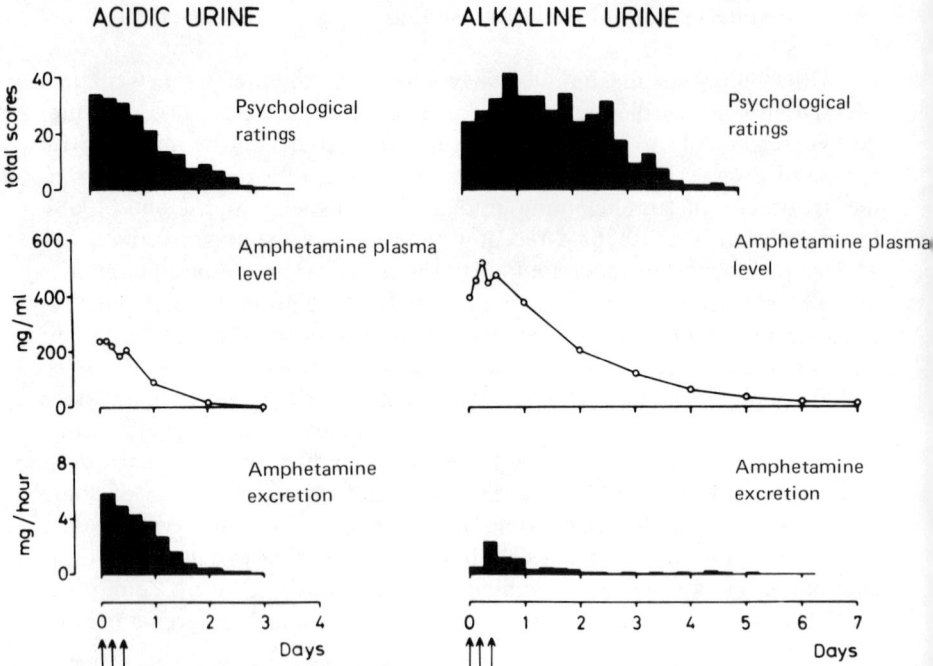

Fig. 4. Psychological ratings of amphetamine psychosis and mean blood and urine levels of amphetamine in conditions of acidic urine (left) and alkaline urine (right). Arrows denote administration of 50 mg of d,l-amphetamine sulfate.

4). The highest plasma amphetamine levels were 269 ng/ml. The elimination of amphetamine from plasma approximately paralleled the disappearance of the psychotic behavior. In the patients with alkaline urine, the psychotic symptoms were aggravated and the mean duration of the illness prolonged to 4.5 days. The mean peak plasma level in this group was 461 ng/ml and the elimination rate was considerably prolonged.

These results show that the psychosis was in some way drug-related, since all subjects had amphetamine in the urine and plasma on admission, and their condition improved when the plasma elimination rate was increased and deteriorated when it was decreased. The psychosis apparently is not a withdrawal phenomenon, since no improvement was observed on administration of moderate doses of d,l-amphetamine sulfate.

Somewhat surprisingly, no correlation was found to exist between the plasma levels of amphetamine and the intensity of the psychosis at any given time point during the first 24 hr after admission. In Fig. 5 the total rating score (i.e., the sum of fifteen psychological variables) was plotted against the plasma concentration of amphetamine. The correlation coefficient was 0.08. That no immediate relationship exists between the degree of the psychosis and the plasma level was also supported by experiments in nonpsychotic individuals receiving 200 mg of d,l-amphetamine sulfate intravenously. In these subjects no signs of psychosis were seen at plasma levels exceeding those found on admission in the psychotic subjects.

At the outset of this study (Änggård et al., 1970b) no reports were available on amphetamine plasma levels and plasma elimination rates in

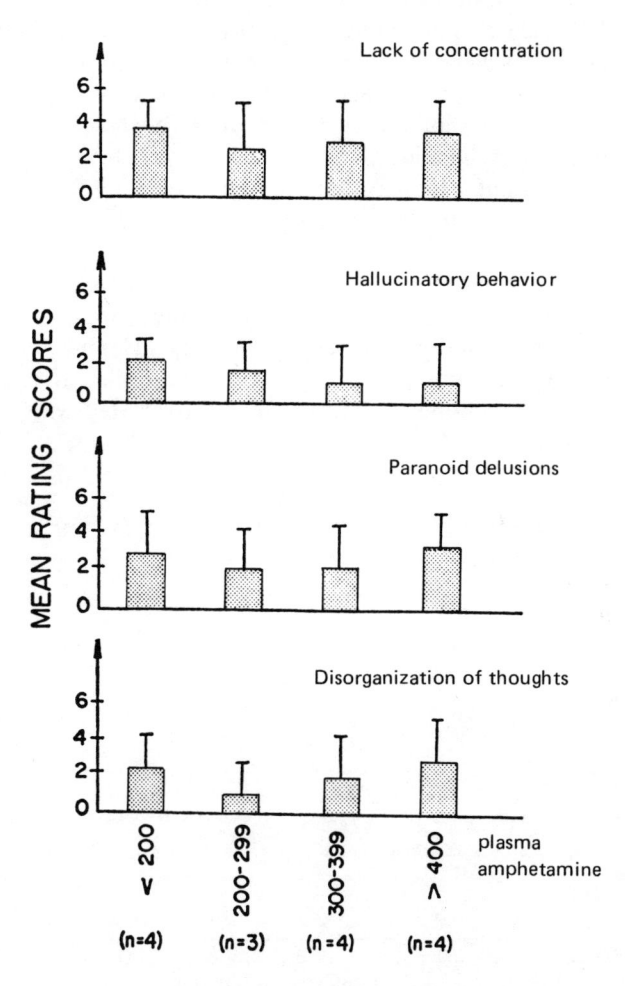

Fig. 5. Lack of correlation between the rating score for amphetamine psychosis and the plasma level of amphetamine observed during the first 24 hr after admission.

man. The urinary excretion of the drug was known to be subjected to the nonionic diffusion mechanism shown to exist for many organic bases (Milne et al., 1958). Thus the amphetamine excretion in urine is facilitated by an acidic urinary pH and depressed by an alkaline urine (Asatoor et al., 1965; Beckett and Rowland, 1965). However, a suppression of the urinary excretion of the unchanged drug during conditions of an alkaline urine might conceivably be compensated for by an increased rate of elimination by metabolism.

In the present study of psychotic amphetamine abusers, the elimination rate of labeled amphetamine was measured, while the body content (and plasma levels) were still high. When the plasma half-life ($T_{1/2}$) was plotted against the mean urinary pH during the first 24 hr, a striking correlation ($r = 0.91$) was obtained (Fig. 6). At a pH of 5.0 the $T_{1/2}$ was about 5 hr. For every increase in unit of urinary pH there was an increase in plasma $T_{1/2}$ of about 7 hr. Thus, at a urinary pH of 7.3 the $T_{1/2}$ was about 21 hr, e.g., more than four times that observed at pH 5. In studies on three drug naïve subjects receiving small doses of amphetamine, evidence for a pH-sensitive plasma elimination rate was obtained (Beckett et al., 1969). Our data confirm these findings and extend them to give quantitative information on the relationship between urinary pH and $T_{1/2}$ in tolerant subjects receiving large doses. It is important to make this distinction, since there is evidence indicating an increase in $T_{1/2}$ associated with the chronic use of the drug.

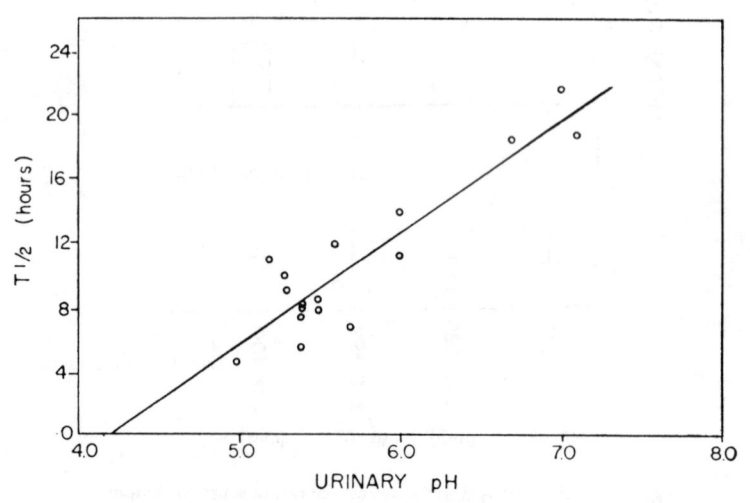

Fig. 6. The relationship between plasma elimination rate of amphetamine ($T_{1/2}$) and urinary pH in seventeen cases of amphetamine psychosis.

When the $T_{1/2}$ was measured in separate experiments in nonpsychotic chronic abusers receiving 20 to 200 mg of unlabeled d,l-amphetamine, it was found to be constant in a given individual at the different doses. The decline in plasma amphetamine was monoexponential over at least three half-lives.

The renal clearance of amphetamine was found to be influenced not only by the urinary pH but also to some extent by the urinary volume. Thus, in the pH range 5.2–6.0, at a low output of urine (< 30 ml/hr), the clearance was about half that observed during conditions of average urine production (30–125 ml/hr). During water diuresis (> 125 ml/hr), the clearance of amphetamine was further increased. These observations may be of importance for the development of toxic symptoms during a period of abuse. Since the amphetamine intake leads not only to anorexia but also to a reduced water intake and increased insensible loss of water from body surfaces, the subjects may become dehydrated during a "run."

In our study most subjects were dehydrated on admission, in extreme cases up to 5–7% of the body weight. Serum electrolytes (K^+, Na^+, Cl^-) were, however, within normal limits. Restlessness and delirium occurs when dehydration amounts to over 5% of the body weight in humans (Bland, 1956). It appears, therefore, that in some cases of amphetamine psychosis, dehydration may contribute to aggravate the symptoms, and by a decreased urine production also reduce the elimination of the drug. In the clinical management of patients with amphetamine psychosis, the administration of ammonium chloride and large amounts of fluid is recommended.

One interesting finding emerging from this study was that the plasma $T_{1/2}$ of amphetamine in chronic amphetamine abusers was significantly longer than in drug naïve control subjects. This difference was not noticeable when the urine was kept acidic but appeared under conditions of alkaline urine (Fig. 7). Comparisons between amphetamine-dependent and drug-naïve subjects indicate that the relative distribution of drug and metabolites are of the same order of magnitude. The increased plasma $T_{1/2}$ in the dependent subjects might then be a consequence of an increased affinity of the tissues for the drug. In accordance with this hypothesis was the finding that the apparent volumes of distribution were high in our patients compared with reports in the literature of studies on nondependent subjects (Rowland, 1969).

Our data permit the calculation of the approximate contribution of renal excretion and metabolism to the clearance of the drug from the body. Assuming no dehydration and an acidic urinary pH, body clearance of amphetamine is about 500 ml/min, of which 370 ml/min is renal and 130 ml/min is metabolic. At alkaline pH (> 7.5), the renal clearance drops to insignificant values and the body clearance equals the metabolic clearance.

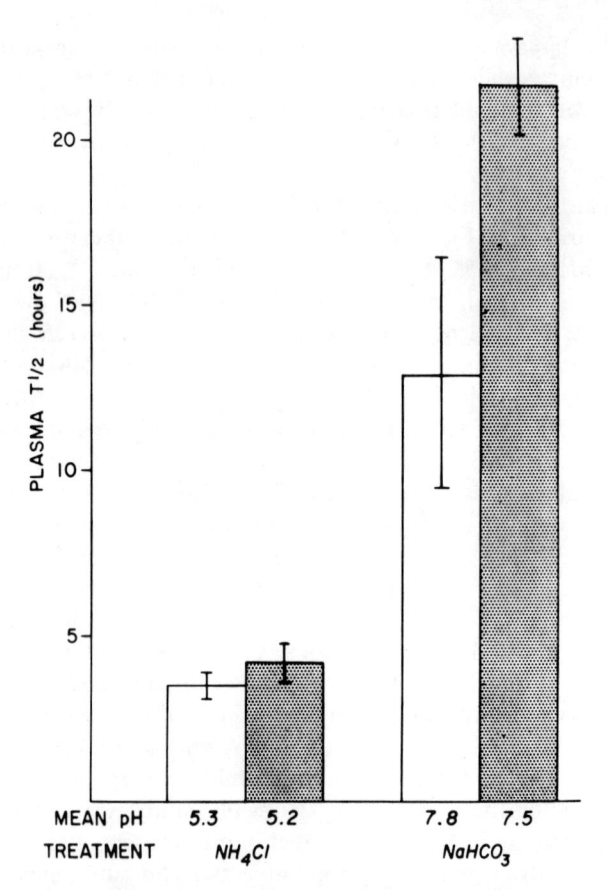

Fig. 7. Comparison of plasma elimination rates of d,l-amphetamine (20 mg p.o.) between a group of chronic abusers of central stimulants (shaded columns) and a group of drug-naïve subjects (white columns).

Several authors (Costa et al., 1970; Angrist et al., 1970) have suggested that metabolites of amphetamine may be responsible for the psychotic symptoms after prolonged use of high doses. p-Hydroxynorephedrine (p-OHNE), is a metabolite of amphetamine in man (Cavanaugh et al., 1970; Davis et al., 1971), and has been shown to function as a false transmitter in the rat.

p-Methoxy-amphetamine has been implied in human amphetamine psychosis on the basis of alleged psychotomimetic properties in the rat. Our own studies indicated that basic metabolites of amphetamine may have contributed to the psychosis since (1) the psychosis was increased in patients with alkaline urine, (2) the proportion of the amphetamine metabolized increased under these conditions, and (3) no immediate relationship could be established between plasma amphetamine and the intensity of the psychosis. We therefore performed a detailed investigation into the metabolism of amphetamine in a group of nine psychotic amphetamine abusers, five with acidic urine and four with alkaline urine.

> Nine psychotic subjects were given 0.2 mC ^{3}H-labeled or ^{14}C-labeled *d,l*-amphetamine sulfate together with 50 mg of unlabeled *d,l*-amphetamine sulfate at 8 a.m. and the excretion of radioactive metabolites were followed for 4–6 days. The subjects were the same as those taking part in the study described above. The urine was subjected to acid hydrolysis and then extracted with toluene at *p*H 12 (= unchanged amphetamine). The residue was adjusted to *p*H 6 and run through a Dowex 50W-X4 column. The fraction remaining on the column (basic metabolites) was eluted with HCl in MeOH. The effluent was adjusted to *p*H 3 and extracted with ethyl acetate to yield acidic metabolites and an aqueous residue. The quantitative composition of the radioactive fractions were examined by thin-layer chromatography (Ellison *et al.*, 1969) and gas chromatography in combination with either flame ionization detection,, radioactivity detection, or mass spectrometry (Änggård and Gunne, 1969). The level of p-hydroxyamphetamine in the fraction of basic metabolites was determined by gas chromatography of the trifluoroacetate derivative using 3-methoxy-4-hydroxy-α- methyl-phenethylamine as an internal standard.

As described earlier (Änggård *et al.*, 1970; Davis *et al.*, 1971) the metabolism of amphetamine was dependent on the urinary *p*H. At an acidic *p*H, 68% of the total excreted urinary radioactivity was present as unchanged amphetamine, 4% as basic metabolites, and 17% as acid metabolites. At an alkaline urinary *p*H the unchanged amphetamine was 27%, basic metabolites 9%, and acidic metabolites 37%. These relationships are further illustrated in Fig. 8 (a) and (b). These figures are essentially in agreement with those obtained by Davis *et al.*, (1971) in drug naïve subjects indicating that there are no dose-dependent changes in the metabolic fate of amphetamine. Nor are there any major changes between dependent and nondependent humans.

The basic metabolites of amphetamine were particularly examined since psychotomimetic metabolites might be expected to appear in this fraction. Since *p*-hydroxyamphetamine (*p*-OHA) would be expected to be the precursor of both *p*-OHNE and methoxy-amphetamine we were interested to note evidence of an accumulation of this metabolite in the psychotic subjects. During 4 days after amphetamine withdrawal the relative urinary content of *p*-OHA (% *p*-OHA/*p*-OHA+A) was gradually increasing from 2.5–4.5% on the first day, up to 14% in the group with acidic urine, and 43% in the alkaline group (Fig. 9). The finding suggests a *p*H-dependent excretion of *p*-OH-amphetamine and also a slower rate of elimination of *p*-OHA as compared with the parent compound. Our data do

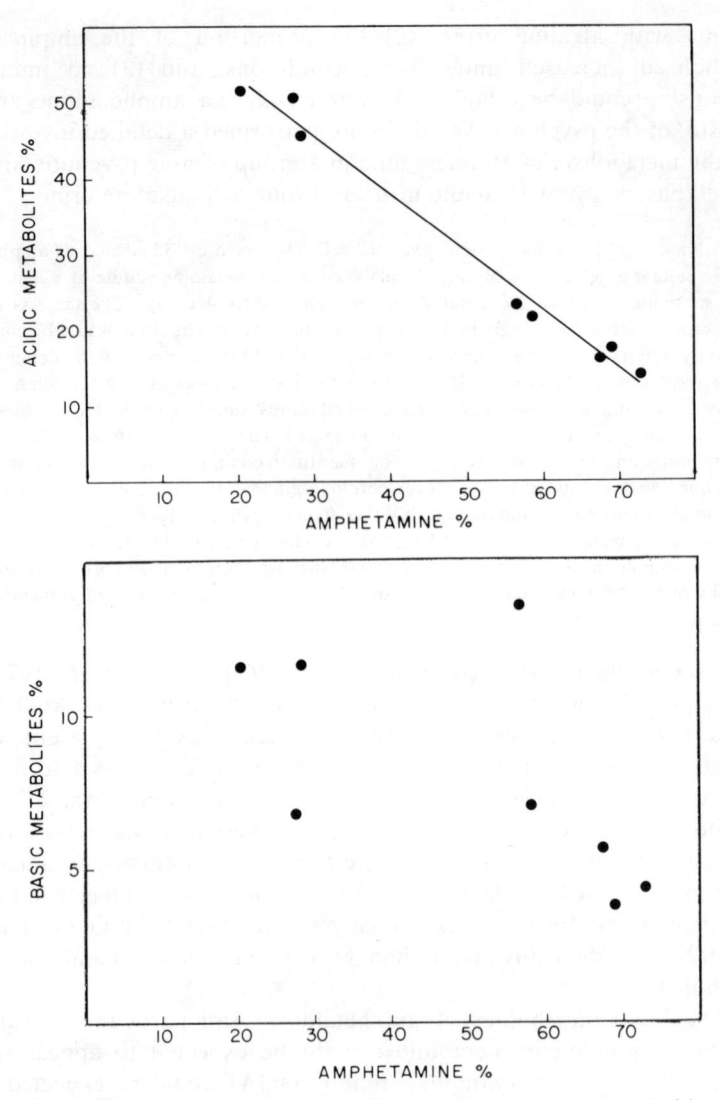

Fig. 8. The relationship between excretion of amphetamine and acidic (a) and basic (b) metabolites.

not support the idea of an induction of *p*-hydroxylation in human amphetamine dependence.

The quantitative composition of the metabolites in the basic fraction was examined by thin-layer chromatography, radio gas chromatography, and mass fragmentography of the trifluoroacetylated metabolites. The

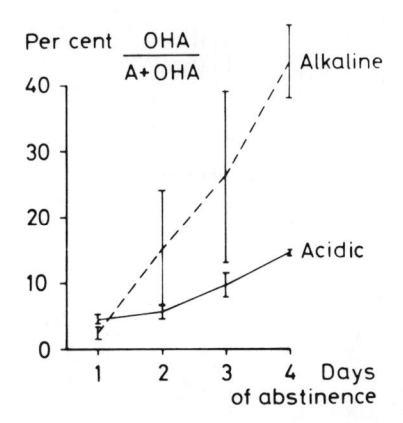

Fig. 9. The relative urinary content of *p*-hydroxyamphetamine (OHA) during 4 days of withdrawal from amphetamine in the psychotic addicts.

major metabolite was p-OHA and norephedrine (NE). Smaller amounts of p-OHNE were also observed. A mass fragmentogram of the basic fraction is shown in Fig. 10. Here the mass spectrometer was focused on the fragment with m/e of 140. This is common for all the basic metabolites and occurs by the elimination of

$$\begin{array}{c} \text{CH-NHCOCF}_3 \\ \parallel \\ \text{CH}_2 \end{array}$$

by β-cleavage. In addition each metabolite was identified by a complete mass spectrum recorded over the peak.

The finding that norephedrine is a metabolite of amphetamine was somewhat unexpected in the light of the work of Goldstein and others (1962) showing that the phenolic phenylethylamines were better substrates for the dopamine β-hydroxylase than compounds lacking the oxygen functions in the ring. Perhaps the high body concentrations of amphetamine found in the abusers as compared to the better substrate OHA might lead to the β-hydroxylation of the parent drug also. An alternative explanation suggested by Caldwell *et al.*, 1972, who recently independently demonstrated norephedrine as a human metabolite of amphetamine, was that this compound might be an intermediate in the formation of benzoic acid.

Some years ago the β-hydroxylation of amphetamine was anticipated, due to some studies of the urinary excretion of the *d*- and *l*-isomers during daily administration of racemic amphetamine (Gunne and Sandberg, 1969). It was found that the *d/l* ratio of amphetamine, measured after resolution in a gas chromatographic system (Gunne, 1967), showed a characteristic pattern in this experiment. On the first days of a given dose, racemic

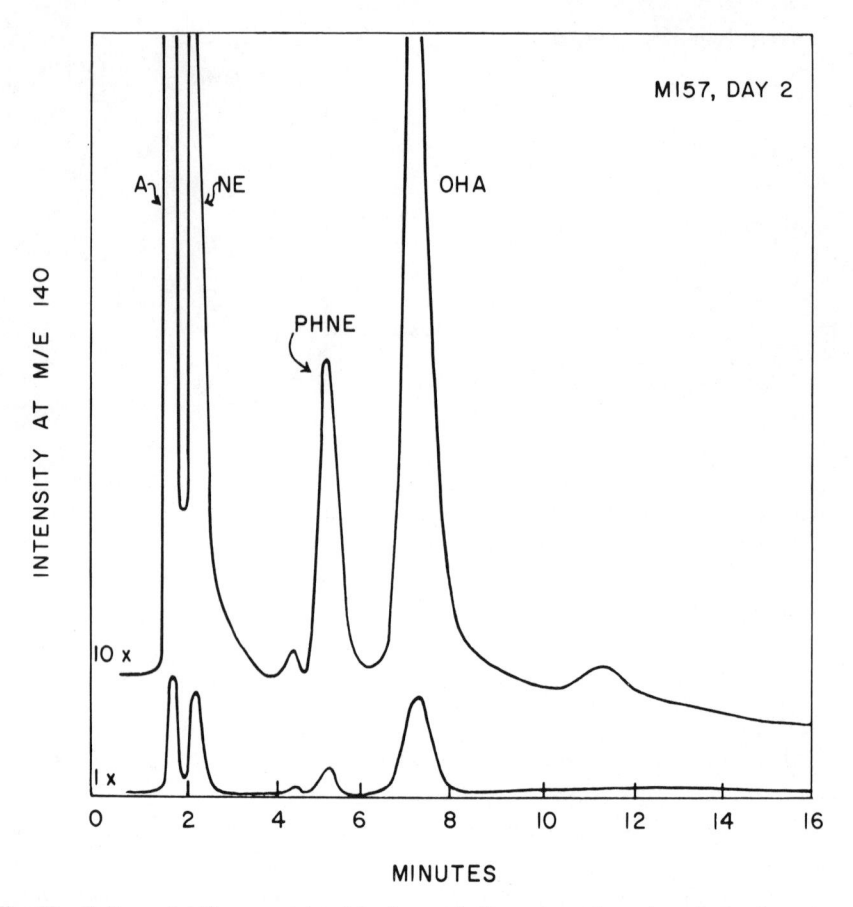

Fig. 10. Pattern of trifluoroacetylated basic metabolites of amphetamine obtained on the second day of withdrawal from amphetamine. The mass fragmentogram was obtained by focusing a LKB-9000 gas chromatograph mass spectrometer on the fragment having an m/e value of 140. This fragment is common for all metabolites of amphetamine retaining the isopropylamine side chain. Except for traces of amphetamine (A) remaining, the fraction is composed of norephedrine (NE), p-hydroxyamphetamine (OHA) and p-hydroxynorephedrine (PHNE).

amphetamine was excreted, but when the same dose had been administered for some days there was a reduction of the d/l ratio, possibly due to some mechanism which selectively eliminated d-amphetamine. It was suggested that the β-hydroxylating enzyme of the sympathetic neuron system might represent this mechanism, although at that time the β-hydroxylation of amphetamine or its metabolites in man was unknown.

CONCLUDING REMARKS

A few practical conclusions have emerged from the present studies. The simultaneous registration of the two opposite subjective effects, euphoria and dysphoria, in combination with studies of drug pharmacokinetics will likely improve our understanding of the mechanisms involved in the drug-induced change from a normal mental state into a schizophrenialike psychosis. Further, our experiments with amphetamine blocking agents have shed some light on the catecholamine mediation of amphetamine-induced euphoria. At present, clinical trials with alphamethyltyrosine are being undertaken in order to explore the therapeutic possibilities of this powerful amphetamine antagonist in drug-dependent subjects.

Since intravenous amphetamine addiction is a serious condition with a relapse rate comparable to heroin addiction (Gunne *et al.*, 1970) the development of a pharmacological antagonist may be of value to combat outbreaks of this kind of dependence, for which we have a great deal of respect in Sweden.

REFERENCES

Angrist, B. M. and Gershon, S., 1970, "The phenomenology of experimentally induced amphetamine psychosis-preliminary observations," *Biol. Psychiat.* **2**: 95–107.
Asatoor, A. M., Galman, B. R., Johnson, J. R., Milne, M. D., 1965, "The excretion of dexamphetamine and its derivatives," *Brit. J. Pharmacol.* **24**: 293.
Änggård, E., Gunne, L.-M., and Nicklasson, F., 1970a, "Gas chromatographic determination of amphetamine in blood, tissue and urine," *Scand. J. Clin. Lab. Invest.* **26**: 137.
Änggård, E., Gunne, L.-M., Jönsson, L. E., and Nicklasson, F., 1970b, "Pharmacokinetic and clinical studies on amphetamine dependent subjects," *European J. Clin. Pharmacol.* **3**: 3–11.
Beckett, A., and Rowland, M., 1965, "Urinary excretion kinetics of amphetamine in man," *J. Pharm. Pharmacol.* **17**: 628.
Beckett, A. H., Salmon, J. A., and Mitchard, M., 1969, "The relation between blood levels and urinary excretion of amphetamine under controlled acidic and under fluctuating urinary *pH* values using ^{14}C-amphetamine," *J. Pharm. Pharmacol.* **21**: 251.
Bland, J. H., 1956, *Disturbances of Fluid Balance.* W. B. Saunders, Philadelphia and London.
Caldwell, J., Dring, L. G., and Williams, R. T., 1972, "Norephedrine as metabolites of ^{14}C amphetamine in urine in man," *Biochem. J.* **129**: 23–24.
Cavanaugh, J. H., Griffith, J. D., and Oates, J. A., 1970, "Effect of amphetamine on the pressor response to tyramine. Formation of *p*-hydroxynorephedrine from amphetamine in man," *J. Clin. Pharmacol. Therap.* **11**: 656.
Costa, E. and Groppetti, A., 1970, "Biosynthesis and storage of catecholamines in tissues of rats injected with various doses of *d*-amphetamines," in: *International Symposium on Amphetamines and Related Compounds* (Costa, E., and Garattini, S., eds.) Raven Press, New York.
Davidoff, E., and Reifenstein, E. C., 1937, "The stimulating action of benzedrine sulfate," *J. Am. Med. Assoc.* **108**: 1770–1776.
Davis, J. M., Kopin, E. J., and Axelrod, J., 1969, "Effects of urinary *p*H on plasma levels and metabolism of ^{3}H-amphetamine in man," *Pharmacologist* **11**: 2.

Davis, J. M., Kopin, E. J., Lemberger, L., and Axelrod, J., 1971, "Effects of urinary pH on amphetamine metabolism," *N.Y. Acad. Sci.* **179**: 493.
Espelin, D. E., and Done, A. K., 1968, "Amphetamine poisoning," *New Engl. J. Med.* **278**: 1361.
Goldstein, M., and Contrera, J. F., 1962, "The substrate specificity of phenylethylamine β-hydroxylase," *J. Biol. Chem.* **237**: 1898.
Griffith, J. D., Cavanaugh, J., Held, J., and Oates, J. A., 1970, *Experimental Psychosis induced by the Administration of d-Amphetamine*, International Symposium on Amphetamines and Related Compounds (Costa and Garattini, eds.) Raven Press, New York.
Gunne, L.-M., 1967, "The Urinary output of *d*- and *l*-amphetamine in man," *Biochem. Pharm.* **16**: 863–869.
Gunne, L.-M., and Sandberg, C. G., 1967, Stereoselective metabolism of amphetamine in man., in: *Abuse of Central Stimulants*, Sjöqvist and Tottie, eds., Stockholm, p. 445–448.
Gunne, L.-M., Änggård, E., and Jönsson, L. E., 1970, *Blockade of Amphetamine Effects in Human Subject.*, I.C.A.A. Tongue and Tongue, Lausanne. p. 249–255.
Haertzen, C. A., Hill, H. E., and Belleville, R. E., 1963, "Development of the Addiction Research Center Inventory CARCI. Selection of items that are sensitive to the effects of various drugs," *Psychopharmacologia* **4**: 155.
Hansson, L. C. F., 1967, "Evidence that the central action of (+)-amphetamine mediated via catecholamines," *Psychopharmacologia* **10**: 289–297.
Inghe, G., 1969, "The present state of abuse and addiction to stimulant drugs in Sweden," in: *Abuse of Central Stimulants*, p. 187 (Sjöqvist, F., and Tottie, M., eds.) Almqvist & Wiksell, Stockholm.
Janssen, P., Niemegeers, C., and Schellekens, K., 1965, "Is it possible to predict the clinical effects of neuroleptic drugs (major tranquillizers) from animal data?" *Drug Res. (Arsneim.-Forsch.)* **15**: 104–117.
Jönsson, L. E., Gunne, L.-M., and Änggård, E., 1969, "Effects of alphamethyltyrosine in amphetamine-dependent subjects," *European J. Clin. Pharmacol.* **2**: 27–29.
Milne, M. D., Scribner, B. H., and Crawford, M. D., 1958, "Non-ionic diffusion and the excretion of weak acids and bases," *Am. J. Med.* **24**: 709–729.
Randrup, A., and Munkvad, I., 1966, "Role of catecholamines in the amphetamine excitatory response," *Nature* **211**: 540.
Rosenberg, D. E., Wolbach, A. B., Miner, E. J., and Isbell, H., 1963, "Observations on direct and cross tolerance with LSD and d-amphetamine in man," *Psychopharmacologia* **5**: 1–15.
Rowland, M., 1969, "Amphetamine blood and urine levels in man," *J. Pharmacol.* **58**: 508.
Stolk, J. M., and Rech, R. H., 1969, "Effect of reserpine on accumulation and removal of *d*-amphetamine-^{3}H.," *Biochem. Pharmacol.* **18**: 2786.
Taylor, K. M., and Snyder, S. H., 1970, "Amphetamine differentiation by *d*- and *l*-isomers of behavior involving brain norepinephrine and dopamine," *Science* **169**: 147.
Weissman, A., Koe, B. K., and Tenen, S., 1966, "Antiamphetamine effects following inhibition of tyrosine hydroxylase," *J. Pharmacol. Exp. Therap.* **151**: 339–352.

DISCUSSION SUMMARY

The subjects used to study amphetamine pharmacokinetics and its euphoric/dysphoric effects were addicts who were detoxified for 1 to 2 weeks. Hinderling asked whether such subjects, accustomed to taking at least 1 g of the drug per day, responded like normal individuals to the smaller (200 mg or less) doses given for study purposes. Gunne responded that former addicts have a decreased drug response which includes the lack of hyperthermia, a phenomenon normally experienced by drug-naive subjects. Such tolerance appears to last at least half a year after detoxification.

Axelrod commented concerning the two types of effects produced by amphetamine. Since the dysphoria lasts much longer than the euphoria (see Fig. 1), it is possible that the beta-hydroxyl metabolite, norephedrine, might be causing the dysphoria. This is reasonable because norephedrine appears to be a major metabolite in these subjects and it is likely to be excreted more slowly than amphetamine. A second point concerned the observation that d-amphetamine is four times more potent in producing euphoria than its levo-isomer. Other studies have indicated that there is no difference between these isomers in producing paranoid psychosis and, on this basis, some important conclusions have been made concerning the mechanism of psychosis. It was queried whether Gunne's research included study of the effects of the two isomers on paranoid psychosis. Gunne replied that it remains an open question whether both isomers are equally active in producing psychosis. The possible effects of the beta-hydroxylated metabolites may be resolved by on-going studies of spinal fluid content of these compounds in patients with amphetamine-produced psychotic effects.

Rowland noted that small doses of amphetamine are known to have a diuretic effect, including an increase in sodium output in urine, which could be partly responsible for the dehydration often seen in amphetamine addicts. Gunne's observation was that amphetamine not only blocks hunger, but very conspicuously abolishes subjective thirst, a factor more likely than mild diuresis to result in severe dehydration.

Further discussion was stimulated by a practical question from Teorell whether or not amphetamines should be considered of more harm than value in general use. Gunne responded that they are useful at least for treating narcolepsy, but he doubted their use in most other cases, since amphetamine is a very strongly addictive drug. When Brown was concerned about treatment of hyperactive children in the United States with small doses of amphetamine over a 6- to 10-year period, Gunne replied that child psychiatrists in Sweden seem to be content with their results from similar use of the drug. Rapoport noted that methylphenidate, a very similar medication, is perhaps more widely used these days for hyperactive children. Children, starting at age 7 or 8 when the teacher becomes concerned about hyperactivity in the classroom, receive doses of 10 or 20 mg a day, and a third of such treated children seem to stay on the drug for 4 to 6 years or more. The dose is increased in relation to body weight and tolerance is extremely rare. There are exceptional cases of escape phenomena, and beyond 50 to 60 mg doses, the side effects prevent further dosage increases. An additional problem with amphetamine was noted by Azarnoff. Tolerance to amphetamine occurs when body weight losses are measured, but the appetite suppressing effect appears to continue. Thus, the situation which results is that appetite suppression lowers the calories, but sooner or later a constant-weight equilibrium occurs again. In essence, no one at the meeting was willing to strongly advocate the continued use of amphetamines for any unique pharmacologic purposes other than treatment of narcolepsy.

A Pharmacokinetic Approach to the Treatment of Depression*

Folke Sjöqvist

Department of Clinical Pharmacology
Karolinska Institutet
Stockholm, Sweden

Treatment with standard doses of the tricyclic antidepressants nortriptyline (NT) and desmethylimipramine (DMI) results in 10- to 30-fold interindividual differences in their steady-state plasma concentrations (Hammer and Sjöqvist, 1967a; Alexanderson and Sjöqvist, 1971).

Studies of NT in identical and fraternal twins have shown that most of this variability between persons is genetically determined although treatment with other drugs will also influence the steady-state plasma concentration (Alexanderson et al., 1969). The mode of inheritance of NT plasma levels is likely to be polygenic (Åsberg et al., 1971b), i.e., controlled by an unknown number of allelic genes at an unknown number of loci.

The relationship between plasma concentration and the biological effects of NT has been studied in model experiments. The inhibition of noradrenaline uptake in rat irides and slices of cerebral cortex, incubated in plasma from patients treated with nortriptyline, is linearly correlated to the plasma level of the drug (Borgå et al., 1970; Hamberger and Tuck, 1973). The blockade of amine uptake in patients treated with nortriptyline, as evidenced by reduced pressor effect of *in vivo* administered tyramine is also correlated to the concentration of drug in plasma (Freyschuss et al.,

---

* This discussion remark was aided by the Swedish Medical Research Council (B73-14X-1021-08, and B74-04X-3902-02) and by NIH, Bethesda, Maryland, U.S.A. (GM 13978-06). Reprint requests should be sent to Huddinge University Hospital, S-141 86, Huddinge, Sweden.

1971). Subjective side effects have repeatedly been found to be associated with high plasma concentrations of nortriptyline (Åsberg et al., 1971b; Åsberg et al., 1970; Hammer et al., 1967), and in the case of disturbed accommodation, a side effect which can be measured objectively, there is a significant correlation to the plasma level of the drug (Åsberg and Germanis, 1972).

In a pilot study by Åsberg et al. (1971) of 30 patients with endogenous depression, the relationship between plasma concentration and therapeutic effect of NT appeared to be complex. The best result was obtained on an intermediate plasma level (50–140 ng/ml) while concentrations above or below this level seemed to be of little benefit to the patient (i.e., the relationship between plasma level and drug response was curvilinear). This finding has recently been confirmed in a joint Danish–Swedish investigation (Kragh–Sørensen, Eggert-Hansen, and Åsberg, 1973). In a recent paper Braithwaite et al. (1972) reported a significant correlation between the antidepressant effect and plasma levels of amitriptyline and its main metabolite NT.

In relation to these findings it seemed to be of clinical importance to further investigate the reasons behind the variability in steady-state plasma concentrations of tricyclic antidepressants and to explore kinetic methods for predicting their plasma levels in a given subject. Kinetic studies after single and multiple oral doses have therefore been performed in unrelated, healthy volunteers (Alexanderson, 1972a) and in twins (Alexanderson, 1973).

These studies can be summarized accordingly (Alexanderson and Borgå, 1973; Alexanderson, Borgå, and Alvan, 1973; Alexanderson, 1972b). It is possible to accurately predict steady-state plasma concentrations of both NT and DMI from single oral dose plasma level data and thereby bring the patient into the therapeutic plasma level range (Fig. 1). Moreover, the steady-state plasma concentration of these drugs is a reproducible kinetic variable (Alexanderson, 1973). There are significant differences in the disposition plasma half-life of NT as well as in the estimated apparent volume of distribution between subjects (Table I). These variations are mainly genetically determined and both parameters may independently contribute to the total variability in steady-state plasma concentrations. This would be consistent with a polygenic mode of inheritance. The parenteral single-dose studies indicate true interindividual differences in the apparent volume of distribution of NT, but the variations may be due to some extent to variations in the availability. No attempt has been made to assess the relative contribution of $(t_{1/2})_\beta$ and $(V_d)_\beta$ to the total variation in steady-state levels. However, it seems as if the range in $(t_{1/2})_\beta$ predominates

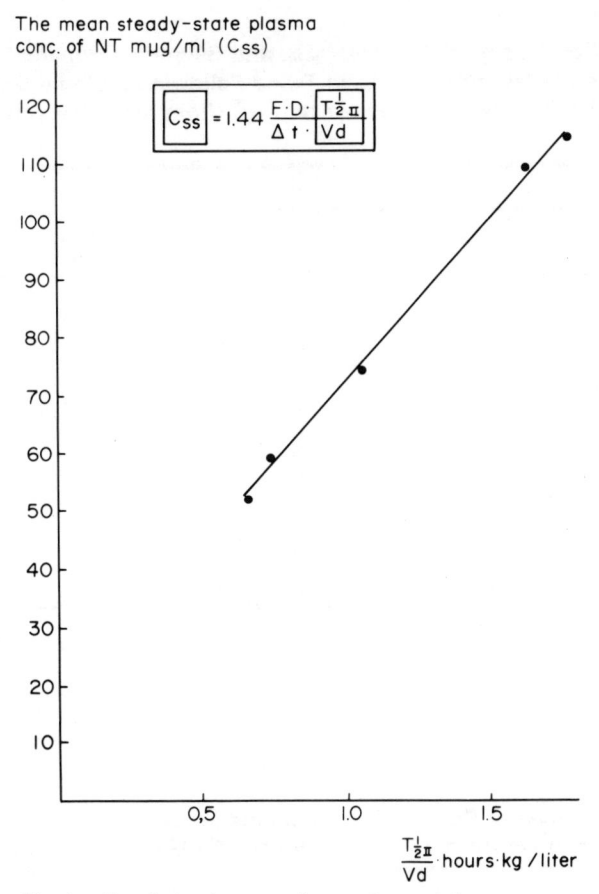

Fig. 1. Correlation between the steady-state plasma concentration of NT (C_{ss}) in five healthy humans given NT for 14 days and the ratio between the plasma half-life (β-slope $= T_{1/2}$ II) and apparent volume of distribution (V_d) of a single oral dose of NT in the same individuals (Alexanderson and Sjöqvist, 1971). The plasma clearance of a drug is equal to ($V_d \cdot 0.693/T_{1/2}$ II). Hence the steady-state plasma concentration of NT will be proportional to the inverse plasma clearance of a single oral dose.

quantitatively. It may be added that the above studies in our laboratory also revealed that the plasma protein binding of NT is under genetic control in man.

The conformity between the steady-state plasma concentrations (Hammer *et al.*, 1969) and the plasma clearances (Alexanderson, 1972c) of NT and DMI (Table II) suggests that their plasma kinetics might be regulated

TABLE I
Disposition Plasma Half-Lives, $(t_{1/2})_\beta$, and Estimated Apparent Volumes of Distribution, $(V_d)_\beta$, in Twins Following a Single Oral Dose of Nortriptyline Hydrochloride (1 mg/kg) (from Alexanderson 1972b, 1973).

	Monozygotic twins			Dizygotic twins	
Subject code No.	$(t_{1/2})_\beta$ hr	$(V_d)_\beta$ liter/kg	Subject code No.	$(t_{1/2})_\beta$ hr	$(V_d)_\beta$ liter/kg
15	21.5	34.6	9	36.2	40.7
16	18.3	34.8	10	19.4	20.6
25	30.4	32.5	27	42.1	32.3
26	27.5	29.0	28	56.5	22.6
39	28.8	32.2	31	26.8	49.4
40	27.6	32.3	32	31.6	49.8
47	25.0	24.8	68	25.7	22.5
89	21.3	22.7	81	37.3	40.8
78	47.9	29.8	74	47.7	41.0
84	55.1	36.5	80	93.3	33.7
—	—	—	92	39.7	56.9
—	—	—	94	67.8	42.2

TABLE II
Linear Regression of Certain Measurements (x) and (y). Computed from the Single and Multiple Dose Studies of DMI and NT (from Alexanderson, 1972c)[a]

Measurements	x		y	n	r	t	$P <$
Observed peak levels	DMI	vs.	NT	8	0.85	3.91	0.01
Plasma half-lives $(t_{1/2})_\beta$	DMI	vs.	NT	8	0.88	4.35	0.005
Apparent volumes of distribution, $(V_d)_\beta$	DMI	vs.	NT	8	0.55	1.60	N.S.
Plasma clearance	DMI	vs.	NT	8	0.90	4.94	0.005
Post steady-state plasma half-lives, $(t_{1/2})_{ss}$	DMI	vs.	NT	6	0.56	1.34	N.S.
Apparent volumes of distribution at steady-state, $(V_d)_{ss}$	DMI	vs.	NT	6	0.53	1.25	N.S.
Plasma half-lives, $(t_{1/2})_\beta$ of DMI		vs.	C_{ss} of DMI	8	0.85	3.99	0.01

[a] C_{ss} is the apparent mean steady-state plasma levels of DMI calculated from day 6 of drug therapy; n is the numbers of pairs of observations; r is the correlation coefficient; t is the test for significance; P is the significance level; N.S. stands for not significant at 5% level.

by common genetic factors. And once the plasma clearance rate is known for one of these two drugs in a subject, it will be possible to predict the subject's steady-state levels of the other drug.

A single oral dose study aimed at predicting steady-state levels will last for about 4 to 5 days (Alexanderson, 1972a). Under certain circumstances such a predictive test will be the most efficient way to unravel an individual's steady-state level for a given maintenance dose. It will also avoid the time-consuming trial-and-error technique, where the dose is adjusted according to subsequent plasma determinations or the appearance of side effects. Moreover, the information from a predictive test may be valid for years provided that the patient is not heavily exposed to other drugs. This is advantageous in patient management, since endogenous depression is often a recurrent disease.

REFERENCES

Alexanderson, B., Evans, D. A. P., and Sjöqvist, F., 1969, "Steady-state plasma levels of nortriptyline in twins: Influence of genetic factors and drug therapy," *Brit. Med. J.* **4:** 764–768.

Alexanderson, B., and Sjöqvist, F., 1971, "Individual differences in the pharmacokinetics of monomethylated tricyclic antidepressants: Role of genetic and environmental factors and clinical importance," *Ann. N. Y. Acad. Sci.* **179:** 739–751.

Alexanderson, B., 1972a, "Pharmacokinetics of nortriptyline in man after single and multiple oral doses: The predictability of steady-state plasma concentrations from single dose plasma-level data," *European. J. Clin. Pharmacol.* **4:** 82–91.

Alexanderson, B., 1972b, On interindividual variability in plasma levels of nortriptyline and desmethylimipramine in man: A pharmacokinetic and genetic study, Linköping University Medical Dissertations No. 6.

Alexanderson, B., 1972c, "Pharmacokinetics of desmethylimipramine and nortriptyline in man after single and multiple oral doses—a cross-over study," *European J. Clin. Pharmacol.* **5:** 1–10.

Alexanderson, B., 1973, "Prediction of Steady-State Plasma Levels of Nortriptyline from Single Oral Dose Kinetics: A Study in Twins," *European J. Clin. Pharmacol.* **6:** 44–53.

Alexanderson, B., and Borgå, O., 1973, "Urinary Excretion of Nortriptyline and Five of its Metabolites in Man after Single and Multiple Oral Doses," *European J. Clin. Pharmacol.* **5:** 174–180.

Alexanderson, B., Borgå, O., and Alvan, G., 1973, "The Availability of Orally Administered Nortriptyline," *European J. Clin. Pharmacol.* **5:** 181–185.

Åsberg, M., Cronholm, B., Sjöqvist, F., and Tuck, D., 1970, "The correlation of subjective side effects with plasma concentrations of nortriptyline," *Brit. Med. J.* **4:** 18–21.

Åsberg, M., Cronholm, B., Sjöqvist, F., and Tuck, D., 1971a, "Relationship between plasma level and therapeutic effect of nortriptyline," *Brit. Med. J.* **3:** 331–334.

Åsberg, M., Evans, D. A. P., and Sjöqvist, F., 1971b, "Genetic Control of nortriptyline kinetics in man: A study of the relatives of propositi with high plasma concentration," *J. Med. Genet.* **8:** 129–135.

Åsberg, M., and Germanis, M., 1972, "Ophthalmological effects of nortriptyline-relationship to plasma level," *Pharmacology* **7**: 349–356.

Borgå, O., Hamberger, B., Malmfors, T., and Sjöqvist, F., 1970, "The role of plasma protein binding in the inhibitory effect of nortriptyline on the neuronal uptake of norepinephrine," *Clin. Pharm. Therap.* **11**: 581–588.

Braithwaite, R. A., Goulding, R., Theano, G., Bailey, J., and Coppen, A., 1972, "Plasma concentration of amitriptyline and clinical response," *Lancet* **1**: 1297–1300.

Freyschuss, U., Sjöqvist, F., and Tuck, D., 1971, "Tyramine pressor effects in man before and during treatment with nortriptyline or ECT: Correlation between pharmacokinetics and effect of nortriptyline," *Pharmacol. Clin.* **2**: 72–78.

Hamberger, B., and Tuck, D., 1973, "Effect of Tricyclic Antidepressants on Uptake of Noradrenaline and 5-hydroxytryptamine into Rat Brain Slices Incubated in Buffer of Human Plasma," *European J. Clin. Pharmacol.* **6**: 1–7.

Hammer, W., and Sjöqvist, F., 1967a, "Plasma levels of monomethylated tricyclic antidepressants during treatment with imipramine–like compounds," *Life Sci.* **6**: 1895–1903.

Hammer, W., Ideström, C. M., and Sjöqvist, S., 1967b, "Chemical control of antidepressant drug therapy," In Proceedings of the First International Symposium on Antidepressant Drugs. Milano, 1966, Ed. by S. Garattini and M. N. G. Dukes, *Excerpta Med. Intern. Congr. Ser. No. 122*: 301–310.

Hammer, W., Mårtens, S., and Sjöqvist, F., 1969, A comparative study of the metabolism of desmethylimipramine, nortriptyline and oxyphenylbutazone in man. *Clin. Pharmacol. Therap.* **10**: 44–49.

Kragh-Sørensen, P., Eggert-Hansen, C., and Åsberg, M., 1973, Plasma levels of nortriptyline in the treatment of endogenous depression. I: 113–115.

Kinetics of Drug-Drug Interactions

Malcolm Rowland

School of Pharmacy
University of California
San Francisco, California

Open any current medical journal and one is reminded that the coadministration of two or more drugs can either cause deleterious effects or lead to ineffective therapy. Those concerned with drug therapy are increasingly aware of this phenomenon but are confronted with the problem that a patient may be taking three, four, and, on occasion, even more drugs simultaneously. The computer will aid in the storage and retrieval of such information and act as a useful early warning signal, but prudent multiple drug therapy, if deemed necessary, can only be achieved with a better understanding of the nature and quantitative aspects of drug interactions. A drug interaction might broadly be defined as any reaction between one drug and another substance within or out of the body. In this review, the definition is restricted to events occurring within living systems with major emphasis on the alteration by one drug on the rate and extent of absorption, distribution, metabolism, and excretion of another. Prescott (1969) has called these "pharmacokinetic interactions" to distinguish them from the numerous interactions between drugs at their sites of action (Morrelli, 1970). This distinction is somewhat arbitrary as any or all possibilities can occur *in vivo*. The interaction may be direct, such as the competitive inhibition of drug metabolism and the displacement of a drug from binding sites, or it may be indirect. One example of the latter is the decreased renal clearance of acids, whose renal clearance is sensitive to urinary pH, produced when the urine is rendered alkaline using either the carbonic anhydrase inhibitor, acetazolamide, or sodium bicarbonate. Another example is the prolongation of the elimination half-life of lidocaine by *d*l-propranolol. The elimination of lidocaine, primarily by hepatic metabolism, is hepatic blood flow limited which propranolol diminishes (Branch *et al.*, 1972).

Many review articles (e.g., MacGregor, 1965; Melmon *et al.*, 1967; Hartshorn, 1968; and Azarnoff and Hurwitz, 1970) and books (e.g., Hansten, 1973; Martin, 1971) cover the whole array of drug interactions. While useful, many, however, are little more than topographical maps with little weighting as to the quantitative significance of any cited interaction.

Our knowledge of the pharmacokinetics of drugs in animals and man has increased substantially over the past few decades (Wagner, 1968). Models have been developed which accurately describe the concentration profile of drugs in various biological fluids following drug administration. Considerable success has also been gained in relating the kinetics of a graded pharmacologic response to a drug with its pharmacokinetics (Levy, 1966; Levy and Gibaldi, 1972). Since many drug–drug pharmacokinetic interactions are dependent on the concentration of the interacting species, the degree of interaction should also be a grade phenomenon varying with drug (and metabolite) concentrations and therefore drug administration and time. Hence, one should be able to develop predictive kinetic models for such drug interactions. Although awareness of this fact exists, there have been relatively few systematic attempts to establish these models. The careful studies on the kinetics of the interaction between salicylate and acetaminophen (Levy and Regardh, 1971) and between acetaminophen and salicylamide (Levy and Yamada, 1971) indicate some of the complexities. Sellers and Koch–Weser (1971) have discussed several quantitative aspects of the augmentation of warfarin anticoagulation induced by concomitant chloral hydrate administration, which might result from displacement of this anticoagulant from binding sites, but theirs were equilibrium rather than kinetic considerations. The intent of the present review is to illustrate how pharmacokinetic analysis leads to further insights regarding the causes, possible mechanisms, and design of future experiments aimed at elucidating various facets of drug interactions. It is also the intent to illustrate how predictive pharmacokinetic models of drug interactions can be developed, and the potential utility of such models in deciding appropriate dosage regimens when a combination of drugs is deemed a therapeutic necessity. For the most part, the examples chosen are from the author's own research experience.

Much of the interpretation of drug–drug interactions arises from careful measurements of the concentration time course of a drug or its metabolite. A decrease in drug plasma levels when administered as a single dose together with another drug could arise either from a reduction in absorption (if drug is given other than intravenously), displacement from plasma proteins, hastening of its elimination, or a combination of any or all of these possibilities. Kinetic analysis has helped greatly in the interpretation of such data and has suggested the design of further experiments. The interaction between the sparingly soluble oral antifungal agent, griseofulvin, and phenobarbital is one example. Bushfield *et al.* (1963) had noted that the plasma levels of griseofulvin following a single dose of this drug were reduced in subjects coadministered with phenobarbital. Griseofulvin is primarily *O*-demethylated to 6-demethylgriseofulvin in man, and it was proposed that phenobarbital had stimulated this oxidative pathway. Analysis by Riegelman *et al.* (1970) showed that there was no change in the elimination half-life of griseofulvin and led them to design a study to prove that phenobarbital reduced the extent of griseofulvin absorption, rather than enhanced its elimination (Fig. 1). The reduced absorption was

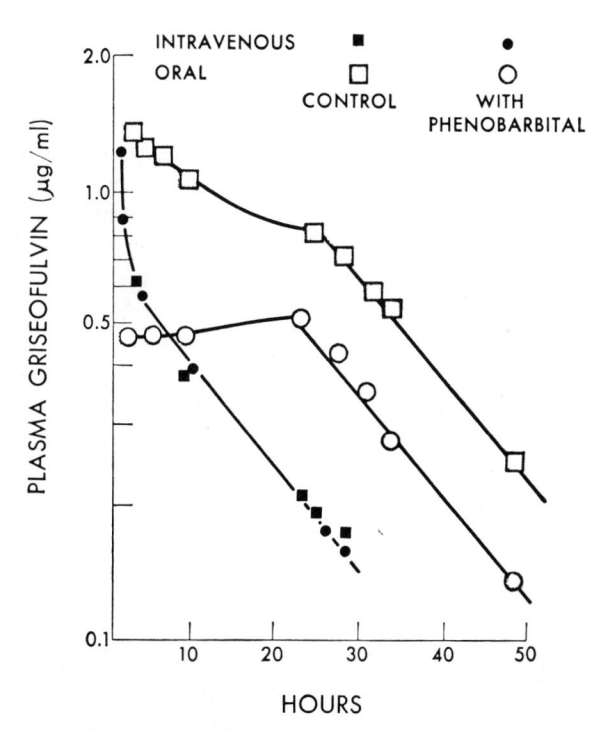

Fig. 1. Griseofulvin-phenobarbital interaction in man. Note that the disposition kinetics of griseofulvin given intravenously are unaffected by phenobarbital administration. In contrast, both the rate and extent of oral griseofulvin are depressed following phenobarbital. (Riegelman *et al., J. Amer. Med. Assoc.* **213**: 426, 1970. Reproduced with permission of the copyright authors.)

complemented by a proportional reduction in the cumulative urinary excretion of 6-demethylgriseofulvin. The mechanism of the interaction is poorly understood. Presumably, phenobarbital diminishes the rate of dissolution of this sparingly soluble and incompletely absorbed drug, perhaps by decreasing gut motility or intestinal transit time. These data would suggest that a more rapidly dissolving griseofulvin formulation should obviate the problem. Probably, by the same or a similar mechanism, barbiturates decrease the absorption of the sparingly soluble anticoagulant, dicoumarol (Aggeler and O'Reilly, 1969). Clinically, the danger arises when the barbiturate is withdrawn from a patient stabilized on this anticoagulant-barbiturate combination. In none of these studies were plasma barbiturate concentrations determined and hence it is difficult to know whether the severity of the depression of the extent of absorption of either griseofulvin or dicoumarol among or within subjects could be correlated with the amount of barbiturate in the body. Nonetheless, some relationship between the effect and the body burden of barbiturate is anticipated.

A more clearly defined and more readily modeled interaction is that between the oral hypoglycemic agent, tolbutamide, and a variety of drugs. Together with the anticoagulants, the interactions with the oral hypoglycemic agents constitute some of the most adverse clinical cases of drug interactions. Hypoglycemic crises have been reported when patients, stabilized on tolbutamide, have added sulfaphenazole, dicoumarol, phenylbutazone, or phenyramidol to their drug therapy (Christensen, 1969; Hussar, 1970). In each case cited, clear chemical data exist showing a slowing of tolbutamide elimination. Many of these interactions appear to involve inhibition of tolbutamide oxidation to hydroxytolbutamide which is virtually obligatory for tolbutamide elimination in man (Thomas and Ikeda, 1966). Hydroxytolbutamide is partially excreted unchanged and the majority is further oxidized to carboxytolbutamide which is excreted intact. The oxidation of tolbutamide is the rate-limiting step in the elimination of the drug and its metabolites. Subsequent oxidation steps are very rapid (Schulz and Schmidt, 1970). Accordingly, a short time after tolbutamide administration, the rate of excretion of the sum of the two metabolites equals the rate of tolbutamide oxidation and offers a very sensitive measure of changing tolbutamide oxidation.

The best studied interaction is that between the sulfonamide, sulfaphenazole, and tolbutamide. While not widely prescribed, sulfaphenazole is reported to increase the half-life of tolbutamide from the normal 4–8 hr to values ranging from 24–70 hr (Christensen *et al.*, 1963; Schulz and Schmidt, 1970). The clinical crises probably arise when tolbutamide accumulates upon chronic administration in the presence of sulfaphenazole. Figures 2 and 3 illustrate the situation we found when sulfaphenazole is given orally

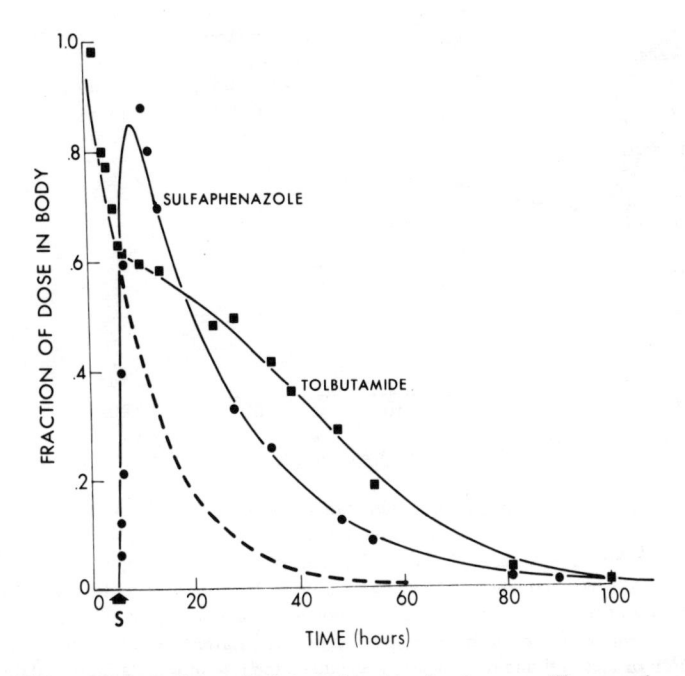

Fig. 2. Tolbutamide-sulfaphenazole interaction kinetics in man. The experimental data (tolbutamide, sulfaphenazole) and the analog computer generated curves (solid lines) describe the interaction between sulfaphenazole and tolbutamide. The subject received an i.v. bolus of 1-g tolbutamide and a 1-g oral suspension of sulfaphenazole (Sulfabid^R) 5½ hr later. For convenience the amount of the two drugs in the body is expressed as a percentage of the administered dose. The half-life of tolbutamide in the absence of sulfaphenazole is approximately 7 hr. The dotted lines depict the anticipated rapid decline of tolbutamide when administered alone. The degree of inhibition of tolbutamide oxidation continuously changes with the amount of sulfaphenazole in the body. Block is maximal at peak sulfonamide plasma levels. The half-life of sulfaphenazole in this subject is 12 hr.

to a subject approximately 5 hr after receiving an i.v. bolus of tolbutamide. Sulfaphenazole markedly prolonged tolbutamide plasma levels with an anticipated sudden drop in the excretion rate of the metabolites at maximum sulfonamide plasma levels, associated with an almost complete block of tolbutamide oxidation. The half-lives from this sharply descending portion of the hydroxy and carboxytolbutamide urinary excretion rate plot approximated the half-lives of these metabolites reported by Schulz and Schmidt, (1970). As the ratio of hydroxy to carboxytolbutamide in the urine remained unchanged in the presence of sulfaphenazole, it appears that this sulfonamide does not influence the oxidation or renal clearance of hydroxytolbutamide in the dose range studied. Separate studies by us confirmed

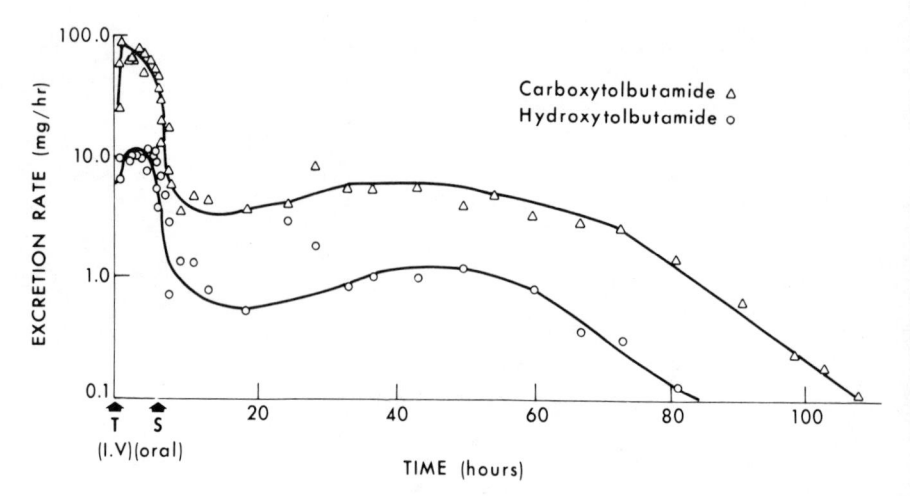

Fig. 3. Tolbutamide-sulfaphenazole interaction kinetics in man. The excretion rate data are of hydroxytolbutamide and carboxytolbutamide for the same subject whose plasma data are portrayed in Fig. 2. At peak plasma sulfaphenazole levels the inhibition of tolbutamide oxidation is almost complete and with essentially no formation of hydroxytolbutamide, the excretion rate of both this metabolite and carboxytolbutamide rapidly fall, reflecting the very short, 20–40 min, half-lives of these species. Beyond 10 hr after the tolbutamide bolus the rate of excretion of these tolbutamide metabolites equals the rate of tolbutamide oxidation. As the sulfaphenazole body levels decline the degree of inhibition of tolbutamide oxidation diminishes and the excretion rate of the metabolites increases. However, even though the inhibition continually diminishes, so also does the amount of tolbutamide in the body, and after 50 hr the excretion rate of metabolites continually declines, albeit slowly.

that tolbutamide (1 g) did not influence sulfaphenazole elimination kinetics, which is principally by N^1-glucuronidation and N^4-acetylation (Riess et al., 1965).

Human in vitro liver microsomal studies confirmed that sulfaphenazole blocks tolbutamide oxidation (Christensen, 1969), which, at least in the rabbit (Matin et al., 1973), is by competitive inhibition. The kinetics of competitive inhibition of a given metabolite step are generally given by (Gillette, 1970):

$$\text{Rate of metabolism} = \frac{V_m \cdot S}{S + K_m(1 + I/K_I)} \quad (1)$$

where V_m is the maximal velocity of the reaction, K_m is the Michaelis–Menten constant, S is the substrate concentration, I is the inhibitor concentration, and K_I is the inhibitor constant, given by the value of I which increases the apparent K_m of the system by twofold. In the particular case of tolbutamide the rate of oxidation to hydroxytolbutamide virtually equals the rate of tolbutamide elimination. Also, as tolbutamide half-life does not change over 0.5–6.0 g dose range (Duncan and Baird, 1957), the concentration of drug at the metabolic site must always be much smaller than its K_m. These facts, and knowing that in the absence of sulfaphenazole the decay of tolbutamide can be described by a first-order process, rate constant k_T, allow the following simple description for the elimination kinetics of tolbutamide in the presence of the inhibitor, sulfaphenazole:

$$\text{Rate of tolbutamide elimination} = \frac{k_T T}{1 + I/K_I} \qquad (2)$$

where T and I are the amounts of tolbutamide and sulfaphenazole in the body, and K_I may now be defined as the amount of inhibitor which diminishes the effective k_T by one-half (or prolongs the half-life twofold). By measuring all chemical species only K_I remains unknown. In the present data, an excellent fit is obtained when K_I is 200 mg sulfaphenazole (Fig. 2). This value of 200 mg is small compared to the 1–2 g daily dose usually recommended for this sulfonamide.

Knowing the K_I for sulfaphenazole and the other relevant pharmacokinetic data, the clinical situation can be modeled. Usually, 0.5 g tolbutamide and 1.0 g sulfaphenazole are given orally twice daily. Initially when only tolbutamide is given, expected plateau levels are reached within 3–4 half-lives (Rowland, 1970) or 30 hr (Fig. 4). When sulfaphenazole is also given, it accumulates and also blocks tolbutamide oxidation, causing a rise in the level of the sulfonylurea to approximately seven times its usual level. A time period of 2 or 3 days is required before this elevated tolbutamide level falls to the level in the absence of sulfaphenazole, regardless of whether only sulfaphenazole or both drugs are stopped. These data can adequately explain the elevated tolbutamide levels seen when these two drugs are administered concomitantly for extended periods (Christensen et al., 1963; Christensen, 1969).

The exact estimate for the new half-life of tolbutamide, and the degree of accumulation in the presence of a steady level of the inhibitor, is gained from two equations (Wagner, 1965):

$$\overline{A} = \frac{1.44 \times \text{Dose} \times \text{Half-life}}{\text{Dosing interval}} \qquad (3)$$

where $\overline{A}$ is the average amount of drug in the body at the plateau. The new steady-state tolbutamide half-life is

$$t_{1/2(\text{inhibited})} = t_{1/2(\text{normal})} \times \left(1 + \frac{\text{Average amount of inhibitor at plateau}}{K_I}\right) \qquad (4)$$

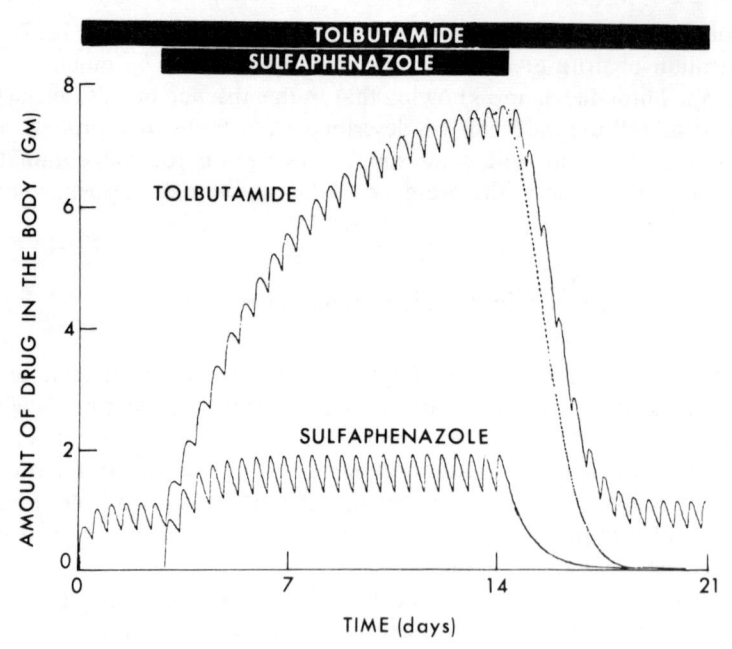

Fig. 4. Tolbutamide-sulfaphenazole interaction kinetics in man. Analog computer simulations of the clinical situation when tolbutamide (0.5 g, twice daily) is given in the absence and presence of sulphenazole (1 g twice daily). The solid black bars denote the duration of each drug regimen. Having a short half-life (4–8 hr) plateau levels of tolbutamide are reached within 2 days. The sulfaphenazole also rapidly reaches plateau concentration (half-life 10–12 hr). In the presence of sulfaphenazole, the amount of tolbutamide in the body continues to rise until output once again equals input. Upon cessation of sulfaphenazole, the decline of tolbutamide, whether continued (solid line) or stopped at the same time as sulfaphenazole (dotted line), is primarily controlled by the rate of removal of sulfaphenazole. Consequently, it takes several days before tolbutamide levels would once again fall into the accepted therapeutic range.

If sulfaphenazole ($t_{1/2}$ = 10 hr, K_I = 200 mg) (Matin *et al.*, 1973) is given 1.0 g twice daily, according to the first equation, 1.5 g is the average amount of inhibitor at the plateau and is reached within 2 days (4 × $t_{1/2}$). Substituting this amount of the inhibitor into the second equation indicates that the new half-life for tolbutamide is 7 to 8 times longer than normal (i.e., from 35–40 hr instead of 5 hr). Now it will take approximately 6 days (4 × 1.5 days) to reach the new plateau when the average amount of tolbutamide is 7 to 8 times the average plateau level in the absence of the inhibitor. It was gratifying to note that these predictions, when appropriately scaled down, were observed in a subject who received the same multiple dose schedule as depicted in Fig. 4 with the exception that 0.1 g rather than 0.5 g tolbutamide was ingested each day (Matin et al., 1973). If it were necessary to give these two drugs in combination it is apparent that the dosage schedule of tolbutamide would have to be reduced one-eighth to maintain essentially the same amount of tolbutamide in the body. In any individual the degree of interaction will depend upon the dosage regimen of each drug and the half-life for each drug, and the K_I in that individual. At this stage the variation of K_I within the population is unknown.

The elimination of tolbutamide in man is a special case of the more general situation where drug is eliminated by several instead of one pathway. Considering the more general situation, one can develop a model of drug inhibition interactions in an analogous manner to the tolbutamide-sulfaphenazole-man model. The equations are similar to those derived for schedules of drugs in patients with varying degree of renal impairment. One needs to know the fraction of the dose in the body eliminated by a particular pathway of interest in the absence of inhibitor (f_m), the amount of inhibitor (I), and the inhibitor constant (K_I). The ratio of the new half-life of the drug in the presence of inhibitor ($t_{1/2\text{inhibited}}$) to the normal half-life ($t_{1/2\text{normal}}$) and the ratio of the steady-state amount of drug after inhibition ($\overline{Ab}_{\text{inhibited}}$) and before ($\overline{Ab}_{\text{normal}}$) when a fixed regimen is administered is given by

$$R = \frac{(t_{1/2\text{inhibited}})}{(t_{1/2\text{normal}})} = \frac{\overline{Ab}_{\text{inhibited}}}{\overline{Ab}_{\text{normal}}} = \frac{1}{f_m/(1 + I/K_I) + (1 - f_m)} \quad (5)$$

The influence of f_m and I/K_I on these parameters is illustrated in Figs. 5. and 6. Unless the therapeutic index of the drug is small, an alteration in the

Fig. 5. The effect of inhibition on the ratio (R) of the new half-life of a drug in the presence of the inhibitor to the normal half-life, or to the ratio of the average amount of drug at the plateau in the absence and presence of the inhibitor. When all the drug is eliminated by the inhibited route ($f_m = 1$), the ratio changes dramatically with changes in inhibitor. Below $f_m = 0.5$, the maximum increase in the ratio is twofold and is inconsequential unless the drug has a narrow therapeutic index or the metabolite affected plays an important pharmacological role.

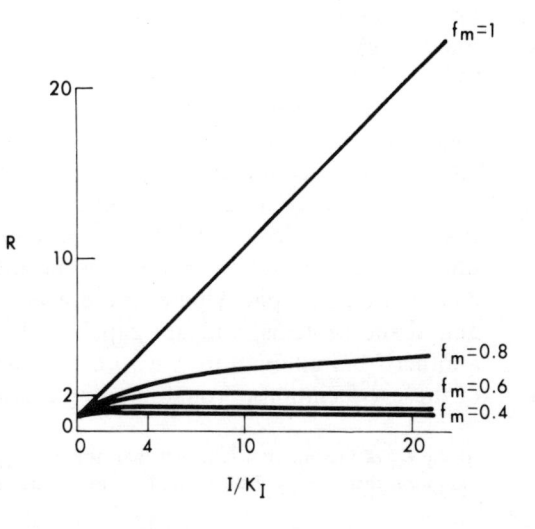

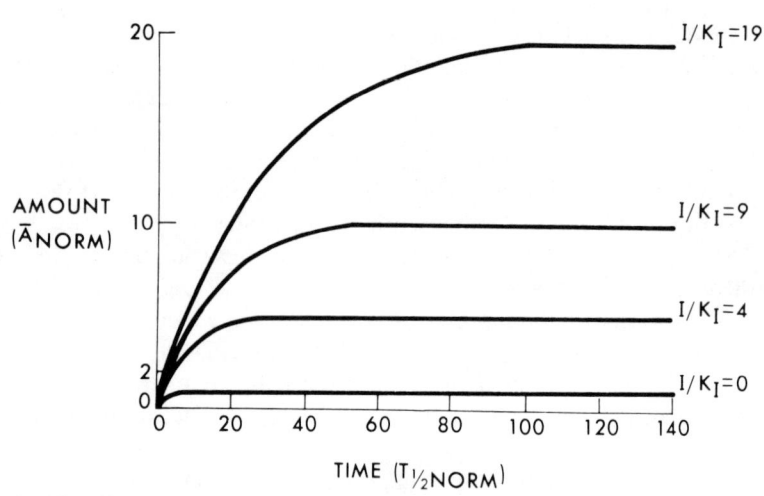

Fig. 6. The effect of inhibition on the rate of accumulation of a drug given on a fixed dose–fixed interval regimen when $f_m = 1$. Note that time for accumulation is expressed in units of the normal half-life and that the amount is expressed as a ratio of the average amount in the body in the absence of inhibitor. The more complete the block, the longer the half-life (Fig. 5) and the longer it takes to reach the new plateau. In clinical practice, toxicity may be noted before the new plateau is reached. These calculations assume that the inhibitor amount in the body is immediately attained and maintained constant.

dosage schedule of a drug is unwarranted for $f_m < 0.5$, even when inhibition of the particular pathway is complete (Fig. 5). Also, if the dosage schedule is maintained and $f_m > 0.5$, an adverse reaction may be seen before the new plateau is reached or, if seen at the plateau, it may take some time ($4 \times t_{1/2\text{ inhibited}}$) after initiation of the inhibitor regimen.* Alternatively, to prevent drug accumulation the dosage schedule of the drug will have to be reduced by $1/R$. The situation will be more complex when the concentration of drug at the metabolic site is greater than its K_m, and when both drugs are competitors of one or more of the other's pathway(s).

Tolbutamide, an acid, is significantly bound to plasma and presumably tissue proteins. Its hypoglycemic activity probably is a function of the unbound concentration in the plasma and tissue waters. Sulfaphenazole, dicoumarol, and phenylbutazone are also acids, highly bound to plasma and tissue proteins, and are capable of displacing tolbutamide and one another from albumin in *in vitro* experiments (Christensen, 1969). Because of these associations, protein binding displacement has been intimated as a

---

*If the $t_{1/2}$ of the inhibitor is longer than the new $t_{1/2}$ of the drug at the plateau level of the inhibitor, then the $t_{1/2}$ of the inhibitor controls the rate of accumulation of the drug.

contributory cause of the enhanced hypoglycemia experience when these drugs are used in combination with tolbutamide. However, in the case of tolbutamide, the contribution of displacement is probably minor compared to inhibition of oxidation, as many other sulfonamides, which displace tolbutamide from albumin *in vitro* produce neither prolongation of its half-life nor increase its effect (Christensen *et al.*, 1963; Dubach *et al.*, 1966). Nonetheless, it is worthwhile to consider when displacement will significantly influence the pharmacologic effect of a drug. To answer this question, one must know whether displacement is from both plasma and tissue proteins, whether drug clearance depends on the total (bound and unbound) or unbound plasma concentrations and whether the drug is given on a single occasion or continually.

Appreciable drug displacement occurs when a major portion of the same binding sites are occupied by the displacing agent. Consequently, to displace drugs from plasma albumin requires that the plasma concentration of the displacer approaches or exceeds 0.6 mM, the concentration of plasma albumin. For a substance of molecular weight of 300, this corresponds to 180 mg/L. These plasma concentrations are seen with sulfonamides and salicylates, which are commonly given in gram doses and which possess small volumes of distribution. They are also reached with phenylbutazone. Although the normal dose of this anti-inflammatory agent is 100 mg, owing to its long half-life, phenylbutazone accumulates to well over 1 g in the body when given three times daily.

Plasma concentrations exceeding 0.6 mM are also probably achieved following the rapid intravenous bolus ($<$ 10 sec) of quite modest doses. These events are likely fleeting, however, as displacer mixes with the vascular system and distributes out into the tissues. The rapid injection of even larger doses ($>$ 14 mg/kg) of drugs which reside primarily in plasma, may still only produce significant rises in the unbound concentration transistently as displaced drug moves down the newly created concentration gradient out into the large tissue water space (McQueen and Wardell, 1971). Indeed, as the following calculation will show, drug displacement is unlikely to be clinically significant unless it is displaced from and substantially bound to both plasma and tissue binding sites. Thus, the fraction of drug in the body bound to plasma proteins is $3\beta/V_d$, where 3 is the plasma volume in liters, V_d the volume of distribution of the drug, also expressed in liters, and β is the fraction of drug in plasma bound to plasma proteins. For a drug like the anticoagulant warfarin, which is highly bound ($\beta = 0.995$) and with a very small V_d, around 10 L, this means that as much as 30% in the body resides on the plasma proteins. Nonetheless, even if it were completely displaced off its plasma binding sites ($\beta \rightarrow 0$), with a dramatic drop in the total plasma concentration, this 30% added to the remaining

70% would only increase the unbound concentration in the body 42%. This increase is small compared to the normal changes in the unbound concentration as drug is eliminated. Any substantial increase in unbound concentration above that anticipated from plasma displacement automatically implies that tissue binding is significant and that displacement from these sites must also have occurred.

The preceding comments refer to situations where the drug is given only once in the absence or presence of the suspected displacer. In drug therapy it is more common to give both drug and displacer on a multiple dose regimen. The changes in the unbound concentration (C_f) depend on whether drug clearance depends on C_f or total plasma concentration (C_p). Upon a constant drug intake (R^0), the steady state plasma concentration ($C_{p_{ss}}$) is defined by

$$R^0 = CL C_{p_{ss}} \qquad (6)$$

where CL is the clearance of the drug, or

$$R^0 = CL \frac{C_{f_{ss}}}{\alpha} \qquad (7)$$

where α is the fraction of drug unbound in plasma. For drugs which are solely cleared by glomerular filtration or for drugs which have very low extraction ratios across the liver, clearance is dependent on the unbound plasma concentration such that

$$CL = CL_{\max} \cdot \alpha \qquad (8)$$

where $CL_{\max}$ is either the glomerular filtration rate or the maximum metabolic clearance when $\alpha = 1$. Displacement, by increasing α, increases clearance. But, substitution of Eq. (8) into Eq. (6)

$$R^0 = CL_{\max} C_{f_{ss}} \qquad (9)$$

indicates that at steady state, when rate out balances rate in, the unbound concentration should be constant and independent on the degree of protein binding. Between steady states, the unbound concentration may be greater or lesser than the $C_{f_{ss}}$, depending upon whether the concentration of the displacing agent is rising or falling. In those cases where changes in the displacing agent are slow, relative to the elimination kinetics of the displaced drug, the drug may be regarded as being at pseudosteady state. Then, upon constant drug therapy, the unbound concentration (and presumably pharmacologic effect) should remain constant and apparently unaffected by the displacing agent.

Both lidocaine (Rowland et al., 1971) and penicillin G are appreciably bound to plasma proteins ($\beta > 0.5$) and yet each is highly cleared by the liver and kidney, respectively. Evidently removal of unbound drug is so effective that the drug–protein complex dissociates almost completely before leaving the eliminating organ. For drugs like these, which have an extraction ratio approaching one, clearance is unaffected by protein binding and for a given constant input (R^0), $C_{p_{ss}}$ must be the same regardless of the degree of binding [cf, Eq. (6)]. However, now $C_{f_{ss}}$ (and presumably activity) will increase dramatically with drug displacement [Eq. (7)].

In practice, the situation can be much more complicated than that envisioned during the foregoing theoretical discussion. An excellent example is the potentiation of the anticoagulant effect of warfarin in patients receiving phenylbutazone (Aggeler et al., 1967). Warfarin is very highly bound to albumin and tissue sites, and the pharmacologic effect probably is related to the unbound circulating drug. Phenylbutazone can displace warfarin from albumin *in vitro* (Solomon and Schrogie, 1967) and this displacement has been suggested as the cause of phenylbutazone augmentation of warfarin activity *in vivo*. Indeed, when subjects receiving phenylbutazone ingest a single dose of warfarin, the percent of warfarin unbound in plasma increases from a control value of 0.4% to 1.0% (personal observation). However, the effects on warfarin disposition by phenylbutazone are far more complex (Fig. 7). These data suggest an additional mechanism for phenylbutazone potentiation (Lewis, R. J., et al., submitted for publication). Warfarin is administered as a racemic mixture. The more potent isomer is eliminated primarily by oxidation to 7-hydroxywarfarin and is partially reduced to the SS warfarin alcohol (alcohol 2). The less potent R warfarin is primarily reduced to the RS (alcohol 1) (Lewis et al., 1973). Present chemical assays measure the sum of S and R warfarin in plasma, while the pharmacologic effect primarily reflects the S warfarin concentration. The decreased production of the 7-hydroxywarfarin and increased production of the alcohol 1 (Fig. 7) prompted the suggestion that phenylbutazone (or its metabolites) might, in addition to displacement, slow S warfarin and hasten R warfarin elimination. Hence, this interaction may alter the isomeric composition and potency of the drug in plasma, without materially changing the total concentration–time profile of the mixture.

The warfarin-phenylbutazone interaction study stresses the importance of measuring metabolites as well as intact drug. Pharmacokinetic analysis aids in the interpretation of this information. At present, one cannot model the expected chemical and pharmacologic sequelae resulting from this interaction. Nonetheless, it is hoped that with careful experimental design the quantitative interrelationships can be ascertained. Then, when consid-

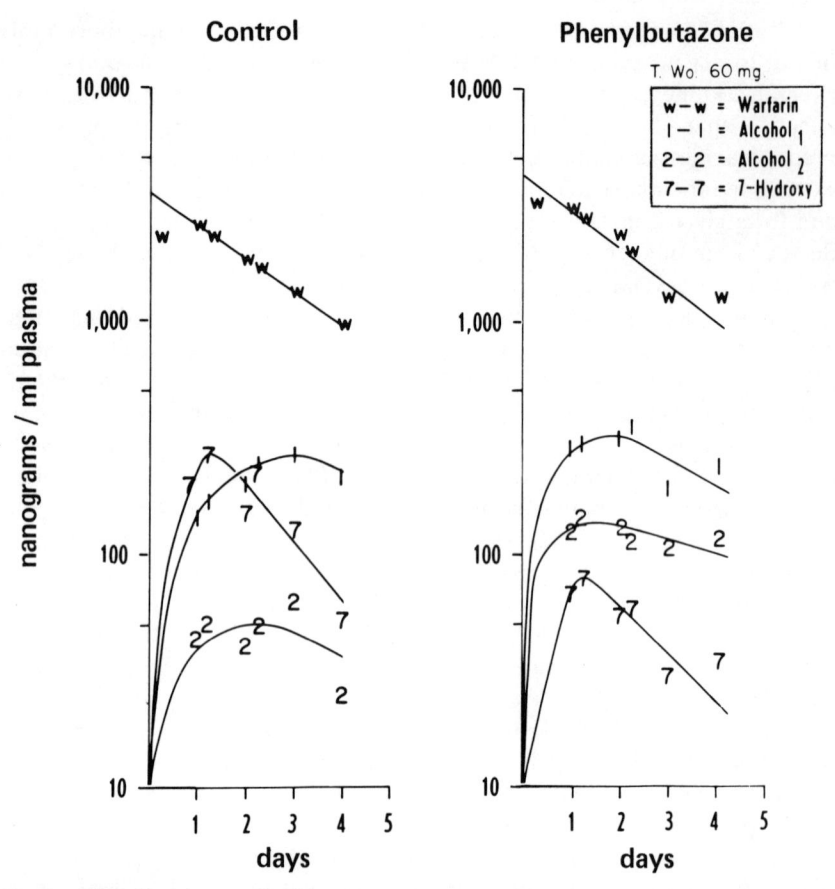

Fig. 7. Phenylbutazone-warfarin interaction in man. In this subject the total plasma warfarin concentration did not change, but the metabolite pattern did. Production of 7-hydroxywarfarin was depressed, but production and elimination of Alcohol 1 was increased (courtesy J. R. Lewis).

ered necessary, appropriate dosage schedules of two such drugs in combination may be predicted that would achieve the desired therapeutic response with minimal toxicity.

ACKNOWLEDGMENT

Much of the work reported in this manuscript was supported by a grant from the National Institutes of Health, Bethesda, Maryland, NIGMS 16496.

REFERENCES

Aggeler, P. M., O'Reilly, R. A., Leong, L., and Kowitz, P., 1967, *New Engl. J. Med.* **271**: 496.
Aggeler, P. M., and O'Reilly, R. A., 1969, *J. Lab. Clin. Med.* **74**: 229–238.
Azarnoff, D. L., and Hurwitz, A., 1970, *Pharmacology for Physicians* **4**.
Branch, R. A., Shand, D. G., Wilkinson, G. R., and Nies, A. S., 1973, *J. Pharm. Exp. Therap.* **184**: 515–519.
Bushfield, D., Child, K. J., Atkinson, R. M., 1963, *Lancet* **2**: 1042–1043.
Christensen, L. K., 1969, Third International Diabetic Symposium. Pharmacokinetics and Mode of Action of Oral Hypoglycemic Agents, Capri. *Acta Diabetologica Lat.* **6** (Supp. 1), 143.
Christensen, L. K., Hansen, J. M., and Kristensen, M., 1963, *Lancet* **2**: 1298.
Dubach, U. C., Bückert, A., and Raaflaub, J., 1966, *Schweiz. Med. Wochscr.* **96**, 1483.
Duncan, L. J. P., and Baird, J. D., 1957, *Scot. Med. J.* **2**: 171.
Gillette, J., 1971, *Fundamentals of Drug Metabolism and Disposition*, Chapter 19 (La Du, B. N., Mandel, H. G., and Way, E. L. eds.), William and Wilkins, Baltimore.
Hansten, P. D., 1973, *Drug Interactions*, 2nd Edition, Lea and Febiger, Philadelphia.
Hartshorn, E. A., 1968, *Drug Intelligence* **2**: 174.
Hussar, D. A., 1970, *J. Am. Pharm. Assoc.* **NS 10**: 619.
Levy, G., 1966, *Clin. Pharmacol. Therap.* **7**: 362–372.
Levy, G., and Gibaldi, M., 1972, *Ann. Rev. Pharmacol.* **12**: 85–97.
Levy, G., and Yamada, H., 1971, *J. Pharm. Sci.* **60**: 215.
Levy, G., and Regardh, C., 1971, *J. Pharm. Sci.* **60**: 608.
Lewis, R. J., Trager, W. F., Chan, K. K., Breckenridge, A., Orme, M., Rowland, H., and Schory, W., 1974 (submitted for publication).
MacGregor, A. G., 1965, *Proc. Royal Soc. Med.* **58**: 943.
Matin, S. B., Karam, J., Rowland, M. (submitted for publication).
Martin, E. W., 1971, *Hazards of Medication*. J. B. Lippincott and Co., Philadelphia.
Melmon, K., Morelli, H. F., Oates, J. A., Conney, A. H., Tozer, T. N., Harpole, B. P., and Clark, T. H., 1967, *Patient Care*, Nov., 1.
McQueen, E. G., and Wardell, W. M., 1971, *Brit. J. Pharmacol.* **43**: 312.
Morrelli, H. F., 1970, *Drug Interactions in Clinical Pharmacology*, Chapter 17 (Melmon, K. H. and Morrelli, H. F. eds), MacMillan Press, Washington.
Prescott, L. F., 1969, *Lancet, N. American Ed.* **2**: 1239.
Riess, W., Schmid, K., and Keberle, H., 1965, *Klin. Wochschr.* **43**: 740.
Riegelman, S., Rowland, M., and Epstein, W. L., 1970, *J. Am. Med. Assoc.* **213**: 426–431.
Rowland, M., Thomson, P., Melmon, K. H., and Guichard, A., 1971, *Ann. N.Y. Acad. Sci.* **179**: 383–398.
Rowland, M., 1970, *Clinical Pharmacology*, Chapter 2 (Melmon, K. H. and Morrelli, H. F., eds), MacMillan Press, Washington.
Sellers, E. M., and Koch-Weser, J., 1971, *Ann. N.Y. Acad. Sci.* **179**: 213–225.
Schulz, E., and Schmidt, F. H., 1970, *Pharmacol. Clin.* **2**: 150.
Solomon, H. M., and Schrogie, J. J., 1967, *Biochem. Pharmacol.* **16**: 1219.
Thomas, R. C., and Ikeda, C. J., 1966, *J. Med. Chem.* **9**: 507.
Wagner, J. G., Northam, J. I., Alway, C. D., and Carpenter, O. S., 1965, *Nature* **207**: 1301–1303.
Wagner, J. G., 1968. *Ann. Rev. Pharmacol.* **8**: 61.

DISCUSSION SUMMARY

The discussion was opened by Teorell who inquired whether the study subjects were normal or diabetic and how the observed drug interactions might affect therapy in diabetic patients. Rowland's research involved normal volunteers, but he pointed out that the type of inhibitory effect observed in such test subjects fits very well with earlier data found in diabetic patients. Further investigation is needed to determine the variability in K_i (inhibition constant) values among individual subjects.

Levy reiterated an important point concerning the effect of slowed elimination on the accumulation kinetics of drugs. When the elimination rate of a drug is decreased, either by inhibition of biotransformation by a second compound or because of dose-dependent kinetics, both the plateau level and the time required to reach the new plateau will increase more than proportionately to an increase in drug dosage. This has been demonstrated for salicylate and is of considerable importance in clinical pharmacokinetics.

Berman related his experiences in use of a comprehensive model describing ^{131}I kinetics to analyze the effect of lithium in treating patients with thyrotoxicosis. Measurements were made of label in the thyroid, urine, and plasma, as well as stable iodine levels. Lithium, at serum levels of about 1 mEq/L, decreased the loss of label from the thyroid which led to a fall both in serum concentrations and urinary excretion of ^{131}I. Analysis of the experimental data with a pharmacokinetic model based on numerous kinetic studies in man under various abnormal conditions revealed that lithium acts primarily by inhibition of thyroglobulin hydrolysis. These results emphasize the importance and power of building models and accumulating libraries of models for use until enough confidence is gained to permit very careful testing of hypotheses for the actions of drugs.

Segre argued for the use of steady-state levels of drugs in evaluating the effects of drug interactions. This approach allows examination of the net result of the interaction at constant levels of the inhibitor and overcomes complications arising from time-dependence in distribution or elimination of either the primary compound or the inhibitor. Rowland acknowledged that use of steady-state drug levels works extremely well in animals, but in human clinical pharmacokinetics, when one is trying to gain as much information as possible from a minimum number of studies, the application of this method is more difficult.

Dedrick pointed out the possibility of drug interactions among environmental contaminants. Some of these, such as DDT or methyl mercury, have extraordinarily high lipid solubility or protein binding constants, and their environmental accumulation takes place over months and years. Sudden interaction of these accumulated materials with more recently designed compounds such as chelating agents or detergents may lead to serious ecological consequences.

Garratini continued this point by describing an actual site of drug interaction which can occur for drugs which are highly lipid soluble. For a compound such as penfluridal, an appreciable fraction of the body content of the compound is stored in adipose tissue. Drugs such as salicylates which are capable of inducing changes in lipidolysis, or the conditions of fasting versus meal ingestion, can alter the amount of lipid-incorporated penfluridal, in turn modifying the quantity of drug available to the rest of the body. Rowland noted that DDT is also highly accumulated in lipids, and changes in lipidolysis could be a similar problem in this instance.

Plaa inquired whether any other sulfonamide derivatives show an inhibitory effect on tolbutamide metabolism. Rowland didn't think this interaction was characteristic of the sulfonamide group itself. It is a function of the furazole ring and is likely to be restricted to analogs of sulfaphenazole. Azarnoff cautioned that a practicing physician, in selecting one drug from a series of compounds having similar pharmacologic effects, should be cognizant of their chemical structures when the existence of a drug interaction has been demonstrated with particular analogs of these agents.

Gillette commented on the problem of feedback mechanisms which involve endogenous steroid in considering the effects of compounds capable of inducing drug metabolizing enzymes. Phenobarbital treatment increases the rate of metabolism of corticoids but the steady-state level of the corticoids is not changed because of a hypothalamic feedback process which increases ACTH levels. This, in turn, maintains normal plasma levels of the corticoids. Similarly, when animals are treated with methyltestosterone, the natural synthesis of testosterone is reduced markedly, presumably resulting in a less than expected overall effect of the compound.

Comparative Pharmacokinetics of the Anticoagulant Effect of Coumarin Drugs in Man and Rat

Gerhard Levy

Department of Pharmaceutics, School of Pharmacy
State University of New York at Buffalo
Buffalo, New York

The coumarin anticoagulants are a particularly interesting group of drugs for pharmacokinetic study because their concentration in plasma or serum and their anticoagulant effect can be readily measured. In addition, these drugs are widely used and subject to many clinically important interactions with other drugs. Our interest in the pharmacokinetics of warfarin and dicumarol was stimulated largely by the classical investigations by O'Reilly *et al.* (1970) and by a collaborative study with him seven years ago (O'Reilly *et al.*, 1966). We became very intrigued by the unusual dose-dependence of the kinetics of dicumarol elimination in man (O'Reilly *et al.*, 1964) and by the fact that the temporal pattern of the anticoagulant effect of the coumarin drugs *appears* to lag considerably behind the concentrations of these drugs in the plasma. Since nonlinear kinetics of drug elimination (Levy, 1968; Levy *et al.*, 1972; Tsuchiya and Levy, 1972) and kinetics of drug action (Levy, 1966; Levy, 1973) are among our major areas of research, it was only natural to focus on both of these aspects as they pertain to the coumarin anticoagulants. The research on the dose-dependent kinetics of dicumarol elimination has been described in a series of six publications from 1968 (Nagashima *et al.*, 1968) to 1969 (Levy and Nagashima, 1969) and has now been expanded to a general consideration of the role of product inhibition in the dose-dependent elimination of drugs that are subject to hydroxylation (Levy *et al.*, 1972). To be described here are the results of some of our studies on the kinetics of the anticoagulant effect of warfarin and dicumarol in man and rats.

KINETICS OF THE ANTICOAGULANT EFFECT OF WARFARIN IN MAN

The maximum decrease of prothrombin complex activity (PCA) in normal human subjects occurs about two days after administration of a single dose of warfarin. This lag seems unusual unless it is realized that PCA is a function of the rates of synthesis and degradation of various clotting factors and that warfarin (like the other coumarin anticoagulants) inhibits the synthesis of the vitamin K dependent clotting factors II, VII, IX, and X, but that it has no effect on their degradation. Consequently, a possible relationship between drug concentration and effect had to be sought by focusing on the "real" effect of the drug, i.e., on the inhibition of the synthesis of vitamin K-dependent clotting factors. Considering the complexity of the blood clotting process and the limited knowledge of its details, this could have been a formidable task. We elected to try a

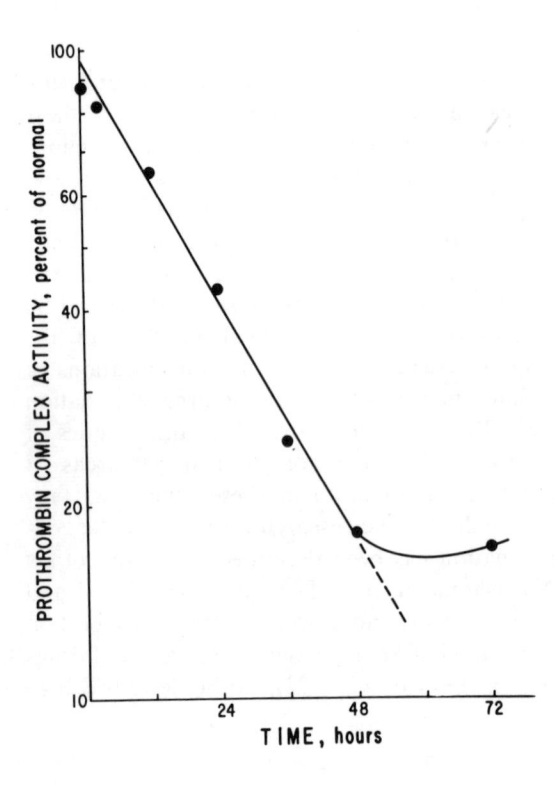

Fig. 1. Plasma prothrombin complex activity in a normal subject as a function of time after oral administration of sodium warfarin, 1.5 mg/kg body weight (from Nagashima, O'Reilly, and Levy, 1969).

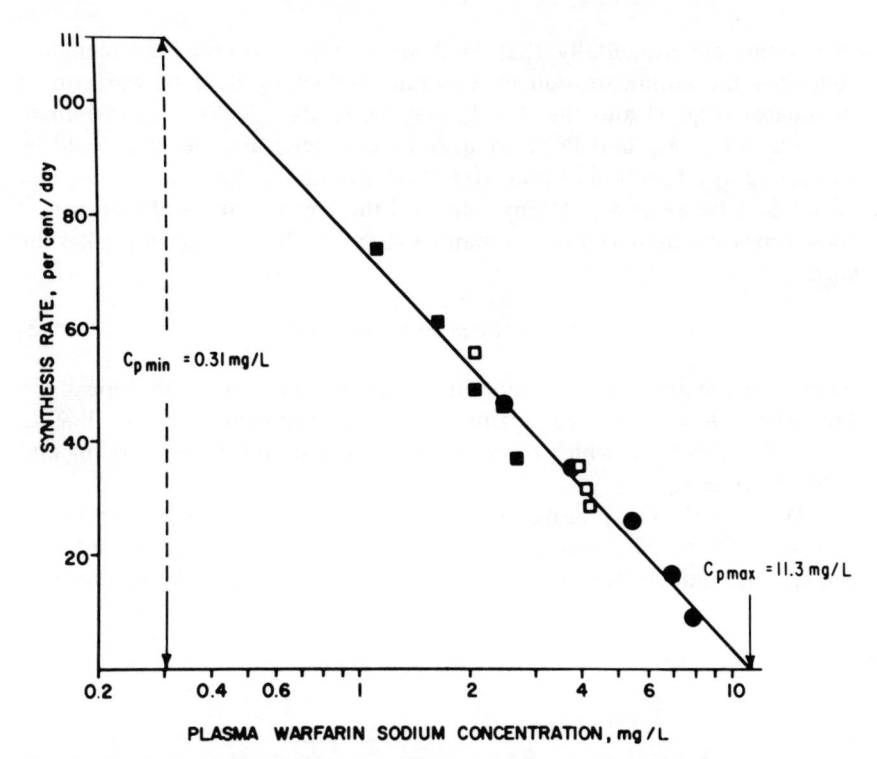

Fig. 2. Synthesis rate of prothrombin complex activity as a function of plasma-warfarin concentration, based on the averaged data from six normal subjects. Sodium warfarin dosing schedules: ●, a single dose of 1.5 mg/kg; ■ 10 mg daily for five days; □, 15 mg daily for four days. All doses were given orally (from Nagashima, O'Reilly, and Levy, 1969).

pharmacokinetic approach where the synthesis and degradation of the several clotting factors are treated as two overall processes (Nagashima *et al*, 1969). Thus, the rate of change of PCA (R_{net}) was considered to be a function of the "rate of PCA synthesis" (R_{syn}) and the "rate of PCA degradation" (R_{deg}):

$$R_{net} = R_{syn} - R_{deg} \tag{1}$$

We also assumed that the degradation of PCA is an apparent first-order process

$$R_{deg} = k_d(\text{PCA}) \tag{2}$$

where k_d is the apparent first-order degradation rate constant. Substituting for R_{deg} in Eq. (1) and rearranging yields

$$R_{syn} = R_{net} + k_d(\text{PCA}) \tag{3}$$

We found experimentally that PCA does indeed decline exponentially following the administration of a synthesis-blocking dose of warfarin or dicumarol (Fig. 1) and that the k_d may be readily determined in human subjects. Since R_{net} and PCA are also directly determinable, R_{syn} could be calculated as a function of time after warfarin administration. An excellent correlation between R_{syn} at any time and the concentration of warfarin at these times was achieved in this manner (Fig. 2). This relationship takes the form

$$R_{syn} = \text{Constant} - m \log C \qquad (4)$$

where C is the drug concentration in the plasma and $-m$ is the slope of the line where R_{syn} is plotted against log C. Extrapolation of this line to $R_{syn} = 0$ yields C_{max}, which is another useful constant for summarizing and comparing data.

We tested our pharmacokinetic model by perturbing one of its components, the elimination rate constant of warfarin. Pretreatment with the enzyme inducer heptabarbital increased the warfarin elimination rate

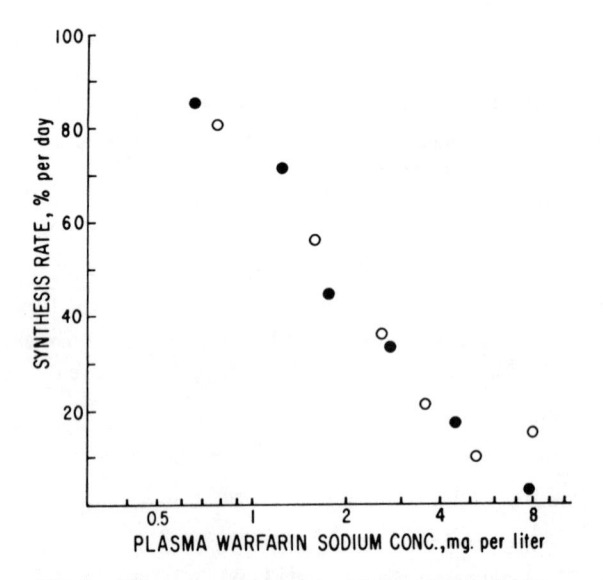

Fig. 3. Effect of pretreatment with heptabarbital (400 mg daily for 10 days) on the relationship between synthesis rate of prothrombin complex activity and plasma-warfarin concentration in a normal subject. ○, control (warfarin half-life, 46 hr); ● with heptabarbital (warfarin half-life, 36 hr) (from Levy, O'Reilly, Aggeler, and Keech, 1970).

constant in most subjects but had no effect on the relationship between R_{syn} and log C (Levy et al., 1970). An example of our results is shown in Fig. 3.

RELATIONSHIP BETWEEN THE ANTICOAGULANT ACTIVITY OF RACEMIC WARFARIN AND THAT OF ITS INDIVIDUAL ENANTIOMERS

It was obviously desirable to test our pharmacokinetic model for the anticoagulant effect of warfarin not only on subjects receiving one or a few doses of the drug, but also on patients being treated with warfarin for long periods of time. Before such a study could be undertaken it was necessary to consider the implications of the fact that warfarin, as used in the clinic, is a racemic mixture of two enantiomers, (+) (R) warfarin and (−) (S) warfarin. Investigations in rats have shown that both enantiomers are active, (−) (S) warfarin being more potent, and that they are eliminated at different rates (Eble et al., 1966; Breckenridge and Orme, 1972; Hewick, 1972). Similar differences were observed by O'Reilly in man (O'Reilly, 1973). If the two enantiomers are eliminated at different rates, then their concentration ratio in the plasma will change with time. Consequently, the relationship between R_{syn} and log C (where C is the sum of the concentrations of both enantiomers) will also change with time. To account for these possible changes it became necessary to determine the relationship between the anticoagulant activity of the individual enantiomers and that of the racemic mixture (Levy et al., to be published). Administration of the individual enantiomers and determination of their concentrations in the plasma as a function of time yields the necessary data to characterize the kinetics of their elimination. Concomitant determinations of PCA make it possible to establish the relationship between R_{syn} and log C for each enantiomer. To predict the relationship between R_{syn} and log C after administration of racemic warfarin, the plasma concentrations of each enantiomer as a function of time are calculated on the basis of their individual elimination rate constants. Then one determines from the R_{syn} − log C relationship (a) the R_{syn} for the concentration of the (−) (S) enantiomer (R_{syn}^1), (b) the concentration (C^1) of the (+) (R) enantiomer equivalent to R_{syn}^1, and finally (c) the R_{syn} for the sum of C^1 and the concentration of the (+) (R) enantiomer at each time.[*] Excellent agreement has been achieved between the thus predicted relationship of R_{syn} and log C for single doses of racemic warfarin and actual experimental results (Fig.

[*] One may also proceed in opposite order, i.e., from (+) (R) to (−) (S). If the two R_{syn} vs. log C regression lines are parallel, the results will be identical. Otherwise, the results will differ slightly, depending on the difference in the slopes.

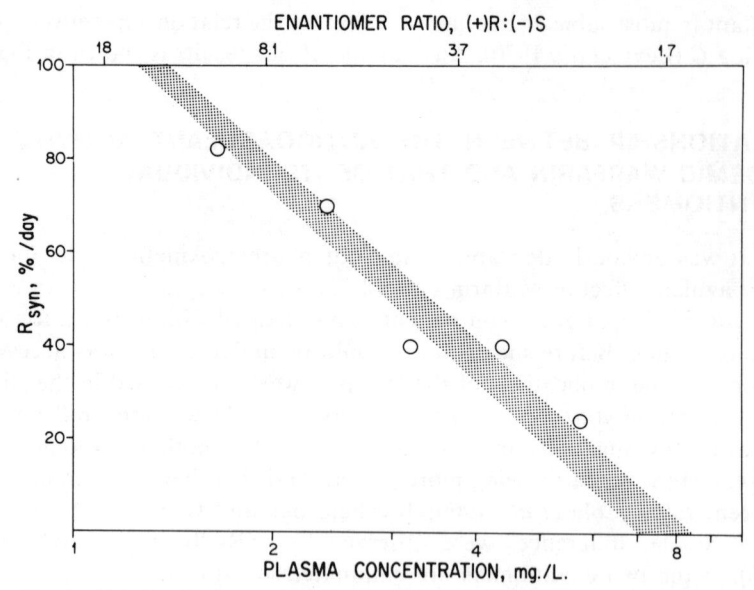

Fig. 4. Relationship between synthesis rate of prothrombin complex activity and plasma-warfarin concentration after oral administration of 1.5 mg/kg racemic sodium warfarin. Shaded line: predicted relationship based on experiments with the individual enantiomers; O, experimental data on racemic warfarin in the same subject.

4). This pharmacokinetic approach may also be useful, in principle, for determining the time course of action of racemic mixtures of other drugs.

KINETICS OF ANTICOAGULANT EFFECT OF MAN IN DICUMAROL

Pharmacokinetic analysis of the anticoagulant effect of dicumarol in man was accomplished by the same methods as were used with warfarin (O'Reilly and Levy, 1970). A typical example of the relationship between R_{syn} and the logarithm of the plasma concentration of dicumarol is shown in Fig. 5. Interestingly, three of the eleven normal subjects in the study exhibited an unusually steep relationship between R_{syn} and log C (Fig. 6 and Table I). This may have important clinical implications; if some patients on dicumarol therapy are similar "steep" responders it will be difficult to maintain their blood clotting times in a safe and effective range. We suspect that the steep R_{syn} − log C relationship may be due to unusual distributional characteristics of dicumarol in the affected individuals. To study this and other distributional effects (such as drug interactions involving displacement of dicumarol from binding sites in the plasma and tissues) in greater detail, it is desirable to have a suitable animal model.

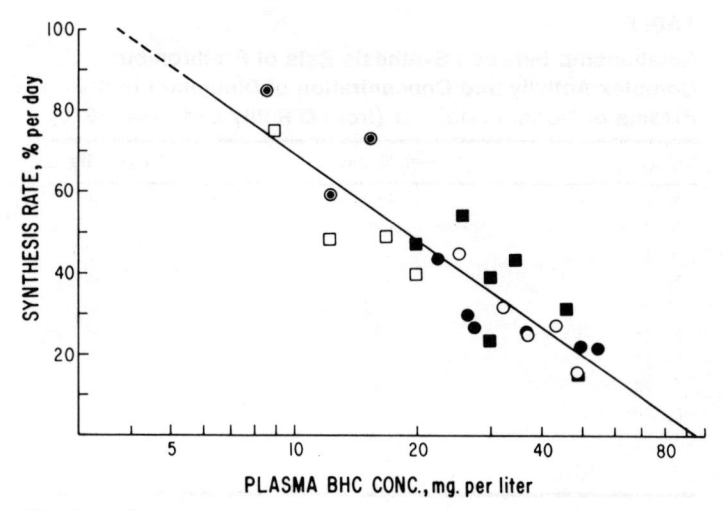

Fig. 5. Relationship between synthesis rate and plasma-dicumarol (BHC) concentration in a normal subject given a 600 mg dose. ○, orally on 7-11-66; ⊙, orally on 8-1-1966; ●, intravenously on 3-6-1967; □, orally after heptabarbital treatment on 8-19-1966; ■, intravenously after heptabarbital treatment on 2-10-1967 (from O'Reilly and Levy, 1970).

KINETICS OF ANTICOAGULANT EFFECT OF DICUMAROL IN RATS

We have been able to develop special techniques to determine the PCA and dicumarol concentration in the plasma as a function of time in individual rats (Wingard and Levy, 1972). The pharmacokinetic methods used to analyze the human data worked equally well in rats. Figure 7 shows

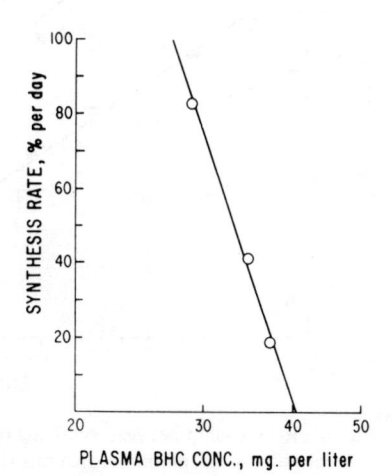

Fig. 6. Unusually steep relationship between anticoagulant effect and plasma-dicumarol (BHC) concentration in a normal subject (from O'Reilly and Levy, 1970).

TABLE I
Relationship between Synthesis Rate of Prothrombin Complex Activity and Concentration of Dicumarol in the Plasma of Normal Subjects (from O'Reilly and Levy, 1970)

Subjects	$-m$, %/day	C_{max}, mg/L
N-1	59	56
N-2	99	68
N-3	127	92
N-17	115	44
N-18	582	40
N-25	71	135
N-27	242	65
N-28	82	80
N-29	150	51
N-31	75	86
N-32	231	57

two typical examples of the relationship between R_{syn} and log C for dicumarol in rats. Interestingly, we found that two out of seven rats were also "steep" responders (Table II) so that we will be able to investigate the mechanism of this phenomenon in some detail. There are some quantitative differences between man and rat (Table III). For example, the k_d is five times higher in the rat than in man, showing that the rat eliminates clotting

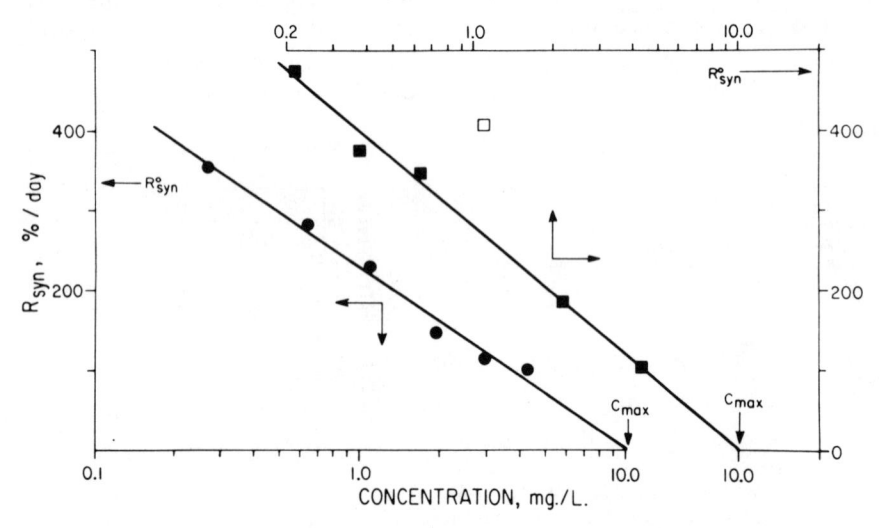

Fig. 7. Relationship between synthesis rate of prothrombin complex activity and dicumarol concentration in the plasma of two rats (from Wingard and Levy, 1972).

TABLE II
Relationship between Synthesis Rate of Prothrombin Complex Activity and Dicumarol Concentration in the Plasma of Adult Male Sprague–Dawley Rats (Wingard and Levy, 1972)

Animal	$-m$, %/day	C_{max}, mg/L
6–1	252	12.2
6–3	224	10.6
6–4	213	6.3
3–3	279	10.2
3–5	370	9.4
3–1	1403	11.0
3–9	1190	10.8

TABLE III
Comparison of k_d Values, and of m and C_{max} Values for Dicumarol in Man and Rats

Species	k_d, days^{-1}	$-m$, %/day	C_{max}, mg/L
Man	1.05 (0.72–1.85)	— (59 to 582)	70 (40–135)
Rat	4.98 (3.96–6.40)	— (213 to 1403)	10 (6.3–12)

factors much more rapidly. Also, C_{max} in the rat is one-seventh that in man. We believe that this is largely due to the more extensive protein binding of dicumarol in human plasma. For example, perfusion of isolated rat livers with human plasma containing 75μg dicumarol per ml yielded a dicumarol concentration of about 0.055 mg/g of liver. The same dicumarol concentration in the liver was obtained with only one-third the plasma concentration (28 μg/ml) when the rat liver was perfused with rat plasma (Nagashima et al., 1968).

CONCLUSIONS

The pharmacokinetic characterizations described here are examples of how one may analyze the time course of an indirect effect (lowering of prothrombin complex activity) having no *apparent* relationship to the drug concentrations in the plasma. Resolution of the data into measures of the "direct" effect (inhibition of synthesis of clotting factors) permits excellent correlation between effect and drug concentration. The parallel development of a suitable animal model has provided the opportunity to study the pharmacokinetics of the anticoagulant effect of the coumarin drugs and of their interactions with other drugs not only in plasma but also at the tissue level. Focusing on the kinetics of drug distribution and elimination as well as on the kinetics of drug action, and carrying out concomitant studies in man and animals (using one to guide or supplement research on the other) provides the necessary dimensions for comprehensive pharmacokinetic investigations.

REFERENCES

Breckenridge, A., and Orme, M., 1972, *Life Sci.* **11**: 337.
Eble, J. N., West, B. D., and Link, K. P., 1966, *Biochem. Pharmacol.* **15**: 1003.
Hewick, D. S., 1972, *J. Pharm. Pharmacol.* **24**: 661.
Levy, G., 1966, *Clin. Pharmacol. Therap.* **7**: 362.
Levy, G., 1968, in: *Importance of Fundamental Principles in Drug Evaluation* (Tedeschi, D. H., and Tedeschi, R. E., eds.) Raven Press, New York.
Levy, G., 1973, *Proc. Fifth Intern. Congr. Pharmacol.*, **3**: 34.
Levy, G., Ashley, J. J., Jähnchen, E., and Perrier, D., 1972, *Abstracts, 13th Nat. Mtg. A.Ph.A. Acad. Pharm. Sci.* **2**: 179.
Levy, G., and Nagashima, R., 1969, *J. Pharm. Sci.* **58**: 1001.
Levy, G., O'Reilly, R. A., Aggeler, P. M., and Keech, G. M., 1970, *Clin. Pharmacol. & Therap.* **11**: 372.
Levy, G., Tsuchiya, T., and Amsel, L. P., 1972, *Clin. Pharmacol. Therap.* **13**: 258.
Nagashima, R., Levy, G., and Nelson, E., 1968, *J. Pharm. Sci.* **57**: 58.
Nagashima, R., Levy, G., and Sarcione, E. J., 1968, *J. Pharm. Sci.* **57**: 1881.
Nagashima, R., O'Reilly, R. A., and Levy, G., 1969, *Clin. Pharmacol. Therap.* **10**: 22.
O'Reilly, R. A., 1973, *Clin. Res.* **21**: 197.
O'Reilly, R. A., and Aggeler, P. M., 1970, *Pharmacol. Rev.* **22**: 35.
O'Reilly, R. A., Aggeler, P. M., and Leong, L. S., 1964, *Thromb, Diath. Haemorrhag.* **11**: 1.
O'Reilly, R. A., and Levy, G., 1970, *Clin. Pharmacol. Therap.* **11**: 378.
O'Reilly, R. A., Nelson, E., and Levy, G., 1966, *J. Pharm. Sci.* **55**: 435.
Tsuchiya, T., and Levy, G., 1972, *J. Pharm. Sci.* **61**: 541.
Wingard, L. B., Jr., and Levy, G., 1972, *J. Pharmacol. Exp. Therap.*, **184**: 253.

DISCUSSION SUMMARY

Wagner was concerned about the decline in total warfarin plasma levels when a mixture of the (−)(R) and (+)(S) enantiomers of warfarin are administered. The data points seemed to be randomly distributed about a certain line for over two half-lives. If the enantiomers are eliminated at different rates, the points should follow a curved rather than a straight line. Levy responded that there are some patients who do show substantial differences in half-lives between the enantiomers and, indeed, a curvilinear decline in total plasma levels may occur. On the other hand, a good number of people show similar half-lives for both enantiomers and, consequently, the ratio of enantiomers in the plasma and on chronic dosing does not change significantly. This leads to the good agreement observed in anticoagulant effect following one-day and five-day warfarin dosing. However, simply knowing that there exist some subjects who will behave differently can enhance the efficacy and safety of anticoagulant therapy with these coumarins. As to the incidence of such abnormal responders, Levy replied that there are abnormal responders in the rat population just as there are for humans.

Condliffe noted that endocrinologists often face the problem of assaying the simultaneous presence of related compounds such as analogs. He suggested that the treatment used in dealing with the effects of warfarin enantiomers (see pages 343 and 344) could probably be similarly applied in such instances. Levy concurred and stated that the notion of adding effects rather than concentrations, when done in a proper manner, should be generally useful because many drugs are administered in the form of racemic mixtures.

Teorell commented that pharmacokinetics, once appearing so uncomplicated, now encounters problems involving drug metabolites, feedback mechanisms, and genetic variability. Complicated feedback schemes have been utilized by physiologists to describe blood pressure control, nerve networks, and hormone pathways. Mathematical treatments of such systems have evolved, and modern regulation theory is now called for.

Garrett submitted the following as a systematic procedure which might be generally useful in evaluating the pharmacokinetics of a drug:

- a. Intravenous administration of several dose levels of a drug in animals and analysis of every possible compartment relative to the amount of drug, drug metabolites, and their time-course, as well as the observed pharmacodynamic effect.
- b. Assumption of simple postulates (e.g., a linear three-compartment model) to functionally describe the system and its properties and examination of the model for deviations to which can be ascribed a known cause (e.g., saturation in metabolism, hepatic drug holdup).
- c. *In vitro* measurement of certain drug properties such as plasma protein binding and red cell drug uptake, and evaluation of the effects thereon of drug metabolites and inhibitors.
- d. Identification and isolation of the metabolites of a drug for toxicology studies in the same animal species and further pharmacokinetic evaluation.
- e. Study of the gastrointestinal absorption of the compound at several doses for evaluation in relation to the data obtained after intravenous injection.
- f. Search for drug interactions by rationalizing which compounds are likely to be administered concomitantly in the clinic.

In general, Garrett proposed use of the simplest model that explains all the data reasonably consistent with physiological reality. Feedback mechanisms would be called on only when needed to explain these systems.

Segre advocated further utilization of pharmacokinetics as a diagnostic tool to determine how different the patient is from the normal state and as a prognostic tool to infer the course of the disease. This might involve further utilization of transfer constants, not only for phenomenological description, but after evaluation of their intrinsic physiological and pathological meaning. A valuable approach involves perturbation of a model system, similar to inducing a disease state, whereby further study could reveal how a drug might best be administered.

Pharmacokinetics and Cancer Chemotherapy

Kenneth B. Bischoff

School of Chemical Engineering
Cornell University
Ithaca, New York

When considering a specific application of pharmacokinetics, a major consideration must be some of the other relevant aspects of the area. We will begin with a few general considerations of cancer chemotherapy in order to set the stage for the role of pharmacokinetics. This will consist of a brief description of cell kinetics and some of the biochemical events involved in cancer chemotherapy followed by a discussion of some aspects of local tissue and cell uptake of drugs. Finally, the combination of cell kinetics and pharmacokinetics will specifically focus on some recent efforts to model this behavior and compare the results with experiment. Many of these topics have not been extensively synthesized into a working quantitative description of cancer chemotherapy, especially for clinical applications. It is hoped that the description of, and references to, these areas will provide a basis for future work.

A very useful overview of the *Chemical Control of Cancer* was provided by Zubrod (1972). One significant general point was that there are about ten types (10-15% of clinical cancer) of disseminated cancer where optimum drug treatment can achieve normal life expectancy for about 50% of the patients. These tumors have a rapid doubling time of 1-4 days rather than the 100 days of more intractable tumors. These two clinical observations immediately lead to considerations of the possible importance of local uptake (disseminated *vs.* solid tumors) and/or cell kinetics aspects. These will each be considered below.

In addition to killing the cancer cells, a successful therapy must naturally avoid excessive toxicity to the normal host cells. Since no "magic bullet" that only affects the tumor and not the normal cells has been found, the only tool is to manipulate the dosage regimen. This again leads to the necessity of being able to predict the pharmacokinetic events—in extended definition to include uptake and other kinetics—in a quantitative fashion:

$$\begin{vmatrix} \text{Dosage} \\ \text{regimen} \end{vmatrix} \rightarrow \begin{vmatrix} \text{Circulatory} \\ \text{transport} \end{vmatrix} \rightarrow \begin{vmatrix} \text{Local} \\ \text{uptake} \end{vmatrix} \rightarrow \begin{vmatrix} \text{Drug effect} \\ \overline{\text{Cell kinetics}} \\ \text{biochemistry} \end{vmatrix}$$

A recent review by Mellett (1972) illustrates some of the striking differences in drug effects that must be due to the above factors. For example, the LD_{10} (I.P.) in mice for the drug cytosine arabinoside (ARA-C) is 3000 mg/kg in a single dose, but a regimen of Q3H (X8) on days 0, 4, 8, and 12 has a total dose LD_{10} = 500 mg/kg (16 mg/kg per dose). On the other hand, the drug cyclophosphamide (CTX) has a (total) LD_{50} = 300–400 mg/kg for several different dosage regimens. Therapeutic trials for the L-1210 leukemia system also showed rather large differences in effect for different schedules. These ranged from 135/155 cures ($>$ 45 days) to almost no increase in life span.

Since our purpose here is not primarily to discuss cancer chemotherapy, but rather the role of pharmacokinetics, more details will not be presented (see Mellett, 1972). However, an important point is that the above results were obtained by extensive trial-and-error experiments, and one would hope that greater knowledge will permit us to do more *prediction* of promising areas to investigate in the laboratory and clinic.

CELL KINETICS

Based on the above considerations, let us briefly consider a few necessary aspects of cell kinetics. Because of the clinical successes and also the rather extensive animal data available, we will only specifically discuss leukemia cells; a more extensive collection of information is given by Skipper (1971) for both human and animal systems.

The cell cycle is usually considered to have four phases: M (mitosis), G_1, S, and G_2. RNA and protein are synthesized in all, but new DNA is *only* synthesized in the S phase. The G_1 phase can be widely variable in length, so that cells can be in a "resting state," and, as we will see in more detail below, often not susceptible to chemotherapy. Thus, there is a distribution of generation times, or this can be stated as a certain fraction of cells essentially nonproliferative.

These effects are usually modeled by keeping track of the number of cells that have a given "biological age." This "age," of course, is the net

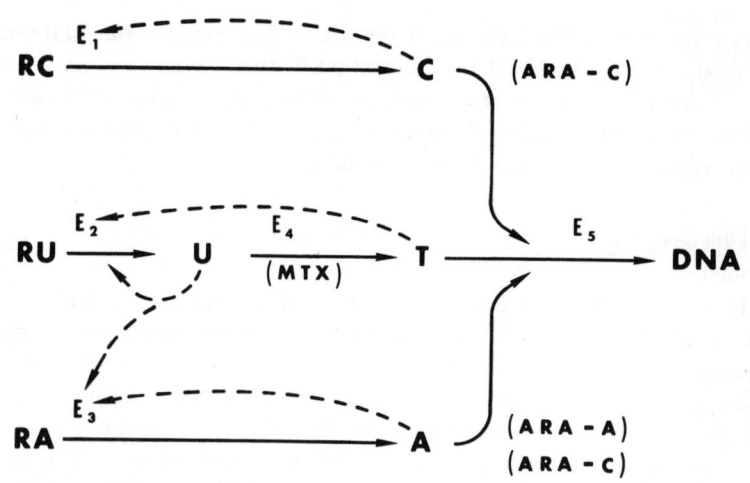

Fig. 1. Simplified DNA synthesis scheme of Werkheiser (1971). A~dATP (adenine); C~dCTP (cytosine); T~dTTP (thymine); U~dUMP (uracil); E_1, E_2, E_3 ~ ribonucleotide reductases; E_4 ~ thymidylate synthetase; E_5 ~ DNA polymerase. The dashed lines signify feedback inhibition. The sites of action of the drugs are signified by ( ).

result of the various biochemical reactions that are occurring, and if the quantitative biochemical kinetics were sufficiently known, could also be predicted. At this time, however, this is not possible, although the qualitative mechanisms are fairly well understood (Mitchison, 1971; Luce et al., 1967, and Mellett, 1972). A significant advance was made by Werkheiser (1971) who reduced the very complicated biochemical pathways to what he considered the minimum essential ones (Fig. 1). These three pathways are those primarily affected by the cancer chemotherapeutic drugs termed antimetabolites. The alkylating agents affect the DNA, and other drugs directly block the mitosis step.

Merely knowing this much of the biochemical events permits rational models to be developed for single and combination drug effects—primarily qualitative at present but hopefully quantitative in the future. Thus, the antimetabolites are active only during the S-phase, and this must be accounted for when describing the drug effect. In other words, a cell kinetic model must be combined with the pharmacokinetics. (Also see Schabel, 1969; De Vita, 1971; and Baserga, 1971).

Models for microbial growth have been used that are intermediate between utilizing the biochemical knowledge or just a biological age (Ramkrishna et al., 1967). Here, just two components of the active biomass are considered, representing essentially (1) the nucleic acids and (2) the other proteins. With this type of model, most of the important features of the usual batch growth curve can be described: lag, exponential, stationary, and decline phases. Some of the interesting features of continuous culture, which in some ways is closer to an organ or tumor, can also be simulated.

The exact use of this cell kinetics and biochemical information in a pharmacokinetic model will be considered shortly.

LOCAL UPTAKE

This last topic we need to consider before looking at the detailed pharmacokinetic models will next be briefly discussed. Physiologists are, of course, also very interested in local uptake of various types of chemical species, and recent work on using indicator-dilution techniques for organs and other tissue areas could provide much useful information. Some very recent references, that also provide an entrée to past work, are: Bassingthwaighte (1970), Goresky et al. (1970), Levitt (1971, 1972), Crone and Lassen (1970), and Bischoff (1967). A general textbook reference that discusses many of these areas is Himmelblau and Bischoff (1968). The text by Middleman (1972) also considers oxygen transport studies, which are again similar.

Figure 2 shows a conceptual view of a local region (the arrows indicate various diffusion and mass transport steps). The general mass balance equations can be written, but are usually far too complex to solve for an application. It is much more usual to ignore the spatial distributions of concentrations, etc., and use lumped or homogeneous compartments. Obviously, these are quite successful for many applications, but the more involved model may be required at times.

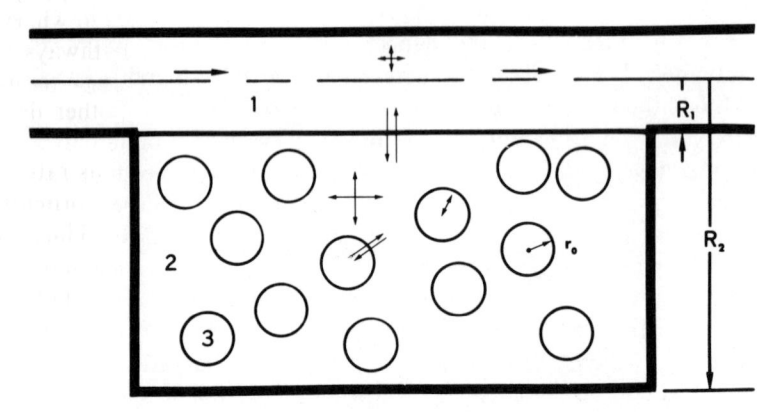

Fig. 2. Schematic diagram of tissue region. 1—blood (capillary); 2—interstitial; 3—cells. The arrows signify various flow, diffusion, and transport steps.

For example, Tannock (1968 and 1970) has found from morphological and other studies that there is a gradient in cell characteristics in the direction away from a capillary for a mouse mammary tumor. The cell cycle lengths were about the same, but the proliferative fraction was smaller and the cell cycle time distribution broader in the outer zones. This gradient could have implications for the design of the chemotherapy, considering possible simultaneous gradients in drug concentration.

On a somewhat less detailed scale, the three regions of intravascular, interstitial, and intracellular, or at least extra- and intracellular, fluid may be required. Using the latter, Zaharko and Dedrick (1972) have provided the simple example shown in Fig. 3 which shows how different relative perfusion rates give different extravascular concentration–time curves. Thus, the plasma concentration would not necessarily be a good measure of the effective drug concentration.

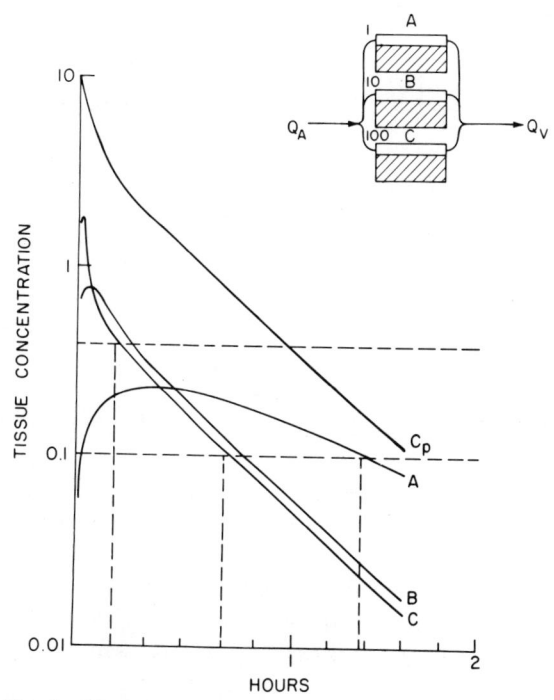

Fig. 3. Model predictions for compartments with widely different blood flows. Arterial blood flow, Q_A; venous blood flow, Q_V. Drug is assumed to distribute into a well mixed fluid which is identical in size in compartments A, B, and C. The ratios of blood flow to compartment size A, B, and C are 1:10:100. From Zaharko and Dedrick (1972).

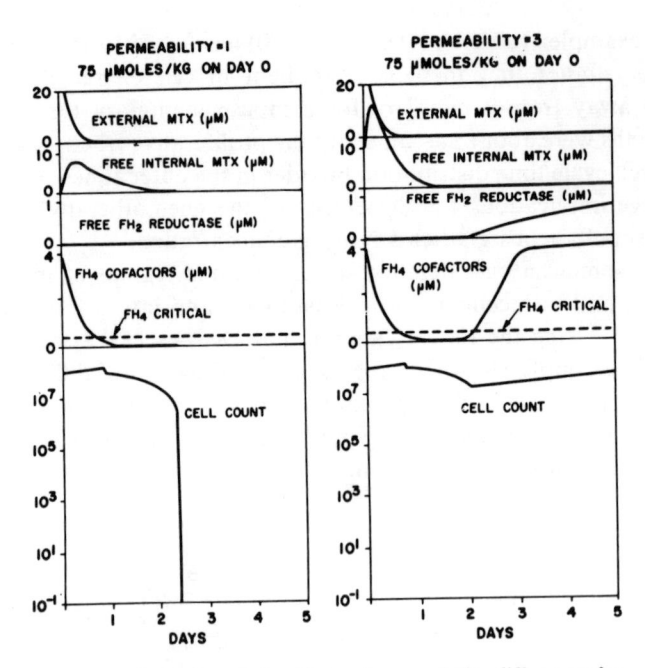

Fig. 4. A simulation of the effects of permeability differences for MTX. From Werkheiser (1971).

A more comprehensive study by Dedrick et al. (1973) has considered the complex interactions of saturable transport, cell binding, and other pharmacokinetic parameters on the concentration levels of methotrexate (MTX) in rat bone marrow and other tissues. Without going into detail, Fig. 4 gives some computed results of the Werkheiser (1971) model that shows the relative effect of the cell permeability on internal MTX and enzyme levels, and the presumed subsequent cell number changes. Most cell uptake data is *in vitro*, but more *in vivo* data will be required in order to be able to quantitatively use this aspect in pharmacokinetic models.

To summarize this section, there exist indicator-dilution techniques and some data. Some beginning work on local uptake of drugs is also available. The integration of this into pharmacokinetics and drug effect predictions, when required, remains for the future.

PHARMACOKINETIC MODELS

We will now finally synthesize the above topics in some pharmacokinetic applications. There are two main levels of this that may be termed semiquantitative and quantitative. By the former is meant that a pharmacokinetics study is made, and the drug effects (cell kinetics) are studied separately, but only the trends of each are utilized to predict the results of a particular therapeutic regimen. The second term will signify attempts to construct a complete model, with all effects included, in order to quantitatively predict results.

Because of the complexities in actually predicting the complete set of events, the semiquantitative method is often highly useful in practice. Examples are given by Skipper et al. (1970), Mellett (1972), and Zaharko and Dedrick (1972). Specifically, it appears that the critical concentration level of MTX below which cell-killing effects are absent is about 0.1–1 μg/ml. (This is actually probably caused by the irreversible binding to the folate reductase enzyme, and its concentration level. Also refer to Fig. 4.) Thus, by using a pharmacokinetic model to predict the time that the local drug concentration is above this minimum, one can deduce (in a semiquantitative way) the extent of cell kill to be expected. This inferential scheme is obviously extremely valuable in planning experiments (especially clinical work), but seems rather clear and so will not be further elaborated upon here.

Examples of quantitative predictions are naturally rare at this point, and, therefore, only two approaches will be summarized. The first is by Jusko (1971 and 1973) and is based on semiempirical formulation of the cell kinetics and the drug effects. The basic idea is shown in the scheme

$$X_t + C_s \xrightarrow{k_s} \atop \downarrow k_d \xrightarrow{k}$$

Pharmacokinetics   Drug effect - Cell kill

where X_t is the tissue drug concentration, C_s is the number of proliferating cells, k_s is the rate of natural mitotic growth, k is the rate of the cell kill, and k_d is the rate of physiologic degradation. For non-cell-cycle-specific drugs (alkylating agents), the details of the cell cycle and/or fraction proliferating cells are not important, and so a cell balance gives

$$\frac{dC_s}{dt} = k_s C_s - k_d C_s - k X_T C_s \qquad (1)$$

Note that the direct proportionality to drug concentration could easily be extended to consider, e.g., saturation effects if the last term were replaced by

$$-k \frac{X_T C_s}{K + X_T} \qquad (2)$$

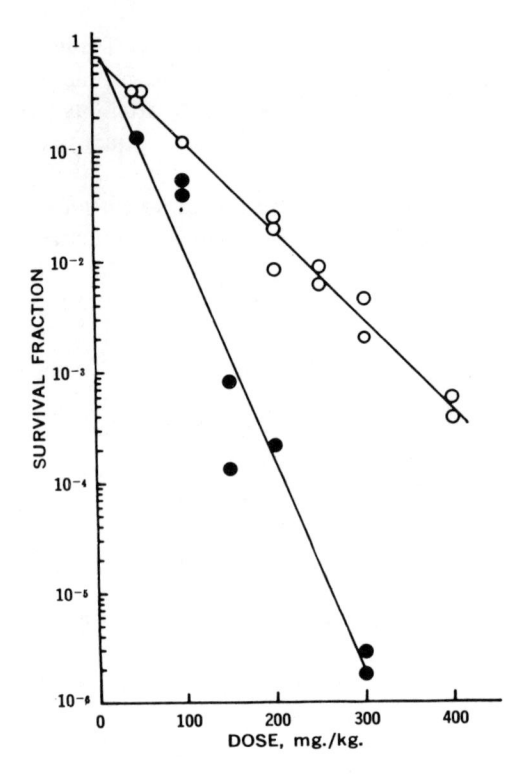

Fig. 5. Survival curves for chimaera spleen cells (0) and osteosarcoma cells (●) after I.P. administration of single doses of cyclophosphamide. From Jusko (1971).

Thus, a pharmacokinetic model is used to determine $X_T(t)$, and this is then substituted into Eq. (1) [or Eq. (2)], and a solution obtained. Thus, if $X_T(t)$ is taken as a known function of time,

$$\ln \frac{C_s}{C_s^0} = (k_s - k_d)t - k \int_0^t \frac{X_T(t)}{K + X_T(t)} dt \qquad (3)$$

where C_s^0 is the initial number of cells. Jusko (1971) used a two-compartment pharmacokinetic model, but, of course, others would also be possible.

Most cancer chemotherapeutic agents have very short half-lives (< 30 min), and so a simplification based on the large difference in time scales (~10-hr cell cycle times) can be used. Thus, the time in the integral of the drug concentration is effectively infinite for its time scale (i.e., the pharmacokinetic events are essentially over before much happens to the cells), and so (neglecting saturation effects):

$$\int_0^t X_T dt \to \int_0^\infty X_T dt \propto \text{(dose)} \qquad (4)$$

Then,

$$\ln \frac{C_s}{C_s^0} = (k_s - k_d)t - K_s(\text{dose}) \tag{5}$$

Figure 5 shows the type of agreement with experimental data that can be obtained.

This was extended to cell-cycle-specific drugs (Jusko, 1973) with the following scheme:

$$X_T + C_s \begin{array}{c} k_s \\ \curvearrowright \\ \xrightarrow{k} \end{array}$$
$$k_{sR} \updownarrow k_{Rs}$$
$$C_R \xrightarrow{k_d}$$

where C_s represents the cells sensitive to the drug (in S-phase, or proliferative) and C_R the insensitive cells (not in S-phase, or nonproliferative). Here the appropriate equations are

$$\frac{dC_s}{dt} = k_s C_s - k_{sR} C_s + k_{Rs} C_R - k X_T C_s \tag{6}$$

$$\frac{dC_R}{dt} = k_{sR} C_s - k_{Rs} C_R - k_d C_R \tag{7}$$

(Note the similarity in concept to that mentioned above for microbial growth.) Usually only the total number of cells can be easily measured

$$C_T = C_s + C_R \tag{8}$$

and this is what is determined by solving Eqs. (6), (7), and (8) and comparing with data. Figure 6 shows this type of comparison for the mitotic inhibitor, vinblastine. Figure 7 illustrates the effect of *not* assuming two different time scales and including the full time behavior of the pharmacokinetics. The main difference is in the "scalloped" shape of the curves; the overall trends are the same.

In order to take the cell cycle kinetics details into account, Himmelstein and Bischoff (1973) used a formal model of Rubinow (1968). [See Fredrickson et al. (1967) for a general treatment of cell kinetic models.] These models consider not only the change with time of the cell number, but also the fraction of cells of a given biological age or maturity. Thus, the number of cells at time t of maturity, μ, is defined: $n(\mu, t)$. The variable(s), μ, are to account for the biochemical events occurring such that:

$$v(\mu, t) = \frac{d\mu}{dt} = \text{Rate(s) of change of biochemical variables} \tag{9}$$

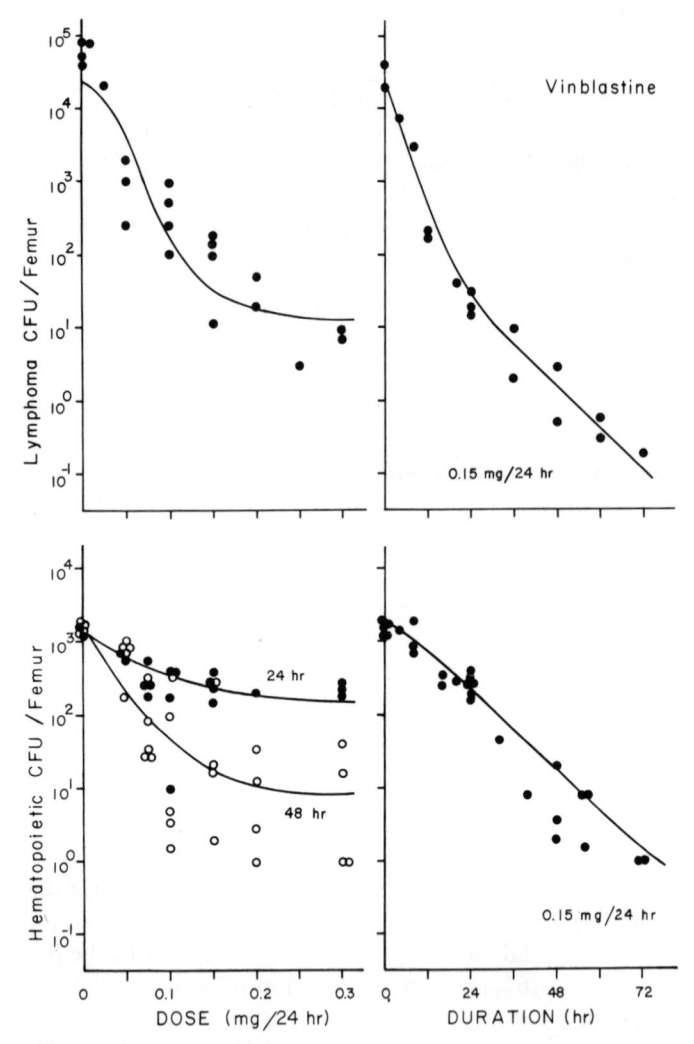

Fig. 6. Dose–time–cell survival curves for the effects of vinblastine on hematopoietic and lymphoma cells in the mouse femur. From Jusko (1973).

At this point, these models are usually simplified to an operational definition that μ is a fraction of the cell cycle.

A balance on $n(\mu, t)$ can be formulated:

$$\begin{pmatrix} \text{Time rate} \\ \text{of change} \end{pmatrix} + \begin{pmatrix} \text{Rate of cell} \\ \text{maturation} \end{pmatrix} = \begin{pmatrix} \text{Rate of} \\ \text{cell death} \end{pmatrix}$$

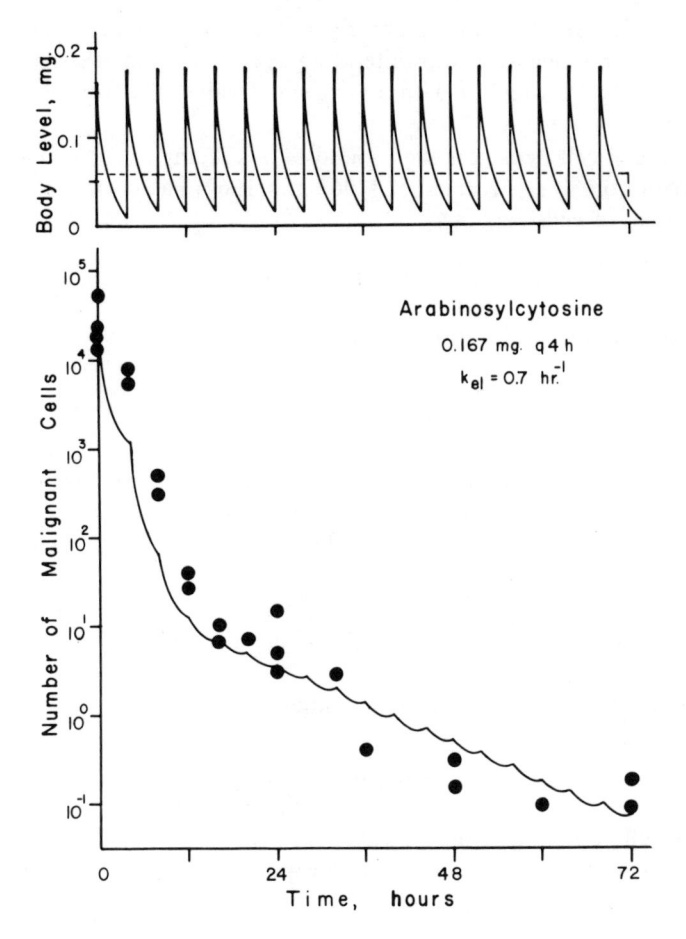

Fig. 7. Cell survival curve for the effect of multiple doses of cytosine arabinoside on lymphoma cells in the mouse femur. From Jusko (1973).

or

$$\frac{\partial n_\nu}{\partial t} + \frac{\partial}{\partial \mu}[\nu v'(\mu, C(t))n_\nu] = -\lambda[\mu, C(t)]n_\nu \tag{10}$$

where λ is the specific cell death rate (function of drug concentration and, for a cell cycle specific drug, the cell maturity) and v is the mean maturation rate, and the subscript ν on n_ν signifies the cell number for a given ν. As briefly described above, real cell populations have a distribution of cell generation times (or inverse mean maturation rate), and this is often a very important consideration in cancer chemotherapy. The cell-cycle-specific agents are only active against proliferating cells actively synthesizing DNA, and those cells "resting" or with a very small value of ν are refractory to treatment.

The mean cell density is then found by averaging over the maturation rate distribution, $W(\nu)$. Kubitshek (1962 and 1967) has correlated data for various types of cells:

$$n(\mu, t) = \int W(\nu) n_\nu(\mu, t) \, d\nu \tag{11}$$

Finally, just as in Eq. (8), the commonly measured entity is the total cell density:

$$N(t) = \int n(\mu, t) \, d\mu \tag{12}$$

At this point, it can be seen that the Himmelstein and Bischoff model is in some respects analogous to the Jusko model in that the continuous distribution $n(\mu, t)$ is used in place of the two discrete fractions, $C_S(t)$ and $C_R(t)$. However, the latter does not consider the cell generation time distribution, which might be very important in applications. This is especially true for significant cell kills, where the timing of the cell cycle (synchrony) is important.

The function λ was also chosen similarly:

$$\lambda[\mu, C(t)] = \frac{K_1 C(t)}{K_2 + C(t)} \tag{13}$$

For large cell populations in exponential growth, an asymptotic solution for Eq. (10) was obtained which for simple exponential decay pharmacokinetics, $C = C_0 \exp(-t/t_d)$, is

$$\frac{N(t)}{N_0} = 2^{\nu t} \left[\frac{K_2 + C_0 e^{-t/t_d}}{K_2 + C_0} \right]^{K_1 t_d} \tag{14}$$

(It should be noted that many other mathematical solutions for more complicated cases were presented.) For small K_2 (i.e., no saturation effects), Eq. (14) reduces to a Gompertz form that is often used empirically to describe tumor growth [see Burton (1966) for an interesting discussion of this].

Himmelstein and Bischoff (1973) used Eq. (14) to attempt to predict the experimental results of Skipper *et al.* (1967) for the ARA-C-mouse L-1210 leukemia system. The pharmacokinetics can be obtained for various animal species as described by Dedrick in this volume, and in detail for MTX by Bischoff *et al.* (1971), so hopefully the results could be scaled up

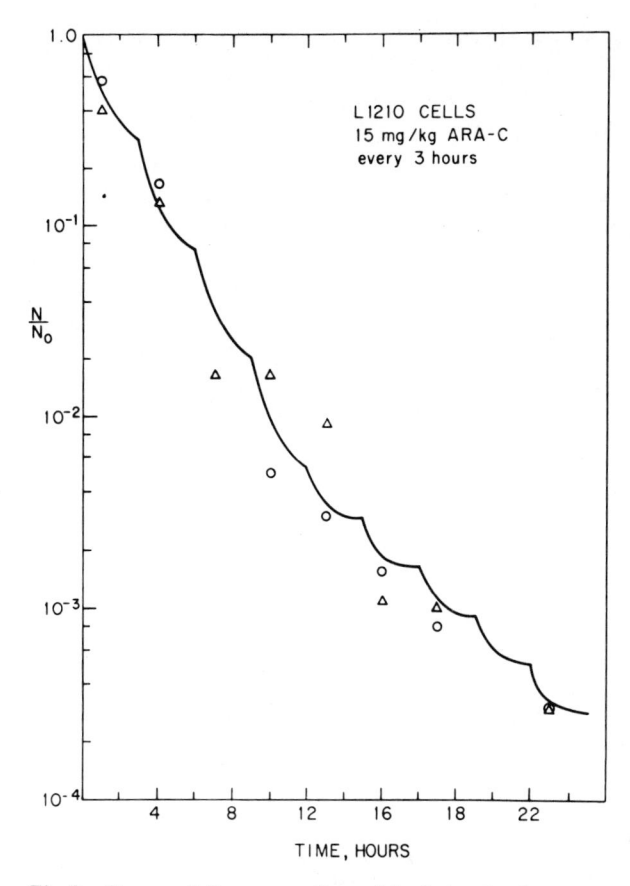

Fig. 8. Exponentially asymptotic model solution fitted to *in vivo* L1210 cell count for multiple injections of 15 mg/kg ARA-C every three hours. From Himmelstein and Bischoff (1973b).

to humans (with the appropriate cell kinetics data). The cell-cycle-specific drugs often show saturation effects, and so the full Eq. (14) was required.

Figure 8 shows the fitting of K_1 and K_2 (all other parameters known independently), and at this point all the model parameters are known. If these models are to be predictive, we should now be able to compute the results for another dosage regimen, *without* modifying the model parameters. The next figures will show some results over a 24-day span: the "scalloped" nature of the cell number curves will no longer be apparent on the size of the drawing, but the pharmacokinetic effects were taken into account. Figure 9 is an example of an "unsuccessful" dosage regimen since the tumor growth ultimately outpaced the drug cell killing effect. Figure 10 is another case, and the model predicted "less" than one cell remaining during the second course (this agreed reasonably well with the 7/10 survivors found experimentally).

Shackney (1970) has given a preliminary report of more complicated models based on direct numerical simulation of cell growth. These have shown similar types of behavior as above, but the extensive details are difficult to present. The efforts of Werkheiser (1971) mentioned earlier are an opening to bringing more of the known biochemistry into the models, and this is probably one of the most important directions for future progress. Finally, such areas as combined radiotherapy and chemotherapy have not been discussed (see the review by Andrews, 1969).

It is hoped that many of the current and possible future methods of modeling pharmacokinetics and cancer chemotherapy have been described here. Many of the main current references, particularly reviews, have been

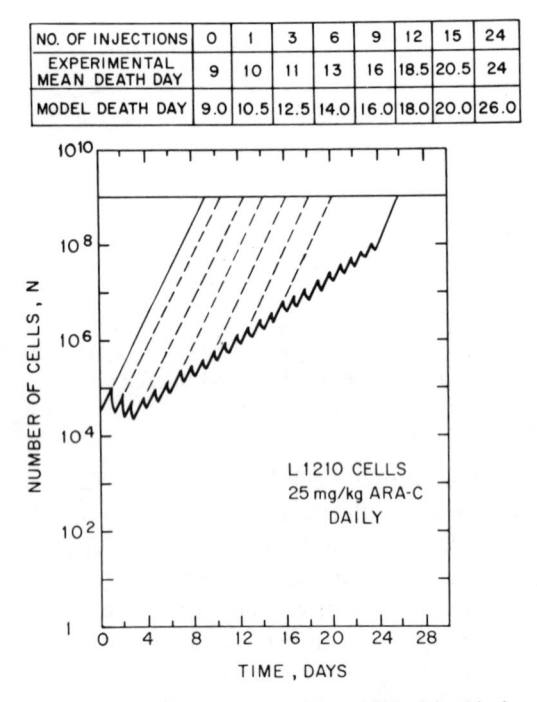

NO. OF INJECTIONS	0	1	3	6	9	12	15	24
EXPERIMENTAL MEAN DEATH DAY	9	10	11	13	16	18.5	20.5	24
MODEL DEATH DAY	9.0	10.5	12.5	14.0	16.0	18.0	20.0	26.0

Fig. 9. Comparison of predictions of model with data for *in vivo* L1210 cells treated with 25 mg/kg ARA-C daily for 0-24 days. From Himmelstein and Bischoff (1973b).

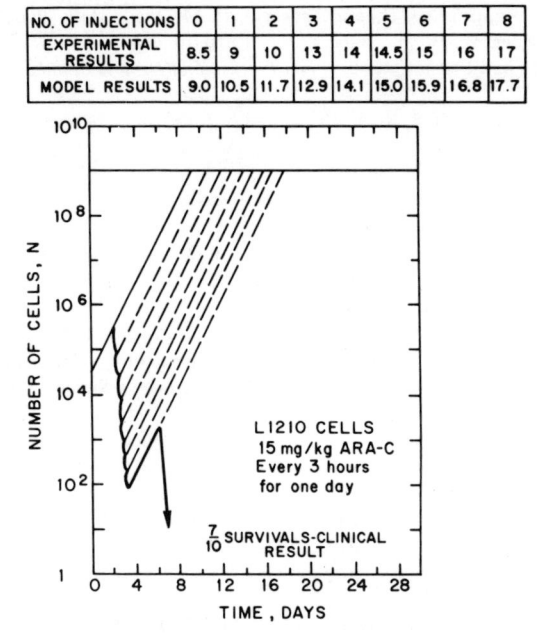

NO. OF INJECTIONS	0	1	2	3	4	5	6	7	8
EXPERIMENTAL RESULTS	8.5	9	10	13	14	14.5	15	16	17
MODEL RESULTS	9.0	10.5	11.7	12.9	14.1	15.0	15.9	16.8	17.7

Fig. 10. Comparision of predictions of model with data for *in vivo* Ll210 cells treated with two courses, separated by three days, of eight injections of 15 mg/kg ARA-C every three hours. From Himmelstein and Bischoff (1973b).

listed as a help to anyone interested in this area. Several of the methods naturally have application to other pharmaceutical agents, but seem to be especially critical for cancer chemotherapy.

REFERENCES

Andrews, J. R., 1969, *Cancer Chemotherapy Rep.* **53**: 313.
Baserga, R. (ed.), 1971, *The Cell Cycle and Cancer*, Marcel Dekker, New York.
Bassingthwaighte, J. B., 1970, *Science* **167**: 1347.
Bischoff, K. B., 1967, in *Chemical Engineering in Medicine and Biology* (Hershey, D., ed.), Plenum Press, New York.
Bischoff, K. B., Dedrick, R. L., Zaharko, D. S., and Longstreth, J. A., 1971, *J. Pharm. Sci.* **60**: 1128.
Burton, A. C., 1966, *Growth* **30**: 157.
Crone, C., and Lassen, N. A. (eds.), 1970, *Capillary Permeability*, Munksgaard, Copenhagen.
Dedrick, R. L., Zaharko, D. S., and Lutz, R., 1973, *J. Pharm. Sci.* **62**: 882.
De Vita, V. T., 1971, *Cancer Chemotherapy Repts., Part 3*, **2**: 23.

Fredrickson, A. G., Ramkrishna, D., and Tsuchiya, H. M., 1967, *Math. Biosciences* **1**: 327.
Goresky, C. A., Ziegler, W. H., and Bach, G. G., 1970, *Circulation Res.* **27**: 739.
Himmelblau, D. M., and Bischoff, K. B., 1968, *Process Analysis and Simulation*, Wiley John & Son, New York.
Himmelstein, K. J., and Bischoff, K. B., 1973a, and b. *J. Pharmacokinetics and Biopharmaceutics*, **1**: 51, 69.
Jusko, W. J., 1971, *J. Pharm. Sci.* **60**: 892.
Jusko, W. J., 1973, *J. Pharmacokinetics and Biopharmaceutics* **1**: 175.
Kubitschek, H. E., 1962, *Exp. Cell Res.* **26**: 439.
Kubitschek, H. E., 1967, *Proc. Fifth Berkeley Symp. Math. Statist. Probab.* **4**: 549.
Leavitt, D. G., 1971, *Am. J. Physiol.* **220**: 250.
Leavitt, D. G., 1972, *J. Theoret. Biol.* **34**: 103.
Luce, J. K., Bodey, G. B., and Frei, E., III, 1967, *Hospital Practice* **2**: 42.
Mellett, L. B., 1972, Fifth International Congress on Pharmacology, San Francisco.
Middleman, S., 1972, *Transport Phenomena in the Cardiovascular System*, John Wiley & Son, New York.
Mitchison, J. M., 1971, *The Biology of the Cell Cycle*, Cambridge University Press.
Ramkrishna, D., Fredrickson, A. G., and Tsuchiya, H. M., 1967, *Biotech. Bioengng.* **9**: 129.
Rubinow, S. I., 1968, *Biophys. J.* **8**: 1055.
Schabel, F. M., 1969, *Cancer Res.* **29**: 2384.
Schackney, S. E., 1970, *Cancer Chemotherapy Rep.* **54**: 399.
Skipper, H. E., 1971, in *Predictions of Response in Cancer Therapy*, p. 2 (T. C. Hall, ed.), Natl. Cancer Inst. Monograph 34.
Skipper, H. E., Schabel, F. M., and Wilcox, W. S., 1967, *Cancer Chemotherapy Rep.* **51**: 125.
Skipper, H. E., Schabel, F. M., Mellett, L. B., Montgomery, J. A., Wilkoff, L. J., Lloyd, H. H., and Brockman, R. W., 1970, *Cancer Chemotherapy Rep.* **54**: 431.
Tannock, I. F., 1968, *Brit. J. Cancer* **22**: 258.
Tannock, I. F., 1970, *Cancer Res.* **30**: 2470.
Werkheiser, W. C., 1971, *Ann. N.Y. Acad. Sci.* **186**: 343.
Zaharko, D. S., and Dedrick, R. L., 1972, Fifth International Congress on Pharmacology, San Francisco, p. 155.
Zubrod, C. G., 1972, *Proc. Natl. Acad. Sci.* **69**: 1042.

DISCUSSION SUMMARY

Jusko elaborated on the pharmacodynamic analysis of the cytotoxic behavior of vinblastine (VB), vincristine (VC), and arabinosylcytosine (Ara-C). He pointed out that the effects of chemotherapeutic drugs on both normal and tumor cells should be considered, and a balance should be sought between killing neoplastic cells and leaving a sufficient number of sensitive normal cells so that the patient survives.

The type of cell survival data shown by Bischoff in Figs. 6 and 7 was analyzed using a two-compartment cell model where cells were assumed to exist either in a drug-sensitive (proliferating) compartment (C_S) or a drug-insensitive (resting) compartment (C_R). Some rate constants of the model which are included in Eqs. (6) and (7) were obtained beforehand by analysis of the normal growth curves of hematopoietic cells and lymphoma cells. Numerical values for the remaining parameters were generated by nonlinear least-square analysis of data for the number of surviving cells as a function of total dose and total duration of drug treatment. Resultant parameters of interest are the chemotherapy constant and the numbers of cells in the C_S and C_R compartments as shown in the table below. The chemotherapy constant contains both the pharmacokinetic parameters and the intrinsic drug–receptor interaction rate constant from Eq. (6). Since the lymphoma cells and hematopoietic cells are both located in the mouse femur, it is assumed that the pharmacokinetics of the drug are identical for both cell types. Thus, the lack of appreciable difference in the chemotherapy constant for a given drug acting on the two cell types suggests that the normal and tumor cells have the same intrinsic sensitivity to the respective anticancer agents. However, examination of the numbers of each cell type which are sensitive to the drug shows that over 99.9% of the lymphoma cells are capable of being affected by the drugs while only 3% of the hematopoietic cells are drug-sensitive at the time of initial drug treatment. This leads to the tentative conclusion that the cell kinetics, rather than the intrinsic properties of the drug itself, determines the therapeutic index of these drugs.

Finally, it was pointed out that the design of optimal dosage regimens for cell-cycle specific chemotherapeutic agents depends on consideration of the rate at which resting cells convert to their proliferative phase. An ideal treatment schedule might involve a priming dose designed to kill the maximum number of proliferating neoplastic cells, followed by administration of smaller maintenance doses at a rate designed to kill the cells as they convert from their resting phase. This treatment has the toxicity restriction that sensitive host cells (e.g., bone marrow) be maintained in adequate numbers for survival of the patient.

Bischoff noted that he has performed similar simulations where comparisons were made of killing effects of drugs on cancerous and normal cells. In many instances there is a reasonably sensitive concentration of a drug where the normal cells are essentially reduced to a lower steady-state number and the neoplastic cell number continues to be depleted. Other dosages cause both cell types to be lost and some doses permit the tumor cell number to increase, but the shift from one type of behavior to the other is fairly sharp. One overall goal is to predict these shifts in order to reduce the amount of clinical experimentation.

Segre inquired whether mutation to resistant cells is a possible limitation to the models. If mutant cells can be generated during time intervals when the drug concentration is low, then the method of drug administration would become very important. Bischoff observed that the genetic time scale is likely to be considerably longer than the cell cycle time scale.

Melmon's comments were directed toward the clinical aspects of cancer chemotherapy. He noted that solid tumors with slow growth and composed of mature cells are considered to be unlikely to respond to antimetabolites, but few studies have been done to legitimately test alkylating agents in relation to tumor size or rate of growth. A system which might be examined in order to test pharmacokinetic models in clinical cancer chemotherapy is a tumor whose size or rate of growth is related to some endocrine function, such as a catecholsecreting

TABLE A
Pharmacodynamic Parameters—Cell Cycle-Specific Model

Drug	Cell	C_S^o	C_R^o	Chemotherapy constant (day^{-1})
VB	Lymphoma	24,300	153	2.85
VB	Hematopoietic	46	1554	1.48
VC	Lymphoma	28,000	587	14.2
VC	Hematopoietic	79	1521	6.42
Ara-C	Lymphoma	19,000	12.4	0.855
Ara-C	Hematopoietic	69	1531	0.850

tumor like pheochromocytoma, a carcinoid tumor that produces serotonin, or a myeloma tumor which produces a variety of light chain immunoglobulins. These products might provide an objective measure of tumor size, particularly when the tumor cannot be detected by any other clinical means. Dosage regimen predictions could then be monitored clinically in treated patients.

Garratini cautioned that destruction of immunocompetent cells should be avoided because of their role in body defense against cancer, especially at the stage when the last few tumor cells are being destroyed. Also, experimental studies are often carried out using tumors present in the peritoneal cavity while, in reality, clinical tumors are often disseminated into different tissues. This creates problems in using pharmacokinetics to predict tumor drug concentrations and, furthermore, the presence of the tumor changes some of the pharmacokinetic parameters of the drug.

Garrett pointed out the similarities which exist in the fields of cancer chemotherapy and microbe chemotherapy. In bacterial cell culture systems, the primary measurement is the concentration dependence of the inhibition of cell proliferation by drugs. The most frequent drug-induced occurrence is inhibition of DNA, RNA, or protein synthesis, resulting in slowed bacterial growth rate rather than direct cell kill. Thus, it is better to conceive of these cells as containing many different internal receptor types and sites in proposing mechanisms of drug action, rather than imposing an oversimplified target theory. In addition, he noted that some of the primary concerns of both pharmacokinetics and chemotherapy include the so-called minimum effective drug concentration and the need to inhibit organisms in their natural environment.

In general agreement with most of these comments, Bischoff outlined some of the factors which complicate the search for ways to make realistic predictions of chemotherapeutic effects of drugs. The need to account for the biochemical events of the system is of special concern. The consideration of the kinetics of interaction of the drug with enzymes, DNA, RNA, or proteins will often involve nonlinear kinetics, including product inhibition and feedback processes. He noted that most cell systems examined to date consist of very large cell numbers because of the difficulty in measuring smaller numbers of cells. The variability in cell cycle times for individual cells in a population is often very large, and the distribution of cell generation times in a cell population gets broader with the higher mammals, making chemotherapy less predictable and more difficult to quantitate in man than in animal systems.

The problem in examining the effects of drugs on cancer cells in their natural habitat may be partially resolved by comprehensive pharmacokinetic models which consider the local uptake of antineoplastic agents. A second helpful approach to this issue may involve studies using recently developed methods for culturing cells at tissue density outside of highly perfused capillaries.

In summary, this discussion tended to preview the exciting possibilities for utilization of pharmacokinetics in quantitating and predicting the clinical effects of cancer chemotherapy while, at the same time, not losing sight of the immediate problems which must be resolved with respect to the limitations of present models.

Concluding Remarks

In our program, these final comments have been given the title "Summary." However, I choose not to attempt any summary, because it would only be a superfluous reiteration of the highlights of all the brilliant presentations of the various reviewers and participants. What I shall do instead is make some general comments.

First to the composition of the program. We were aware at the outset that we had a very diversified program, the purposes of which were to *review the present status, describe or formulate the pertinent problems*, and *finally delineate*, if possible, *the best ways of solving these problems*. In other words, the meeting was intended to be a general, "broad-spectrum" discussion rather than a presentation forum for new results. Now the Conference is over and only time will tell if it fulfilled its purposes. I would think that perhaps the best yield for the future would be not the particular new knowledge that any one individual might have acquired about one aspect of the broad field of pharmacokinetics, but rather, a general stimulus, immediate or latent, toward new research and new concepts beneficial to the medical sciences.

In spite of a generally positive outlook, I cannot help having some misgivings about the present status of pharmacokinetics. Its very essence is the use of mathematical formulations based on certain biophysical or biochemical models of the living body, and we must never forget that we are dealing with models, not necessarily with realistic facts. Although the basic model concepts as used hitherto are quite simple, a combination of them in a mathematical shape may appear to many people as formidable mathematical machinery, which becomes so overpowering, say, to a bedside doctor, that he gets suspicious of the usefulness of the pharmacokinetic approach. And yet, it cannot be denied that classical mathematical pharmacokinetics have been proved to be extremely useful for description, explanation, and even prediction of the distribution of drugs and have helped to "optimize" drug administration.

But sometimes pharmacokinetics in its present state is a failure - where the basic assumptions are not valid or are too simplified. In fact, for an oldtimer it is surprising that such an almost naively simple model as the serial multicompartment governed by Fick's diffusion has survived over the years. One way of explaining this is to state that the model may not represent "a diffusional compartment model" at all, but be rather a special case of "sequential chain of first-order reactions," which has an identical mathematical formalism. We need not commit ourselves to any particular mechanism. There is a somewhat similar situation with the use of irreversible thermodynamics in biophysics. One regards, say, the cell membrane, as a "black box," and yet it is possible to describe flows and fluxes of material implied in the permeability processes without necessarily identifying any detailed invisible force or visible anatomical structure. With such a modified view, modern quantitative pharmacokinetics becomes more abstract. But at the same time it becomes elusive in the sense that the final consumers of the pharmacokinetical products, the bedside doctors, will never acquire understanding, nor interest, nor faith in this particular branch of pharmacy. I have a feeling that here we meet an educational problem which should be handled in our medical schools. We should introduce modern pharmacokinetics there, but prevent overdosing with the mathematical ramifications.

After having listened to the last days' sessions one might get the overall impression that metabolism, enzymes, genes, and antigens must render a realistic use of classical pharmacokinetics almost impossible. Added to that are the species differences in experimental materials and individual patterns among patients. We really learned yesterday that "mice and men can be different."

Now, if we admit that the dangers for pharmacokinetics can arise from oversimplified basic concepts, from overuse of mathematics, etc., what kind of *projections for the future* can be envisaged? To me it appears quite obvious that we have to penetrate deeper into membrane events to incorporate chemical kinetics with classical transport kinetics so that metabolism and enzyme behavior may be better described. The efforts to describe the time course of blood and tissue concentrations will soon also include quantitative treatments of the dose-response relationship in the target organ. The mutual interactions among different organ systems will be dealt with in greater depth, and this will lead to the incorporation of pharmacokinetics into "regulation theory," including "feedbacks" and "loops," as handled by biophysicists and bioengineers. It would not be surprising if these expanded theories of transport and feedback processes lead to an understanding of the *rhythmical* processes so often encountered in the living body, so that even diurnal influences might be successfully described and modified by drugs. If these are possible projections to the organism or organ level, expanded work in the future must also project to

Concluding Remarks 371

the cell level and even to the molecular level, such that "molecular pharmacology" and "pharmacokinetics" can be relevant to one another and, indeed, unified. You may think that this all sounds like a fairytale, and I may then confess that that's exactly the feeling I have gotten myself from all the past and recent wonderful work you participants of this Conference have talked about during the last days. There has been enormous progress during the forty years I have been an observer in this field. Many solid facts of today were unbelievable fairytales in our early days, so it has really been a great pleasure to listen to you all!

This Conference was conceived as an effort by the Fogarty International Center to contribute to the advancement of health sciences. The program would not have been possible if we had not had this Center and the National Institutes of Health as sponsors. There are many people who have contributed to the planning and execution of this program. I wish to thank, in particular, among others, Drs. Axelrod, Berman, Dedrick, the late Dr. Effron, Drs. Garrett, Gillette, Riegelman, Wagner, and Vesell for valuable advice and participation during the planning period. Last, but not least, I wish to convey our thanks to Dr. P. Condliffe on behalf of the Conference. He has had the burden of being the Executive Officer of the Conference. His work has been shared by his deputy, Dr. Maureen Harris, and his very efficient secretary, Mrs. Toby Levin, to whom we are all obliged.

Torsten Teorell

Index

Acatalasia, genetic factors of, 262 (Table I)
Accumulation kinetics, 336
Acetamide, osmolal threshold, 244 (Table I)
Acetaminophen
 interaction of, 332
 nonlinearities in metabolism, 39 (Table III)
 nonlinearities in renal excretion, 44 (Table IV)
Acetanilide, metabolism of, 40 (Table III), 236 (Table I)
Acetazolamide
 indirect drug interaction of, 321
 in treatment of glaucoma, 191–194 (Fig. 1, 191; Fig. 2, 192)
Acetophenetidin
 altered metabolism of, 263 (Table I)
 oxidative dealkalinization of, 103
 side effects of, 254 (Table I)
Acetophenetidine-induced
 methemoglobinemia, genetic factors of, 262 (Table I)
Acetylation, genetic factors of, 256
Acetyl-β-methylcholine, 181, 186
Acetylcholine, 179, 181, 186 (Fig. 11)
 metabolism in lungs, 200, 203
Acetylsalicyclic acid, 87
 metabolism of, 95 (Table II), 263 (Table I)
N-Acetyltransferase activity, (liver) 256, 257
N_2-Acetylsulfanilamide, altered metabolism of, 263 (Table I)
Acid dyes, binding of, 211
Acidic and basic drugs
 nonlinearities in absorption, 29 (Table I)
 nonlinearities in renal excretion, 44 (Table IV)
 pharmacokinetic characteristics, 77
Acid phosphatase in red cells, genetic factors, 258–259 (Figs. 2 and 3)

ACTH (see Adrenocorticotropic)
Adenyl cyclase system, 171
Adrenergic agents, 170
 role in mediator release, 290, 296
α-Adrenergic agents, 176, 177, 180
Adrenocorticotropic, 171
Adverse drug reactions, genetic factors of, 253–260 (Table I, 254), 261, 262–264 (Table I)
Agonists, relationship to drug-receptor interaction, 174–175 (Fig. 6), 176–177, 178 (Fig. 7), 184 (Fig. 10)
Albumins, in drug binding, 212
Aldosterone, luminal and/or mucosal metabolism in, 95 (Table II)
Aldrin, binding of, 214
Allergic sensitization, chemical lesions in, 165
Allopurinol, adverse reaction to, 254 (Table I)
Alphamethyltyrosine, as amphetamine antagonist, 311
Alprenolol, hepatic metabolism in, 96 (Table III)
Amines, distribution in brain tissue, 239
Amines, inactivation of, 203
 in acetylcholine, 200
 in 5-hydroxytryptamines, 195–198
 in catecholamines, 198–200
Amino acids, transport at vascular capillaries, 242
p-Aminobenzoic acid
 acetylation of, 91, 257
 in liver disease, 152
 luminal and/or mucosal metabolism in, 95 (Table II)
 nonlinearities in metabolism, 39, (Table III)

p-Aminohippuric acid
  intestinal amide hydrolysis of, 91
  luminal and/or mucosal metabolism in, 95 (Table II)
Aminopyrine, altered metabolism of, 263 (Table I)
p-Aminosalicylic acid
  altered metabolism of, 263 (Table I)
  dosage, 103
Amitriptyline,
  5-HT inhibition, 196–197
  in treatment of depression, 316
Amphetamines
  abuse of in Sweden, 297
  blocking agents, 299–301, 311 (Figs. 2 and 3, 300)
  dehydration, 313
  elimination rate of, 304, 306, 308
  euphoric and dysphoric effects, 298–301 (Fig. 1, 298), 311, 312–313
  β-hydroxylation of, 309–310, 313
  metabolism of, 305–310
  nonlinearities in renal excretion, 44 (Table IV)
  pharmacokinetic studies in dependent subjects, 301–310 (Fig. 4, 302; Fig. 5, 303; Fig. 6, 304; Fig. 7, 306; Fig. 8, 308; Fig. 9, 309; Fig. 10, 310), 312–313
  plasma and urine levels, 301–303
  relationship to neuropsychiatric disorders, 297–311, 312–313
  renal clearance of, 305–306
  subjective effects of single doses, 297–299
  in treatment of disorders, 313
Amphetamine psychosis
  relationship to elimination rate, 304 (Fig. 6)
  relationship to metabolites, 306–307, 313
  relationship to plasma and urine levels, 301–305
Amylobarbitane, nonlinearities in metabolism, 40 (Table III)
Anaphylactic response, release of vasoactive substances, 202
Anaphylaxis, 296
  activation of, 202
  immulogic release of, 288–289 (Table II), 290
  in mediator release in guinea pig lung, 290–294 (Figs. 4–7, 291–292; Table III, 293)

Angioedema, catabolism of complement components, 287
Angiotensin
  I, 202, 203
  II, 201, 202–204
Aniline antipyrine, absorption of, 93
Anisotropine methylbromide, nonlinearities in renal excretion, 44 (Table IV)
Antagonism, types of, 176–178, (Fig. 7)
Anthropoid scale, 106 (Table II)
Antibiotics, 278–279
Anticholinergic agents, receptor sites for, 179–188 (Fig. 8, 180; Table I, 182; Fig. 9, 183; Table II, 185)
Anticoagulants, 278
  interaction effects, 324
Antigen, in mediator release, 291–294 (Figs. 4–7, 291–292), 296
Antihistaminic activity, 187
Antihypertensive drugs, 278
Antimalarials, altered metabolism of, 263 (Table I)
Antimetabolites, 353, 367
Antineoplastic drugs, 142
  uptake of, in cancer chemotherapy, 368
Antipyrine
  altered metabolism of, 263 (Table I)
  blood tissue distribution of, 238
  clinical applications of, 277
  distribution in brain tissue, 239
  effects of, in older patients, 154
  effects of insecticides on, 155–156 (Fig. 4, 156)
  environmental and genetic factors of, 271 (Table II), 272–273 (Fig. 6), 275 (Table III), 276
  genetic factors of, 269–270 (Fig. 5), 272–273
  metabolism of, 147–148 (Table I)
  thyroid disorders, 162
C-Antipyrine
  nonlinearity in absorption, 29 (Table I)
Antisera, use of as antidotes, 212
Appetite suppressants,
  amphetamines, 313
Aprobit, distribution of, 167 (Fig. 3)
Arabinosylcytosine, cytotoxic behavior of, 366
ARA-C
  in cancer chemotherapy, 363 (Fig. 8), 364 (Fig. 9), 365 (Fig. 10)

Index

ARA-C *(cont'd)*
  effect on lymphoma and hematopoietic cells, 367 (Table A) pharmacokinetics of, 138-140 (Fig. 19, 138)
ARA-U *(see* Uracil arabinoside)
Aspirin
  body clearance of, 95-96
  in drug binding, 213
  nonlinearities in distribution, 36 (Table II)
  nonlinearities in metabolism, 39 (Table III)
Atabrine *(see* Quinacrine)
Atropine, 181
Autoimmune hemolytic anemia, 287
Azulfidine *(see* Salicylazosulfapyridine)

Barbituates
  binding of, 211
  effect in uremic patients, 151
  interaction with dicoumarol, 324
  nonlinearities in absorption, 29 (Table I)
  relationship to drug distribution in brain tissue, 239
Benzilyl esters, 181
Benzylpenicillin, nonlinearities in distribution, 36 (Table II)
Benzoic acid, 107
  nonlinearities in metabolism, 38 (Table III)
Benzopyrene
  nonlinearities in distribution, 37 (Table II)
Benzpyrene
  dietary factors, 159
  metabolism in lungs, 207
Beta adrenergic receptor, 189
Bile acids, nonlinearities in renal excretion, 44 (Table IV)
Bilharziasis, 152-153
Biliary disease, drug absorption in, 154
Biliary excretion
  analysis of, 12, 20
  equation relating to, 6
  nonlinearities in, 45 (Table V)
Bilirubin
  binding of, 211, 212
  conjugation of, 113
Bioavailability
  bioavailability profile, 164
  defined, 164
Biopharmaceutics, 1, 3

Biophase, 19, 22
Biotransformation, genetic factors of, 276, 277
Biscoumacetate
  nonlinearities in metabolism, 39 (Table III)
Bishydroxycoumarin
  clinical applications of, 277
  environmental and genetic factors of, 270 (Fig. 5), 271-272 (Table II), 274-275 (Table III), 276
  interaction with phenobarbital, 155
  metabolism of, 147, 148 (Table I) nonlinearities in distribution, 36 (Table II)
  nonlinearities in metabolism, 39 (Table III)
  polygenic control, 261
  sensitivity to, 262 (Table I)
Bisonium compounds, concentration of, 166, 168 (Fig. 4)
Blood alcohol, relationship to Michaelis-Menten equation, 31, 46 (Table VII)
Blood-brain barrier, 241-250
  diagram at capillary level, 242 (Fig. 1)
  eye barriers, 250
  opening of, 242-243 (Fig. 2), 244 (Table I), 245 (Fig. 3), 246 (Table II), 247 (Fig. 4), 248 (Fig. 5), 249 (Fig. 6)
  osmolal thresholds, 244 (Table I), 245 (Fig. 3), 246 (Table II), 247 (Fig. 4)
  relationship to drug distribution, 238-239
Blood clotting, 340-343
Blood platelets, role in 5-HT uptake, 198
Blood tissue distribution, 233-238 (Fig. 1, 235; Fig. 2, 237)
  relationship to metabolic conversion, 238
  relationship to nonmetabolized substance, 236-237
Blue dextran, circulation of, 200
Body weight relationships in mammals in pharmacologic scaling, 130 (Table II), 131-134
Bradykinin
  activation of, 202
  metabolism of, 200-203
Brain, modification of, as target opening, 241-250
Brain edema, treatment of, 242
Bretylium, effect of kidney disease on, 149
8-Bromo-cyclic GMP, role in mediator release, 290

Bupivacaine, nonlinearities in distribution, 37 (Table II)

Campothecin, binding of, 211
Cancer chemotherapy, 351–365 366–368
  cell kinetics, 352–354, 359–366
  dosage regimen, 352, 363–364
  local uptake, 354–356, 368
  pharmacokinetic models, 356–365, 367–368 (Fig. 5, 358; Fig. 6, 360; Fig. 7, 361; Fig. 8, 363; Fig. 9, 364; Fig. 10, 365)
Carbon monoxide, effect on drug metabolism, 155
Carbon tetrachloride, effect on drug metabolism, 155
Carboxytolbutamide, interaction effects, 325, 326 (Fig. 3)
Carcinogenic actions, chemical lesions in, 165
Carcinoid tumor, use as model in cancer chemotherapy, 368
Cardiac glycosides, absorption of in older patients, 154
Cardiac volume, 12
Catecholamine
  as amphetamine blocking agent, 301
  metabolism of, 198–200
Cell kinetics, 351–354, 359–365, 366–368
  biological age, 352–354
  cell cycle kinetics, 359, 367 (Table A)
  drug effects, 357–358
  phases of cell cycle, 352
Cellular response to drugs, 115
Central nervous system, uptake in, 125 (Fig. 7), 126
Chemical Control of Cancer, 351
Chemical lesions, 164–165
Chloramphenicol
  altered metabolism of, 263 (Table I)
  glucuronide conjugation of, 151
  toxicity to in newborns, 155
Chloride
  distribution of, 121 (Fig. 3), 123–124, 239
  pharmacokinetics of, 126–128 (Fig. 8, 126; Fig. 9, 127)
4-Chlorophenylacetic acid, 107
Chloroquine, in retinopathies, 213, 214
Chlorothiazide, in drug binding, 212–213

Chlorpromazine
  as amphetamine blocking agent, 299, 301
  drug binding, 213
  5-HT inhibition, 197
  interaction with tolbutamide, 155
  metabolism of, 148 (Table I)
  plasma concentrations, 55
Cholecystokinin, inactivation of, 201
Cholinergic agents, 170, 174, 176, 177, 179
  receptor sites for, 179–188 (Fig. 8, 180; Table II, 182; Fig. 9, 183; Table II, 185)
  role in mediator release, 290
Cholinergic receptor, 179, 189
Chromopharmacology, 141–142
Chylomicrons, nonlinearities in distribution, 36 (Table II)
Ciliary epithelium, 192 (Fig. 2)
Clinical metabolic profiles,
  patterns of, 20
Coagulation of colloids, collision theory, 296
Cocaine
  role in catecholamine inhibition, 199
  role in 5-HT inhibition, 197
Colchicine, binding of, 230
Colloidal lanthanum, in blood-brain barrier, 241
Complement-induced cytolysis, 282–285
  one-hit model, 284 (Fig. 2), 285 (Fig. 3), 296
Components of complement, 281
  catabolism of, 287, 296
  metabolism of, 285–287 (Table I, 286)
Conjugation, in primates, 107–111
Convallotoxin, nonlinearity in absorption, 29 (Table I)
Convulsants, pharmacodynamics of, 165
Corticoids, interaction with phenobarbital, 337
Corticosteroids, genetic reaction to, 264 (Table I)
Corticosterone, binding of, 211, 228 (Fig. 8), 229 (Fig. 9)
Cortisol, use in uremic patients, 151
Cortisone, luminal and/or mucosal metabolism in, 95 (Table II)
Coumarin drugs, anticoagulant effect
  in man and rat, 339–349
  of dicumarol in man, 344–345
  of dicumarol in rats, 345–347
  of racemic warfarin and that of its enantiomers, 343–344
  of warfarin in man, 340–343

Index

Curare, 115
Curariform drugs (see Bisonium compounds)
Cyanamide, osmolal threshold, 244 (Table I)
Cyclophosphamide, effects, 352, 358 (Fig. 5)
Cyclopropane, genetic reaction to, 264 (Table I)
Cystic fibrosis, drug absorption in, 154
Cytokinetics, relationship to pharmacokinetics, 142
Cytolytic cell destruction, 281–287
Cytolytic immunologic reaction, 281–282 (Fig. 1)
Cytosine arabinoside, effects, 352, 361 (Fig. 7)
Cytotropic reaction, 282

Dapsone, reaction to, 262 (Table I)
DDT
  binding of, 214
  effect on drug metabolism, 155–156
  interaction effects, 336
15-Dehydrogenase, relationship to prostaglandins, 201
Depressants, absorption of, in older patients, 154
Depression, treatment of, 315–319
Desmethylimipramine
  effect on norepinephrine, 200
  effect in uremic patients, 151
  hepatic metabolism in, 96 (Table III)
  inhibition of 5-HT, 197
  metabolism of, 148 (Table I)
  plasma concentration of, 315, 316, 318 (Table II)
Dexamethasone phosphate, luminal and/or mucosal metabolism in, 95 (Table II)
DFP (see diisopropyfluorophosphate)
Diabetes, drug interaction in, 335–336
Diaminodiphenylsulfone, acetylation of, 256–257
Diazepam, 114
Dibutyrl cyclic AMP, role in mediator release, 290
Dicumarol, 68, 211, 339
  anticoagulant effect in man, 342, 344–345 (Fig. 5 & 6), 346
  anticoagulant effect in rats, 345 (Fig. 6), 346 (Fig. 7), 347 (Tables II-III)
  interaction with barbituates, 324
  interaction with tolbutamide, 324, 330

Dietary factors, effect on drug metabolism, 159 (Table VIII)
Diffusion rates
  perfusion models, 145
  vs. perfusion rates, 144
Digitoxin, 175 (Fig. 6), 211, 279
Digoxin, 84, 85
  blood concentration in, 279
  effect of kidney disease on, 149–150 (Fig. 1)
  effect of, in older patients, 155
  nonlinearities in distribution, 37 (Table II)
Diisopropylfluorophosphate inhibitable serine esterase, activation of, 289
Dimercaprol, genetic reaction to, 263 (Table I)
Diphenhydramine, 186–187 (Fig. 12)
  nonlinearities in distribution, 37 (Table II)
  relationship to tissue uptake, 33, 41 (Fig. 4), 42 (Fig. 5)
Diphenylhydantoin, 50, 68
  in uremia, 151
  metabolism of, 113, 148 (Table I), 149
  nonlinearities in metabolism, 39, 40 (Table III)
  plasma levels of, 84
  relationship to enzyme system, 46 (Table VII)
  relationship to plasma concentrations, 59 (Fig. 10)
Diphenylhydantoin toxicity
  blood concentration in 278
  genetic factors of, 262 (Table II)
  plasma half-life in, 266–267
DNA
  inhibition of, 368
  relationship to drug binding, 213, 214
  synthesization of, 352, 353 (Fig. 1)
L-Dopa, 90
  liminal and/or mucosal metabolism in, 95 (Table II)
Dopamine
  as amphetamine blocking agent, 301
  hepatic metabolism in, 96 (Table III)
  metabolism of in lungs, 199
Dosing regimens, 21, 22, 84–85
Drug, pharmacokinetic definition of, 71
Drug absorption, 14–18 (Fig. 4, 16), 20, 21, 28, 62–63, 145
  factors affecting, 87–88, 90–100, 154
  genetic factors of, 276

Drug absorption *(cont'd)*
  in primates, 106, 111
  nonlinearities in 29-30 (Table I)
Drug accumulation, 71-73 (Table I)
Drug action
  pharmaceutical phase, 163 (Fig. 1), 164
  pharmacodynamic phase, 165-172
  pharmacokinetic phase, 164-165
  receptor sites, 18-20
Drug binding, 79-80
  in multicompartment systems, 217-219, 220-22, 226, 227
  in plasma 211-213, 216 (Table III)
  measurement of, 216, 217-220 (Fig. 3), 225-226 (Fig. 6)
  to tissues, 213-216 217
Drug bioavailability, 87, 101, 103
  determining, 4, 13-16 (Fig. 4), 18-19, 23-24
  dosage form factor, 89 (Table I)
  physiological factors of, 89 (Table I)
  rate of, 88 (Fig. 1), 91, 98-99 (Fig. 6), 100 (Fig. 7)
Drug clearance
  determination of, 94-98
  relation to body weight, 133
Drug concentration
  applied to cancer chemotherapy, 355 (Fig. 3), 357, 368
  genetic factors, 277-279
  in drug—drug interactions, 322
  in target conpartments, 166-167 (Fig. 3), 168 (Fig. 4), 169 (Fig. 5), 170 response of, 170-172
Drug disposition
  effect of route of administration, 87-101, 103
  polygenic factors, 265-266
Drug distribution
  genetic factors, 276
  measurement of, 217-230
  mechanisms of, 209-211
  nonlinearities in, 28, 36-37 (Table II)
  physiological and physical factors of, 233-239
  relationship to interspecies scaling, 118-143, 144-145 (Table I, 118; Table II, 130)
Drug–drug interactions, 321-334, 335-337
  defined, 321
  environmental contaminants, 336

Drug–drug interactions *(cont'd)*
  in diabetes, 335-336
  inhibition effects, 329-330, 336
  kinetic analysis of, 322-323
  plasma concentration in, 330-333
  steady-state drug levels, 336
Drug excretion
  genetic factors of, 276
  in primates, 106, 111-112
Drug interactions, 115, 170
  with receptor sites, 276, 278-279
  (*see also* Drug—drug interactions and Drug—receptor interaction)
Drug localization, 216-230
Drug metabolism, 55-58, 147-160, 162
  chemical lesions in, 164-165
  dietary factors of, 159 (Table VIII)
  effect of age, 154-155
  effects of drug interaction on, 155, 337
  effect of environmental chemicals, 155-159 (Fig. 4, 156; Tables IV-VII, 157-158)
  effect of kidney disease on, 149-151 (Table II, 149; Table III, 150; Fig. 1, 150)
  effect in liver disease, 151-154 (Fig. 2, 152; Fig. 3, 153)
  effect in uremia, 151
  environmental factors, 162, 267, 272-273
  genetic factors, 112-113, 159, 253-260, 267-268, 273-274, 275 (Table III), 276
  in primates, 107-115
  interindividual variations in, 147, 148 (Table I), 149
  nonlinearities in, 28, 30, 32 (Fig. 1), 38-40 (Table III)
  rates of, 265-267 (Figs. 1 and 2), 274
  thyroid disorders, 162
Drug-receptor interaction
  rate of diffusion, 174
  rate of dissociation, 174
  receptor activation, 174
  receptors and receptor sites, 177, 179-189, 276, 278-279
  relationship to drug action, 171-172, 172-188 (Fig. 6, 175)
Drug receptors, 172-173
Duanomycin, nonlinearities in distribution, 37 (Table II)

ECF-A (*see* Eosinophil chemotactic factor of anaphylaxis)
Emboli, filtering of, 195

Index

Endothilial cells, 241, 242–243 (Fig. 2)
Enterohepatic circulation, analysis of, 13
Environmental chemicals
  effect on drug metabolism, 155–159 (Fig. 4, 156; Tables IV-VII, 157–158
  interaction of, 336
Enzyme-substrate interaction, 173
Enzyme system, 46 (Table VII)
Eosinophil chemotactic factor
  of anaphylaxis, immulogic release of, 288-289 (Table II)
  in mediator release in guinea pig lung, 290–294 (Figs. 4–7, 291–292; Table III, 293)
Epinephrine, metabolism of in lungs, 198–199, 203
Erythrocytes, 192–193
Erythromycin acid erythromycin-2′-propionate ester, nonlinearities in distribution, 37 (Table II)
17β-Estradiol, 5-HT inhibition, 197
Estrogens
  binding of, 211
  luminal and/or mucosal metabolism in, 95 (Table II)
Ethanol
  availability, 98
  blood tissue distribution, 237–238
  genetic factors, 270–272, 275 (Table III)
  osmolal threshold, 244 (Table I), 245, 246 (Table II), 247–248
Ether, genetic reaction to, 264 (Table I)
Ethyl alcohol
  nonlinearities in metabolism, 38 (Table III)
  relationship to enzyme system, 46 (Table VII)
Ethyl biscoumacetate
  metabolism of, 148 (Table I)
  plasma half-life of, 265-267 (Fig. 2)
Ethyl carbamate, osmolal threshold, 244 (Table I)
Ethylene glycol, osmolal threshold, 244 (Table I)
Excretion, in one- and two- compartment models, 27 (see also Renal excretion)

Fat emulsions, nonlinearities in distribution, 36 (Table II)
Fatty acids, binding of, 211, 212

Favism, genetic factors of, 263 (Table I)
Fibrinopeptides, inactivation of, 201
Flufenamic acid, in drug binding, 213
Fluorescein, effect in uremic patients, 151
Folic acid, nonlinearities in absorption, 29 (Table I)
Food additives, effect on drug metabolism, 155
Food constituents, effect on drug metabolism, 155
Formamide, osmolal threshold of, 244 (Table I)
Furadantine (see Nitrofurantoin)
Furazolidone, genetic factor of, 263 (Table I)

Gantrisin (see Sulfacetamide sulfisoxazole)
Gastrectomy, drug absorption in, 154
Gastrin, inactivation of, 201
Genetic effects in drug metabolism (see Drug metabolism, genetic factors)
Gentamycin, 84
  in kidney disease, 81 (Fig. 1), 149 (Table II)
Glaucoma
  acetozolamide, use of, 191–194 (Figs. 1 and 2)
  genetic factors of, 264 (Table I)
Glomerulonephritis, 287
Glucagon, metabolism of, 201
Glucose, 242
  osmolal threshold of, 244 (Table I)
Glucose-6-phosphate dehydrogenase deficiency, genetic factors, 263 (Table I)
Glucuronic acid, conjugation of, 107–108, 113, 114
Glucuronide
  absorption of, 93
  availability, 97
  plasma concentration, 97 (Fig. 5)
Glutamine, conjugation of, 107–108, 111 (Table VII)
Glycerol, osmolal threshold, 244 (Table I)
Glycine, conjugation of, 107, 113
Griseofulvin
  interaction of, 323–324 (Fig. 1)
  nonlinearities in absorption, 29 (Table I)
  nonlinearities in distribution, 37 (Table II)
Guanethidine
  nonlinearities in absorption, 29 (Table I)
  nonlinearities in distribution, 36 (Table II)

Halothane, genetic factors of, 264 (Table I), 270–271, 275 (Table III)
Hematopoietic cells, effect of vinblastine on, 360 (Fig. 6), 366–367 (Table A)
Hemoglobins, drug sensitivity to, 264 (Table I)
Hemolytic anemia, genetic factors, 263 (Table I)
Heparin, nonlinearities in metabolism, 40 (Table III)
Hepatic clearance, 94
  (*see also* Drug clearance)
Hepatic disease (*See* Liver disease)
Hepatic extraction ratio, 94
Hepatic necrosis, 153
Hepatitis, use of prednisolone in, 152
Heptabarbital, in test of anticoagulant effect of warfarin, 342–343 (Fig. 3)
Heptachlor, binding of, 214
Herbicides, effect on drug metabolism, 155
Hexobarbital
  differences in response to, 268
  metabolic effects, 162
Hippuric acid, 109
  in conjugation, 107
  luminal and/or mucosal metabolism in, 95 (Table II)
  (*see also* Quinic acid)
Histamine, 175 (Fig. 6)
  activation of, 202, 203
  binding of, 211
  5-HT uptake, 198
  immulogic release of, 288–289 (Table II), 290
  in mediator release in guinea pig lung, 290–294 (Figs. 4–7, 291–292; Table III, 293)
Histamine-releasing agents, 170
Histaminergic agents, 176, 177, 181
Histaminergic receptors, 187
5-HT (*see* 5-Hydroxytryptamine)
Hydralazine
  acetylation of, 256–257
  reaction to, 262 (Table I)
Hydrocarbons, effect on drug metabolism, 155
Hydrochlorthiazide, 115
Hydrocortisone
  5-HT inhibition, 197
  luminal and/or mucosal metabolism in, 95 (Table II)

Hydrogen, in blood tissue distribution, 235–236
Hydrogen peroxide, reactions to, 262 (Table I)
p-Hydroxyamphetamine, in amphetamine withdrawal, 309 (Fig. 9)
p-Hydroxynorephedrine, metabolite of amphetamines, 306, 307, 308
Hydroxytolbutamide, inhibition of tolbutamide oxidation, 324–325, 326 (Fig. 3)
5-Hydroxytryptamine, 195–198, 203
  activation of, 202
  in catecholamine inhibition, 199
Hyperactive children, treatment of with amphetamines, 313
Hyperthermia
  genetic factors of, 264 (Table I)
  in amphetamine abuse, 312
Hypochloremia, 123
Hypoglycemic agents, interaction effects, 324–325, 330

IgE antibody, in sensitization of human lung, 288
Ileitis, drug absorption in, 154
Imipramine, binding of, 210–211, 214–215 (Table I and Table II)
  5-HT inhibition, 197
Immune hemolysis, 282–283
Indocyanine green, nonlinearities in distribution, 37 (Table II)
Indoleacetic acid, 107
Indomethacin
  binding of, 211
  nonlinearities in absorption, 30 (Table I)
  nonlinearities in biliary excretion, 45 (Table V)
Industrial chemicals, effect on drug metabolism, 155
Inhibition effects in drug interaction, 329–330 (Figs. 5 and 6), 336
  (*see also* Drug—drug interaction, Tolbutamide)
Insecticides
  effect on drug metabolism, 155–156 (Fig. 4)
  relationship to drug binding, 214
Insulin receptor, 189
Interspecies scaling, 105–115
  (*see also* Drug distribution)

Index

In vitro—in vivo correlations in drug distribution, 140–141
  in vivo effects, 141
Isoniazid, 91
  acetylation of, 113, 256–257 (Fig. 1)
  genetic factors, 273 (Fig. 6)
  metabolism of, 148, 151–152
  nonlinearities in metabolism, 39 (Table III)
  slow inactivation of, 262 (Table I)
Isoniazid-diphenylhydantoin, side effects of, 254 (Table I)
Isoniazid polyneuritis, adverse reaction to, 254 (Table I)
Isopropamide, 181
Isoproterenol, chromotropic potency of, 90
Isosorbide, 115

Kallikrein, 203
Kanamycin, 84
  effect of in older patients, 155
  effect of kidney disease on, 149 (Table II)
  nonlinearities in distribution, 36 (Table II)
Kidney disease
  effect on drug metabolism, 149–151 (Table II, 149; Table III, 150; Fig. 1, 150) relationship to pharmacokinetics, 80–82 (Fig.1)
Kidneys, active tubular secretion of, 30–31, 32 (Fig. 1)
Kinetic linearity (*see* Linear and nonlinear pharmacokinetics)
Kinetics, in drug distribution, 125–126
Kinetics of competive inhibition of metabolite step, 326
Kinetics of drug action, 339–349
Kinetic variables of mediator release, 293 (Table III), 296
Kinin-forming factors, 288–289
Krueger-Thiemer's dosage theory of bacteriostatic agents, 73–75
  in sulfonamides, 76 (Table III)
Kynex (*see* Sulfamethoxypyridazine)

Lactamide
  effect on blood-brain barrier, 246 (Table II)
  osmolal threshold, 244 (Table I)

Langmuir-type tissue binding, 48 (Fig. 7), 49, 60
Lanthanum, 243 (Fig. 2)
Leukemia cells, 352–65
Lidocaine, 87, 94–95, 101
  blood concentration in, 279
  body clearance of, 95–96
  hepatic extraction ratio of, 94–95
  hepatic metabolism in, 96 (Table III)
  in heart disease, 154
  in liver disease, 154
  interaction of, 322
  metabolism of, 148–149
  plasma concentration of, 333
Lincomycin, 68
Lindane, effect on drug metabolism, 155–156 (Fig. 4)
Linear and nonlinear pharmacokinetics, 27–68
  active tubular secretion in kidneys, 30–31, 32 (Fig. 1)
  biliary excretion, 45 (Table V)
  causes of nonlinearities, 58–60, 68
  drug absorption, 28–30 (Table I)
  drug action, 45 (Table VI)
  drug distribution, 36–37 (Table II)
  drug metabolism, 28, 38–40 (Table III), 55–58
  Michaelis-Menten equation, 31, 46 (Table VII), 48 (Fig. 7)
  nonlinear models, 52–53
  recognition of nonlinearities, 51–52
  renal excretion, 44 (Table IV)
  tissue binding, 54–55
  tissue uptake of drugs, 31, 33–35 (Figs. 2 and 3), 41 (Fig. 4), 42 (Fig. 5), 44–45
Lipid-soluble substances, effect on cells, 242–43 (Fig. 2)
Lithium, 189
  Blood concentration in, 279
  in Graves disease, 24
  inhibition effects, 336
Lithium chloride (LiCl),
  osmolal threshold, 244 (Table I)
Liver, role of in inhibition of 5-HT, 197–198
Liver disease, drug metabolism in, 151–154 (Fig. 2, 152; Fig. 3, 153)
Liver perfusion, 114
Liver plasma flow, relationship to extraction ratio, 225 (Table IV)
Local uptake, 354–356 (Fig. 2, 354)

Lungs
  endocrine function of, 202, 204
  mediator release from in guinea pigs, 288–289 (Table II), 290–294 (Figs. 4 and 5, 191; Figs. 6 and 7, 292; Table III, 293)
  mediator release from in humans, 288–290 (Table II, 289)
  relationship to metabolism of vasoactive substances, 195–204, 206–207
  relationship to other disorders, 203
  respiratory function, 204
Lymphoma cells
  effect of cytosine arabinoside on, 361 (Fig. 7), 366–367
  effect of vinblastine on, 360 (Fig. 6), 366–367

Mannitol, in treatment of brain endema, 242
Marihuana, effect on drug metabolism, 158
Mass balances, in drug distribution, 119 (Fig. 1), 120 (Fig. 2), 121
Mediator compounds, formation of, 170
Melanin granules, in drug binding, 213–214
Meperidine, luminal and/or mucosal metabolism in, 95 (Table II)
Metabolism
  equation, relating to, 6 in one- and two-compartment models, 27
Metabolites, of amphetamines, 306–310, (Fig. 8, 308; Fig. 10, 310), 313
Metabolized substances, in drug distribution, 134–140
Metaraminol, role in catecholamine inhibition, 199
Methacycline, nonlinearities in distribution, 37 (Table II)
Methadone, luminal and/or mucosal metabolism in, 95 (Table II)
Methanol, osmolal threshold, 244 (Table I)
Methotrexate, 54
  cell-killing effects, 357
  in relation to body weight, 131 (Fig. 12), 132, (Fig. 13). 133 (Fig. 14), 134 (Fig. 15), 144
  in vivo, 142–143
  nonlinearities in distribution, 36 (Table II)
  permeability differences in, 356 (Fig. 4)
  pharmacokinetics of, 122 (Fig. 4), 123–124, 128–129 (Figs. 10 and 11), 130

p-Methoxy-amphetamine, metabolite of amphetamines, 306, 307
Methoxyfluorane, genetic reaction to, 264 (Table I)
Methylcarbamate, osmolal threshold, 244 (Table I)
α-Methyldopa, luminal and/or mucosal metabolism in, 95 (Table II)
Methylene blue
  genetic reaction to, 263 (Table I)
  nonlinearities in distribution, 37 (Table II)
  nonlinearities in renal excretion, 44 (Table IV)
  relationship to blood concentration, 55, 56 (Fig. 8)
  relationship to tissue uptake, 35 (Fig. 3), 41, 44
Methylenedioxyphenyl pesticides, effect on drug metabolism, 155
Methylhydroxycoumarin, nonlinearities in distribution, 37 (Table II)
p-Methyl mendelic acid, nonlinearities in renal excretion, 44 (Table IV)
Methyl mercury, interaction effects, 336
Methyl orange, nonlinearities in biliary excretion, 45 (Table V)
Methyltestosterone, 337
5-Methyltetrahydrofolate, nonlinearity in absorption, 29 (Table I)
Methylthiouracil, genetic reaction to, 264 (Table I)
α-Methyltyrosine, as amphetamine blocking agent, 299–300 (Figs. 2 and 3)
Methyl urea, osmolal threshold, 244 (Table I)
Michaelis–Menten kinetics, 31, 46 (Table VII), 48 (Fig. 7), 49, 52, 55, 58, 60, 61, 68, 98
  relation to enzymatic processes, 78
Migraine, 203
Monoamine-oxidase inhibition, relation to 5-HT, 196–197, 198
Morphine, binding of, 211–212
MTX (*see* Methotrexate)
Musculotropic spasmolytic agent, 176
Mutagenic actions, chemical lesions in, 165
Myeloma, use as model in cancer chemotherapy, 368

NaCl, osmolal threshold, 244 (Table I), 245, 246 (Table II)

Index

Naphthalene, altered metabolism of, 263 (Table I)
Narcolepsy, treatment with amphetamines, 313
Na$_2$SO$_4$, osmolal threshold, 244 (Table I), 245 (Fig. 3)
Nicotine, 158
Niridazole, in bilharziasis, 152–153
Nitrazepan, 114
Nitro-furantoin, altered metabolism of, 263 (Table I)
Noncytolytic immunologic reaction, 282 (Fig. 1)
Noncytolytic mediator release, 287–290 (Table II, 289), 296 from guinea pig lung, 290–294 (Figs. 4–5, 291; Figs. 6–7, 292; Table III, 293)
 genetic control, 296
 kinetic variables of, 293 (Table III), 296
Nonelectrolytes
 in treatment of brain endema, 242
 osmotic pressure of, 244
Nonionic diffusion mechanism, in amphetamine abuse, 304
Nonlinear pharmacokinetics (see Linear and nonlinear pharmacokinetics)
Nonmetabolizable drugs, 114–115
Nonmetabolized substances, 126–134
Nonsulfonamide antibacterial agents, genetic factors of, 263 (Table I)
Noradrenaline
 as amphetamine blocking agent, 301
 inhibition of, 315
Norchlorcyclazine, binding of, 215–216
Norephedrine, metabolite of amphetamine, 309, 313
Norepinephrine
 blood concentration of, 204
 5-HT uptake, 198
 metabolism of in lungs, 198–200
Nortriptyline
 clearance of, 96
 clinical applications of, 277, 279
 genetic factors of, 271, 273 (Fig. 6), 276
 hepatic metabolism in, 96 (Table III)
 in polygenic control, 261
 metabolism of, 148 (Table I), 149
 plasma half-life of, 265
 role in catecholamine inhibition, 199
 volume of distribution, 225
Novobiocin, nonlinearities in metabolism, 39 (Table III)

One-compartment system, in drug binding, 219, 221
Onium group
 effect on anticholinergic agents, 183
 effect on cholinergic agents, 179
Opiate receptor, 189
Oral availability, 96–100
Organic acids, nonlinearities in renal excretion, 44 (Table IV)
Organic nitrates, luminal and/or mucosal metabolism in, 95 (Table II)
Organophosphorus insecticides, effect on drug metabolism, 155
Osmolal thresholds, 244 (Table I), 245–246
Osmotic pressure, 242, 244
Oxazepam, 114
Oxyphenbutazone, hepatic metabolism in, 96 (Table III)
Oxytocin, inactivation of, 201, 203
Ozone, effect on drug metabolism, 155

PAH, nonlinearities in renal excretion, 44 (Table IV)
Pamaquine, genetic factor of, 263 (Table I)
Pancreatic insufficiency, drug absorption in, 154
Pancreozymin, inactivation of, 201
Paracetamol, in liver disease, 153
Parathion, distribution of, 123 (Fig. 5), 124, 125
Pempidine, binding of, 212–213
Penfluridal, interaction of, 336
Penicillin, adverse reaction to, 254 (Table I)
Penicillin-G, 115
 effect of kidney disease of, 149 (Table II)
 plasma concentration of, 333
Pentaquine, altered metabolism of, 263 (Table I)
Pentazocine
 effect of cigarette smoking, 158
 effect of environment, 162
 luminal and/or mucosal metabolism in, 95 (Table II)
Pentobarbital
 in blood tissue distribution, 237 (Fig. 2), 238
 nonlinearities in absorption, 30 (Table I)
Peptides, inactivation of, 200–201, 203
Peroxidase, in blood-brain barrier, 241
Pesticides (see Insecticides)
Phagocytosis by alveolar macrophages, 195

Pharmacodynamics, 70
  of drug action, 165-169 (Figs. 2-5). 170-172
  parameters, 367 (Table A)
Pharmacogenetics, 1, 75
  clinical applications, 276-279
  environmental factors in, 267-274
  polygenically controlled effects, 261-280
  single gene effects, 253-260
  twin studies, 268-275
Pharmacogens, 164
Pharmacokinetic interaction (see Drug—drug interactions)
Pharmacokinetics,
  analyses, 10-13
  clinical applications, 22, 24
  definition of, 3, 70
  equations relating to, 5-6, 15, 18
  models, 4-7 (Fig. 1), 8 (Fig. 2), 9 (Fig. 3), 10, 356-365
  of drug action, 45 (Table VI), 164-165
  origins of, 27
  problems of, 47-52
  profiles, 20-24
  relationship to patient treatment, 75-84
Pharmacokinetics and clinical medicine, 69-82, 84-85
  kidney disease, 80-82
  saturation effects, 78-80
Pharmacokinetics of drugs, evaluation of, 349
Phenacetin
  effect of cigarette smoking on metabolism of, 156-158 (Tables IV-VII)
  in uremia, 151
  metabolism of, 113
Phenelzine
  acetylation of, 256-257
  reaction to, 262 (Table I)
Pheniprazine, hepatic metabolism in, 96 (Table III)
Phenobarbital
  concentration in brain, 210
  environmental factors, 274-275
  interaction of, 155
  interaction of, with griseofulvin, 323 (Fig. 1), 324
  interaction with corticoids, 337
  in uremia, 151
Phenol, 107

Phenothiazine, in retinopathies, 213
Phenoxybenzamine
  as amphetamine blocking agent, 301
  role in catecholamine inhibition, 199
Phenylacetic acid, 107
  conjugation in primates, 108 (Table IV)
Phenylbutazone, 68, 210
  binding of, 211-213
  clinical applications of, 277
  effect of DDT on metabolism of, 156
  elimination of, 280
  environmental and genetic factors in, 271 (Table II), 272, 274-275 (Table III), 276
  interaction of, 324, 330, 333-334 (Fig. 7)
  metabolism of, 147, 148 (Table I), 268 (Fig. 3)
  metabolism of in liver disease, 151-152 (Fig. 2), 153 (Fig. 3)
  nonlinearities in metabolism, 39 (Table III)
  plasma concentration of, 331
  plasma half-life of, 265, 266 (Fig. 1), 268
  polygenic control, 261
Phenylhydrazine, genetic reaction to, 263 (Table I)
Phenylthiocarbamide, inability to taste, 264 (Table I)
Phenylthiourea, genetic reaction to, 264 (Table I)
Phenyramidol, interaction with tolbutamide, 324
Pheochromocytoma, use as model in cancer chemotherapy, 367-368
Phosphate, distribution in brain tissue, 239
Phosphodiesterase inhibitors, role in mediator release, 290
Phospholipids, in drug binding, 215
Photosensitization, chemical lesions in, 165
Pimozide, as amphetamine blocking agent, 301
Plasma concentration, 87, 330-333 (Fig. 7)
Plasma kinetics, genetic factors, 317-318 (Table II), 319
Plasma level-time curves, 9 (Fig. 3)
Plasma protein binding, 52-53
Plasma pseudocholinesterase, in uremia, 151
Platelet activating factor, 289
Polar compounds, 210
Polygenically transmitted diseases
  causes of, 264-265

Index

Polygenically transmitted diseases *(cont'd)*
  Mendelian law, relating to, 265
Polyphasic systems *(see* Two-compartment system)
Potassium, distribution in brain tissue, 239
Prednisolone, use in hepatitis, 152
PrFM$(e)_3$, 175 (Fig. 6)
Primaquine
  altered metabolism of, 263 (Table I)
  sensitivity to, 257
Primary malabsorption
  disease *(see* Steatorrhea)
Primate scale, 105-106 (Table I)
  metabolism in, 106
Probenecid
  binding of, 211
  genetic reaction to, 263 (Table I)
  nonlinearities in metabolism, 39 (Table III)
Procainamide
  blood concentration in, 279
  in liver disease, 154
  metabolism of, 148-149
  plasma half-life of, 266
Procaine, in uremia, 151
Progesterone, luminal and/or mucosal metabolism in, 95 (Table II)
Promethiazine, distribution of, 167 (Fig. 3)
Propantheline, 181
  nonlinearities in renal excretion, 44 (Table IV)
Propionamide, osmolal threshold, 244 (Table I)
Propoxyphene, luminal and/or mucosal metabolism in, 95 (Table II)
Propranolol, 87
  as amphetamine blocking agent, 301
  blood concentration, 279
  hepatic metabolism in, 96 (Table III)
  interaction of, 322
  oral availability, 96, 98
  plasma half-life in, 266
Propylene glycol, osmolal threshold, 244 (Table I), 246 (Table II), 247-248
Propylthiouracil, genetic reaction to, 264 (Table I)
Prosimian scale, 107 (Table III)
Prostaglandins
  abortifacient action, 203
  activation of, 202, 203

Prostaglandins *(cont'd)*
  immulogic release of, 289
  inactivation of, 201-202 203
  metabolism in lungs, 203
Protein binding, analysis of, 12
Protein synthesis, inhibition of, 368
Prothrombin complex activity, 340, 341 (Fig. 2), 342 (Fig. 3), 343, 344 (Fig. 4), 345 (Fig. 5), 346 (Table I), 347 (Table II)
Pulmonary drug metabolism *(see* Lungs)
Pyramidon *(see* Aminopyrine)
2-Pyridenealdoxime methochloride, nonlinearities in metabolism, 40 (Table III)
Pyridoxine, in steatorrhea, 154
Pyrimidine, 139

Quabain-H^3, nonlinearities in distribution, 36 (Table II)
Quasilinearization, 60
Quaternary ammonium compounds, levels in brain, 210
Quaternary onium compounds, concentration of, 166
Quinacrine, altered metabolism of, 263 (Table I)
Quinic acid, 107, 109
  aromatization of in primates, 110 (Table VI), 111 (Table VII)
  (see also Hippuric acid)
Quinidine
  blood concentration of, 279
  effect in uremic patients, 151
  genetic reaction to, 263 (Table I)
  metabolism of, 148-149
Quinine, genetic reaction to, 263 (Table I)
Quinoline, binding of, 213-214

Rabbit aorta contracting substance, activation of, 202
Racemic warfarin, anticoagulant activity of, 343-344 (Fig. 4)
RCS *(see* Rabbit aorta contracting substance)
Receptor isolation, 179
Red-blood cell partition, analysis of, 12
Red cell glucose-6-phosphate, dehydrogenase deficiency, 257
Renal allograft rejection, 287
Renal clearance, 94

Renal excretion
  analysis of, 12, 20
  equation relating to, 6
  of drugs and metabolites, 44 (Table IV)
Renal impairment, drug interaction in, 329
Reserpine, 278
  as amphetamine blocking agent, 299
  hepatic metabolism in, 96 (Table III)
Reticuloendothelial cells, in removal of 5-HT, 198
Rheumatoid arthritis, 287, 296
Ribitol, absorption of, 93
Riboflavin, 51
  nonlinearities in absorption, 29 (Table I)
  nonlinearities in renal excretion, 44 (Table IV)
  nonlinearities in biliary excretion, 45 (Table V)
RNA
  inhibition of, 368
  relationship to drug binding, 214
  synthesization of, 352

Salicyl acyl glucuronide, 49
Salicylamide, 88, 91 (Fig. 2)
  absorption rate, 93
  interaction of, 322
  luminal and/or mucosal metabolism in, 95 (Table II)
  nonlinearities in absorption, 30 (Table I)
  nonlinearities in metabolism, 39 (Table III)
  oral availability, 96–97, 101 plasma concentration of, 92 (Fig. 3), 93 (Fig. 4), 97 (Fig. 5)
Salicylates, 49–50, 79, 278
  accumulation kinetics of, 336
  binding of, 211
  blood concentration in, 279
  interaction of, 322, 336
  metabolism of, 277
  nonlinearities in distribution, 37 (Table II)
  plasma concentration of, 331
  relationship to "enzyme system," 46 (Table VII)
  with aspirin, 49
Salicylazosulfapyridine, altered metabolism of, 263 (Table I)
Salicylic acid
  absorption of, 93
  adsorption isotherms for, 120 (Fig. 2), 122; 124 (Fig. 6), 125

Salicylic acid (cont'd)
  binding of, 211
  nonlinearities in metabolism, 38 (Table III)
Salicyl phenolic glucuronide, 49
Salicylsalicylic acid
  nonlinearities in metabolism, 39 (Table III)
Salicylurate, 49
Saturation kinetics, 78–80
Secobarbital, nonlinearities in distribution, 37 (Table II)
Sensitization, 287–288
Serotonin, 288–289
  hepatic metabolism in, 96 (Table III)
Serum albumin, in drug binding, 211, 212, 213
Serum cholinesterase, reaction of, to succinylcholine, 254 (Table II), 255
Se^{75}-selenite, nonlinearities in distribution, 36 (Table II)
Side-effects of drugs, 164–165
Sodium, distribution in brain tissue, 239
Sodium bicarbonate, role in drug interaction, 321
Sodium chloride (see NaCl)
Solid-state kinetics, 296
SRS-A (see Anaphylaxis)
Steady-state drug levels, study of, 336
Steatorrhea, drug absorption in, 154
Steroids, metabolization of, 90
S-Thiamine, excretion in steatorrhea, 154
Streptomycin, effect of kidney disease on, 149 (Table II)
p-Substituted acetanilides, nonlinearities in absorption, 30 (Table I)
Succinylcholine, 210
  genetic factors of, 264 (Table I)
  metabolism of, 148
  sensitivity to, 254 (Tables I–II), 255
Sucrose, osmolal threshold, 244 (Table I)
Sulfacetamide sulfisoxazole,
  altered metabolism of, 263 (Table I)
Sulfadiazine
  dosage regimens, 76 (Table II)
  elimination rate, 78 (Table III)
  in liver disease, 151
Sulfadimethoxine, 107–109
  conjugation of, 107–109 (Table V), 111 (Table VII)
  dosage regimen, 76 (Table II)
  elimination rate, 78 (Table III)
  urinary excretion of, 112 (Table VIII)

Index

Sulfadimethoxypyrimidine, urinary excretion in primates, 112 (Table VIII)
Sulfaethidole
  elimination rate, 78 (Table III)
  nonlinearities in absorption, 29 (Table I)
2-Sulfa-5-ethylpyrimidine, elimination rate, 78 (Table III)
Sulfaethylthiadiazole, absorption of, 93-94
Sulfamaprine, adverse reaction to, 262 (Table I)
Sulfamethazine
  acetylation of, 256, 257
  adverse reaction, 262 (Table I)
Sulfamethoxazole, elimination rate, 77, 78 (Table III)
Sulfamethoxydiazine, dosage regimen, 76 (Table II)
Sulfamethoxypyrazine
  dosage regimen, 76 (Table II)
  elimination rate, 78 (Table III)
Sulfamethoxypyridazine
  altered metabolism of, 263 (Table I)
  dosage regimen, 76 (Table II)
Sulfanilamide, altered metabolism of, 263 (Table I)
Sulfaphenazole
  binding of, 212
  interaction with tolbutamide, 324-325 (Fig. 2), 326 (Fig. 3), 327-328 (Fig. 4), 329-330, 336
Sulfapyridine, altered metabolism of, 263 (Table I)
Sulfasymazine, elimination rate, 78 (Table III)
Sulfate, distribution in brain tissue, 239
Sulfisomidine, elimination rate, 78 (Table III)
Sulfisoxozole
  elimination rate, 78 (Table III)
  use in uremic patients, 151
Sulfobromophthalein
  nonlinearities in biliary excretion, 45 (Table V)
  nonlinearities in distribution, 36 (Table II)
Sulfonamides, 77-78
  acetylators of, 113
  altered metabolism of, 263-264 (Table I)
  binding of, 211
  dosage regimens of, 76 (Table II)
  effects in uremic patients, 151
  elimination rate, 78 (Table III)
  evaluation of, 75

Sulfonamides (cont'd)
  evaluation of, 75
  interaction of, 324-329, 330-331, 336
  luminal and/or mucosal metabolism in, 95 (Table II)
  nonlinearities in renal excretion, 44 (Table IV)
  plasma concentration of, 331
Sulfones, altered metabolism of, 263 (Table I)
Sulfonic acid derivatives, levels in brain, 210
Sulfoxone, altered metabolism of, 263 (Table I)
Suxamethonium sensitivity, genetic factors of, 262 (Table I)
Systemic lupus erythematosus, 287

Tachyphylaxis, 170
Target compartment, blood concentration in (see Drug concentration)
Testosterone
  binding of, 211
  luminal and/or mucosal metabolism in, 95 (Table II)
Tetracycline, 94
  absorption of, 145
  binding of, 211
  effect of kidney disease on, 149 (Table II), 150 (Table III)
  nonlinearities in biliary excretion, 45 (Table V)
  nonlinearities in metabolism, 40 (Table III)
Tetrahydrocannabinol,
  metabolism of in lungs, 207
1,2,3,4,5-Tetrahydroxycyclohexanecarboxylic acid
  (see Quinic acid)
Thermodynamics, in drug distribution, 121-125
Thiamine, absorption of in ileitis, 154
Thiazolsulfone, altered metabolism of, 263 (Table I)
Thiopental, 54
  binding of, 214
  nonlinearities in distribution, 36 (Table II)
  pharmacokinetics, 134-135 (Fig. 16), 136 (Fig. 17), 137 (Fig. 18)
Thyroglobulin hydrolysis, inhibition of, 336
Thyrotoxicosis, treatment of, 336
Thyroxine, 189
  binding of, 211
  metabolic effects, 162

Index

Tissue binding, 54–55
Tissue distribution in primates, 106, 111
Tissue necrosis, chemical lesions in, 165
Tissue region, in local uptake, 354 (Fig. 2)
Tissue uptake of drugs, 31, 33–35 (Figs. 2–3), 41 (Fig. 4), 42 (Figs. 5), 43 (Fig. 6), 44–45
Tobacco, effect on drug metabolism, 155, 156–157 (Tables IV-V), 158 (Table VI)
Tolbutamide
  elimination rate, 327, 329
  hypoglycemic activity, 330–331
    in liver disease, 153
    interaction of, 155, 324–325 (Fig. 2), 326 (Fig. 3), 327–328 (Fig. 4), 329, 336 in uremia, 151
Transcortin, binding of, 230
Trichloroethanol, relationship to hypoprothrombinemia, 170–171
Tricyclic antidepressants, in treatment of depression, 316
Trifluoro-iodo-methane, in blood tissue distribution, 235–236
Trinitrotoluene, genetic reaction to, 263 (Table I)
Tryptamine, relationship to 5-HT metabolism, 198
Tryptophan
  binding of, 211, 212
  effect in uremic patients, 151
  hepatic metabolism in, 96 (Table III)
Two-compartment system
  determining volume of distribution, 222–224 (Fig. 5)
  relationship to drug binding, 217–218 (Fig. 1), 219 (Fig. 2), 220 (Fig. 3), 221 (Fig. 4), 222, 226 (Fig. 6), 227 (Fig. 7)
Tyramine
  activation of, 202
  relationship to plasma concentration, 315
Tyrosine hydroxylase, as amphetamine blocking agent, 299

Uracil arabinoside, 139–140
Urea
  effect in blood-brain barrier, 246 (Table II), 247 (Fig. 4), 248 (Fig. 5)
  in treatment of brain endema, 242
  osmolal threshold, 244 (Table I) uptake, 125 (Fig. 7), 126
Uremia, drug metabolism in, 151
Uric acid, binding of, 211

Vancomycin, effect of kidney disease on, 149 (Table II)
Vasoactive substances
  activation of, 202
  metabolism of, 195–204, 206–207
  types of, 203
Vasopressin, inactivation of, 201, 203
Vinblastine
  cytotoxic behavior of, 366
  effects of hematopoietic and lymphoma cells, 360 (Fig. 6), 367 (Table A)
Vincristine
  cytotoxic behavior of, 366
  effect on lymphoma and hematopoietic cells, 367 (Table A)
Virchow-Robin perivascular spaces, 239
Vitamin B_{12}, absorption of in ileitis, 154
Vitamin C, binding of, 211
Vitamin E, absorption of, 154
Vitamin K
  clotting effects, 340
  genetic reaction to, 263 (Table I)
Volatile anesthetics
  in blood tissue distribution, 234–235 (Fig. 1)
  relationship to blood-brain barrier, 239
Volume of distribution
  defined, 222–224 (Fig. 5), 227–228
  equations for determining, 222–224

Warfarin
  adverse reaction to, 254
  anticoagulant effect in man, 340 (Fig. 1), 341 (Fig. 2), 342 (Fig. 3), 343–344 (Fig. 4), 348–349
  binding of, 212
  nonlinearities in metabolism, 39 (Table III)
  pharmacokinetics of, 339
  plasma levels of, 348
  relationship to tissue distribution, 44
Warfarin anticoagulation, 322
  plasma concentration of, 331
  interaction of with phenylbutazone, 333–334 (Fig. 7)
Warfarin resistance, genetic factors, 263 (Table I)

Zoxazolamine, metabolism of, 162